# NEUROLOGICAL COMPLICATIONS OF HIV AND AIDS

*Volume 34 in Series*

Major Problems in Neurology
PROFESSOR CP WARLOW, BA, MB, BChir, MD, FRCP
PROFESSOR J VAN GIJN, MD, FRCPE
*Consulting Editors*

OTHER MONOGRAPHS IN THE SERIES

Hutchinson and Acheson: **Strokes**
Gubbay: **The Clumsy Child**
Hankinson and Banna: **Pituitary and Parapituitary Tumours**
Behan and Currie: **Clinical Neuroimmunology**
Cartlidge and Shaw: **Head Injury**
Lisak and Barchi: **Myasthenia Gravis**
Johnson, Lambie and Spalding: **Neurocardiology: The Interrelationships between Dysfunction in the Nervous and Cardiovascular Systems**
Parkes: **Sleep and its Disorders**
Hopkins: **Headache Problems in Diagnosis and Management**
Wood and Anderson: **Neurological Infections**
Critchley: **Neurological Emergencies**
Ross: **Syncope**
Donaldson: **Neurology and Pregnancy** SECOND EDITION
Porter: **Epilepsy: 100 Elementary Principles** SECOND EDITION
Harper: **Myotonic Dystrophy** SECOND EDITION
Sjaastad: **Cluster Headache Syndrome**
Hodges: **Transient Amnesia: Clinical and Neuropsychological Aspects**
Vermeulen, Lindsay and Van Gijn: **Subarachnoid Haemorrhage**
Bauer and Hanefeld: **Multiple Sclerosis**
Hankey and Warlow: **Transient Ischaemic Attacks of the Brain and Eye**
Zakrzewska: **Trigeminal Neuralgia**
Hilton-Jones, Squier, Taylor and Matthews: **Metabolic Myopathies**
Hoogenraad: **Wilson's Disease**
Harper: **Huntington's Disease** SECOND EDITION
Acheson and Sanders: **Common Problems in Neuroophthalmology**
Bousser and Ross Russell: **Cerebral Venous Thrombosis**

# NEUROLOGICAL COMPLICATIONS OF HIV AND AIDS

**G. Said MD**
*Professor*
*Service de Neurologie*
*Centre Hospitalier Universitaire de Bicêtre,*
*F-94275 Le Kremlin Bicêtre Cedex,*
*Paris, France*

**A. G. Saimot MD**
*Professor*
*Service des Maladies Infectieuses,*
*Hopital Bichat Claude Bernard,*
*F-75018,*
*Paris, France*

**M. Tardieu MD**
*Professor*
*Service de Neurologie Pédiatrique,*
*Centre Hospitalier Universitaire de Bicêtre,*
*F-94275 Le Kremlin Bicêtre Cedex,*
*Paris, France*

**C. Lacroix MD**
*Laboratoire de Neuropathologie,*
*Centre Hospitalier Universitaire de Bicêtre,*
*F-94275 Le Kremlin Bicêtre Cedex,*
*Paris, France*

W. B. Saunders Company Ltd
London · Philadelphia · Toronto · Sydney · Tokyo

W. B. Saunders Company Ltd
24–28 Oval Road
London NW1 7DX, UK

The Curtis Center
Independence Square West
Philadelphia, PA 19106–3399, USA

Harcourt Brace & Company
55 Horner Avenue
Toronto, Ontario M8Z 4X6, Canada

Harcourt Brace & Company, Australia
30–52 Smidmore Street
Marrickville, NSW 2204, Australia

Harcourt Brace & Company, Japan
Ichibancho Central Building, 22–1 Ichibancho
Chiyoda-ku, Tokyo 102, Japan



This book is printed on acid-free paper



A catalogue record for this book is available from the British Library

ISBN 0–7020 1836–8

Typeset by Phoenix Photosetting, Chatham, Kent
Printed and bound in Great Britain by The University Press, Cambridge

# Contents

*The authors wish to thank the Association Nationale pour la Recherche Contre le Sicla for its support.*

# *Series Editor's Foreword*

Any hyperbole to introduce a book to do with HIV infection and AIDS would be both unnecessary and repetitive. The subject is important, by definition and is indeed one of the 'Major Problems in Neurology'. It is a complicated problem because HIV infection causes such a large number of clinical problems, in so many different organs, over so many years. No one doctor or scientist can know and understand, in detail, all there is to know and understand about this infection. Infectious disease specialists need the help of many other specialists when managing their patients, and of course neurologists are important in this regard. For the most part however, neurologists do not claim any particular expertise in managing AIDS patients, even with neurological complications, and look for help from their infectious diseases colleagues. This book is for both neurologists who need to know more of AIDS and AIDS specialists who need to know more of neurology. Not surprisingly, and very appropriately, it is written not by one person, but by a small team who bring together their neurological, infectious disease, paediatric and neuropathological knowledge and experience. The result is a useful account of the neurological complications of HIV infection, presented in a readable and concise format, without sacrificing accuracy or disappointing the interested reader. The authors have been comprehensive in their coverage of the subject to date, and, as one would expect, authoritative.

*Charles Warlow*
*Edinburgh, April 1997*

# *Preface*

Human immunodeficiency virus (HIV) is responsible for a number of neurological problems. These range from acute febrile illness at the time of seroconversion, with polymorphic, usually transient, neurological manifestations affecting the central and/or peripheral nervous system, to late onset dementia related to specific brain involvement by the virus. In the interval, a number of neurological complications may occur caused either by HIV infection of the nervous system itself, drug toxicity, or opportunistic infection.

Opportunistic infections of the nervous system, mainly parasitic like toxoplasmosis, but also mycotic, or viral, like progressive multifocal leukoencephalopathy (PML), in addition to the high rate of cerebral lymphomas, all result from decreased cell mediated immunity and represent a major problem. Recent progress in prevention and treatment has seen a remarkable control of toxoplasmosis, once the most common opportunistic infection in HIV infected patients. PML however, and to a lesser extent cerebral lymphoma, remain out of control, while infection of pregnant women and of the newborn has led to previously unknown neurological manifestations.

Since the outbreak of HIV infection, virtually all countries over the world have been involved. Some countries, especially in Asia, which seemed spared ten years ago are among the most affected now. An enormous amount of clinical and basic work has been performed to better understand the pathophysiology of the disease and control HIV replication and penetration to target cells. This has already lead to improvement in the control of HIV infection with dramatic reduction of viral replication and significant increase of life expectancy of HIV infected patients.

We have focused this book on the practical aspects and on the management of patients with neurological problems associated with HIV infection, and hope that it will be useful to the clinicians and pathologists in charge of HIV infected individuals.

GERARD SAID

# 1

# *Introduction*

The nervous system is involved in a number of ways in the course of HIV infection. The virus seems to penetrate the nervous system early in the course of the disease, without inducing clinical manifestations in most cases. In a small proportion of patients, however, early invasion of the central and/or peripheral nervous system can lead to severe, usually self-limited, neurological manifestations, with a more or less complete recovery. The viral load usually remains low until the onset of symptomatic disease. Afterwards, for several years, most patients are asymptomatic, although again a minority of them develop peripheral neuropathy or central nervous system involvement. In most patients, however, it is only at the stage of profound immunodepression that disabling and often life-threatening neurological complications develop. While the neurological complications before the onset of immunodepression are related to HIV itself, either directly or through the immune response of the host, a number of neurological manifestations in immunodepressed individuals are due to opportunistic infections and, less often, to the development of lymphomas. Post-mortem neuropathological studies reveal that opportunistic infections occur in up to 90% of patients with AIDS. The frequency with which an infective agent is responsible for these opportunistic infections varies between countries and the year of the study (Table 1.1). For instance, the frequency of cerebral toxoplasmosis has been found to range from 5% in the study by Lacroix, unpublished data to 41 and 42% in the series of Gray *et al.* (1991) and Hénin *et al.* (1987), all three reports from France. This apparent discrepancy actually reflects the efficacy of prevention and treatment of cerebral toxoplasmosis. In the USA, the incidence of cerebral toxoplasmosis was much lower in 1986 (Anders *et al.*, 1986; Petito *et al.*, 1986) due to a lower endemicity of the parasitic infection in this country. The most common opportunistic infections observed in this context, namely toxoplasmosis and cytomegalovirus infections, are accessible to specific treatment, but no treatment is presently available for infection with the JC papovavirus, the agent of progressive multifocal leucoencephalopathy, which leads to progressive disability and death in a matter of months in most cases. Also, late in the course of HIV infection, the AIDS dementia complex leads to progressive neurological

**Table 1.1** Opportunistic and HIV infection of the central nervous system in post-mortem studies

| Reference | Country (city) | Total cases | HIV (%) | Cytomegalo-virus (%) | Toxo-plasmosis (%) | Lym-phoma (%) | Crypto-coccosis (%) | Progressive multifocal leuco-encephalo-pathy (%) | Others (%) |
|---|---|---|---|---|---|---|---|---|---|
| Moskowitz *et al.* (1984) | USA (Miami) | 52 | 10 | 4 | 30 | 2 | 0 | 4 | 8 |
| Anders *et al.* (1986) | USA (Los Angeles) | 89 | 47 | 16 | 7 | 5 | 14 | 7 | 4 |
| Petito *et al.* (1986) | USA (New York) | 153 | 28 | 26 | 10 | 6 | 2 | 3 | 6 |
| Budka *et al.* (1987) | Austria, Italy | 100 | 38 | 18 | 17 | 6 | 9 | 5 | 2 |
| Hénin *et al.* (1987) | France (Paris) | 31 | 30 | 13 | 42 | 9 | 9 | 0 | 3 |
| Kanzer *et al.* (1989) | USA (Washington) | 156 | 30 | 10 | 21 | 5 | 12 | 3 | 7 |
| Lantos *et al.* (1989) | UK (London) | 26 | 23 | 7 | 7 | 12 | 0 | 0 | 4 |
| Stavrou *et al.* (1989) | Germany | 61 | 18 | 20 | 11 | 6 | 6 | 0 | 1 |
| Lang *et al.* (1990) | Switzerland | 206 | 18 | 7 | 24 | 0 | 4 | 7 | ? |
| Burns *et al.* (1991) | USA (Dallas) | 141 | 38 | 20 | 3 | 6 | 9 | 3 | 8 |
| Gray *et al.* (1991) | France (Paris, Créteil) | 135 | 38 | 15 | 41 | 11 | 4 | <1 | 4 |
| Kure *et al.* (1991) | USA (New York City) | 268 | 26 | 13 | 13 | 7 | 9 | 5 | 7 |
| Chimelli *et al.* (1992) | Brazil | 252 | 10 | 8 | 34 | 4 | 13 | 1 | 14 |
| Cornford *et al.* (1992) | Canada (Vancouver) | 39 | 18 | 23 | 18 | 28 | 0 | 0 | 13 |
| Matthiessen *et al.* (1992) | France (Paris, Bichat) | 174 | 19 | 14 | 37 | 18 | 6 | 3 | 1 |
| Rhodes (1993) | USA (Los Angeles) | 400 | 20 | 8 | 8 | 6 | 6 | ? | ? |
| Lacroix, unpublished data* | France (Paris) | 70 | 33 | 16 | 5 | 16 | 3 | 10 | 17 |

* Data taken from autopsies performed on patients with AIDS, in Bicêtre between 1986 and 1995.

deterioration and death. At this time the viral load is high, and the virus is present in microglia, macrophages, monocytes and possibly astrocytes. Infected cells produce cytokines that may induce further productive infection. The new therapeutic approach to treatment of HIV infection with combined bi- or tri-therapy, and the use of antiproteases, will hopefully reduce the risk of dementia in HIV-infected patients. Management of patients with HIV infection needs a multidisciplinary approach, including psychological support, because of the diversity of medical problems encountered in this context. Our goal in that respect should be not just improvement in survival rate but also in the quality of life, which can be badly impaired by neurological problems.

## REFERENCES

Anders KH *et al.* (1986) *American Journal of Pathology* **124**: 537–558.
Budka H *et al.* (1987) *Acta Neuropathologica* **75**: 185–198.
Burns DK *et al.* (1991) *Journal of Neuropathology and Experimental Neurology* **50**: 323.
Chimelli L *et al.* (1992) *Neuropathology and Applied Neurobiology* **18**: 478–488.
Cornford ME *et al.* (1992) *Canadian Journal of Neurological Sciences* **19**: 442–452.
Gray F *et al.* (1991) *Annales de Pathologie* **11**: 236–247.
Hénin D *et al.* (1987) *Revue Neurologique* **143**: 631–642.
Kanzer MD *et al.* (1989) *Journal of Neuropathology and Experimental Neurology* **48**: 314.
Kure K *et al.* (1991) *Human Pathology* **22**: 700–710.
Lang W *et al.* (1990) *Schweizerische Rundschau fur Medizin Praxis* **79**: 562–568.
Lantos PL *et al.* (1989) *Lancet* **ii**: 309–311.
Matthiessen L *et al.* (1992) *Annales de Medecine Interne* **143**: 43–49.
Moskowitz LB *et al.* (1984) *Archives of Pathology and Laboratory Medicine* **108**: 867–872.
Petito C *et al.* (1986) *Journal of Neuropathology and Experimental Neurology* **45**: 635–646.
Rhodes RH (1993) *Human Pathology* **24**: 1189–1198.
Stavrou D *et al.* (1989) *Neuropathology and Applied Neurobiology* **15**: 207–222.

# 2

# *HIV-1 Associated Dementia Complex*

Impairment of higher cerebral functions, which is among the most troublesome neurological manifestations of HIV infection, may occur at different stages of HIV infection but is more commonly observed late.

## CLINICAL AND EPIDEMIOLOGICAL ASPECTS

### Acute encephalopathy at the time of seroconversion to HIV

Disturbances of higher functions are occasionally observed in association with an acute infectious mononucleosis-like illness, with headache and myalgias, as manifestations of seroconversion to HIV (Cooper *et al.*, 1985; Clark *et al.*, 1991). The inaugural and presenting manifestations of HIV infection may thus include acute encephalopathy with confusion, fever, myalgias, seizures, meningoencephalitis and cognitive deficit persisting for a few weeks (Carne *et al.*, 1985; Hardy *et al.*, 1991). In a review of 139 published cases of symptomatic primary HIV-1 infection, Clark *et al.* (1991) found that 8% of patients presented with peripheral neuropathy and another 8% manifested encephalopathy. Both central and peripheral manifestations may occur simultaneously, as in one of our patients who manifested an acute inflammatory polyneuritis of the Guillain–Barré type and a transient encephalopathy at seroconversion. Early manifestations of HIV infection usually carry a good prognosis and the patient recovers spontaneously. Cerebrospinal fluid (CSF) analysis in early infection shows oligoclonal bands and intrathecal synthesis of antibodies to HIV and viral antigens (Goudsmit *et al.*, 1986).

### Epidemiology

Infection of the central nervous system (CNS) by HIV was recognized early (Snider *et al.*, 1983; Levy *et al.*, 1985; Gabuzda and Hirsch, 1987; Price and Brew, 1988), and the disturbances of higher functions that ensued were given various appellations including AIDS subacute encephalopathy (Brew and Perdices,

1992), AIDS dementia complex (Price *et al.*, 1988a; Ho *et al.*, 1989; Brew, 1993; McArthur *et al.*, 1993), AIDS-related dementia, HIV dementia, HIV associated neurocognitive disorder and HIV associated neurobehavioural abnormalities (Coffin *et al.*, 1986). In 1991, experts of the World Health Organization (WHO) suggested for adults the use of the terms *HIV-1 associated cognitive/motor complex*, which was separated into *HIV-1 associated dementia complex* (*HIV-ADC*), and *HIV-1 associated myelopathy*, the HIV-1 associated progressive encephalopathy of childhood representing a different entity (Budka *et al.*, 1991). HIV-ADC is one of the criteria of AIDS (Price and Brew, 1988), but neuropsychological abnormalities also occur in non-immunodepressed HIV-infected patients (Janssen *et al.*, 1988, 1989; Price *et al.*, 1991; McArthur *et al.*, 1993).

Small series of patients with neuropsychological impairment but otherwise asymptomatic were reported (Bornstein *et al.*, 1993), but other reports did not find significant abnormalities in patients without AIDS-related complex (ARC) or AIDS (Harter, 1989; McArthur *et al.*, 1993). In the USA, the frequency of HIV-ADC in patients with AIDS was 7.3% in a study performed from September 1987 to August 1991 (Janssen *et al.*, 1992). The proportion of patients with HIV-ADC increased with age, from 6% under 34 years of age to 19% after 75 years of age. In 2.8% of the patients, HIV-ADC was the only AIDS-defining illness (Janssen *et al.*, 1992). Working on a clinical basis may overestimate the frequency of HIV-ADC because many patients have cognitive impairments due to other causes, such as cerebrovascular lesions, senility, alcoholism, drug addiction, opportunistic infections or brain lymphoma (Janssen *et al.*, 1992). In another small group of patients with AIDS, the frequency of HIV-ADC was 7.1% (McArthur *et al.*, 1993). In other reports, the prevalence of HIV-ADC is higher, affecting up to 65% of patients with AIDS (Navia *et al.*, 1986a; Gabuzda and Hirsch, 1987; Price and Brew, 1988). It is important to keep in mind that depression, which is common in HIV-infected patients, can lead to pseudodementia and that treatment with antidepressants should be considered in patients with dementia and normal cerebral imaging. HIV-ADC seems more common when the CD4 T-cell count falls (de Martini *et al.*, 1988; Barohn *et al.*, 1990; Brew, 1993). No significant risk factors were found including specific AIDS illness, zidovudine use and CD4 T-cell count before AIDS (McArthur *et al.*, 1993). In Europe, no epidemiological study is presently available on the subject. HIV-ADC could be the presenting or sole manifestation of HIV infection in some patients (Navia and Price, 1987).

**Clinical presentation**

The onset of mental deterioration is usually insidious, occasionally abrupt (Jones *et al.*, 1988). The patient's condition usually worsens within 1–9 months. Fluctuation of symptoms or relapsing encephalitis may occur in some patients (Berger *et al.*, 1992). The first symptoms of HIV-ADC are impairment in behavioural, cognitive and motor functions. Loss of concentration or forgetfulness are common complaints. Changes in social behaviour occur such as irritability, impairment of judgement or socially inappropriate behaviour and disinhibition. Patients develop difficulty in writing and reading, causing them to stop their work. Many patients have temporo-spatial disorientation (Navia *et al.*, 1986a). More than one-third of patients have social withdrawal, apathy and abulia, associated with emotional lability (Ho *et al.*, 1989). A few patients experience hallucinations and psychosis. Chronic headache and generalized seizures are uncommon. Half of the patients have slowing of rapid movements, moderate weakness of lower limbs and incoordination. Gait ataxia is frequent. Tendon reflexes are usually brisk, often with Babinski's sign. Smooth-pursuit eye movements are impaired (Navia *et al.*, 1986a; Price and Brew, 1988). Cognitive, behavioural and motor disorders evolve gradually, but fluctuations and transient spontaneous improvement may occur. Sphincter disturbances, myoclonus, hypertonia, involuntary movements, ataxia, apraxia of walking develop progressively and the patients become bedridden (McArthur *et al.*, 1993). They usually die from general opportunistic infection or pneumonia (Navia *et al.*, 1986a). HIV-ADC usually evolves as a subcortical subacute encephalitis (Navia *et al.*, 1986b). The clinical presentation of HIV encephalitis produces some variations such as involuntary hyperkinetic movements, parkinsonism or status epileptitus. Relapsing multiple sclerosis-like illness (Berger *et al.*, 1989) was reported in this context, but coincidental illnesses are possible.

Staging of AIDS dementia complex can be useful, as suggested by Price and Brew (1988).

Stage 0 (normal): normal mental and motor function.

Stage 0.5 (subclinical): absent, minimal or equivocal symptoms without impairment of work or activities of daily living. Mild signs such as snout response, slowed ocular or extremity movements may be present.

Stage 1 (mild): able to perform all but the most demanding aspects of work or daily living. Evidence of functional intellectual or motor impairment as elicited on history, examination or neuropsychological investigation. Can walk unaided.

Stage 2 (moderate): able to perform basic activities of self-care, unable to work or maintain the more demanding activities of daily living. Ambulatory, but may require assistance.

Stage 3 (severe): major intellectual incapacity (cannot follow news or personal events, cannot sustain a complex conversation, considerable slowing of all cognitive response) or motor disability (cannot walk unassisted, slowing and clumsiness of arms).

Stage 4 (end stage): nearly vegetative state. Intellectual and social comprehension and response are at a rudimentary level. Nearly or absolutely mute. Paraparetic or paraplegic with urinary and faecal incontinence.

## INVESTIGATIONS

### Neuroimaging

Brain computed tomography (CT) and/or magnetic resonance imaging (MRI) are mandatory in patients with HIV-ADC to exclude the possibility of detectable opportunistic infections or lymphomas. In one of the first reports on neuroradiological findings in patients with AIDS, brain atrophy, as established on imaging criteria, was found in 75/200 patients and cerebral mass in 51/200 patients (Levy *et al.*, 1986). Cerebral imaging shows non-specific lesions. On CT, cerebral atrophy with dilatation of the ventricular system and hypointense white matter non-enhancing lesions are common (Chrysikopoulos *et al.*, 1990). MRI can detect brain lesions earlier than CT, showing high-intensity signal abnormalities on $T_2$-weighted images in the periventricular white matter and the centrum semiovale, but is no more specific (Figure 2.1) (Jarvik *et al.*, 1988; Post *et al.*, 1988). In some cases, abnormalities on CT or MRI are detected before the onset of clinical manifestations (Post *et al.*, 1988; Price and Brew, 1988), but systematic brain imaging in asymptomatic HIV-infected patients is not justified since the results do not modify the management of the patients. Quantitative evaluations of MRI findings in patients with AIDS and control patients found that enlargement of the ventricles and atrophy of the caudate region

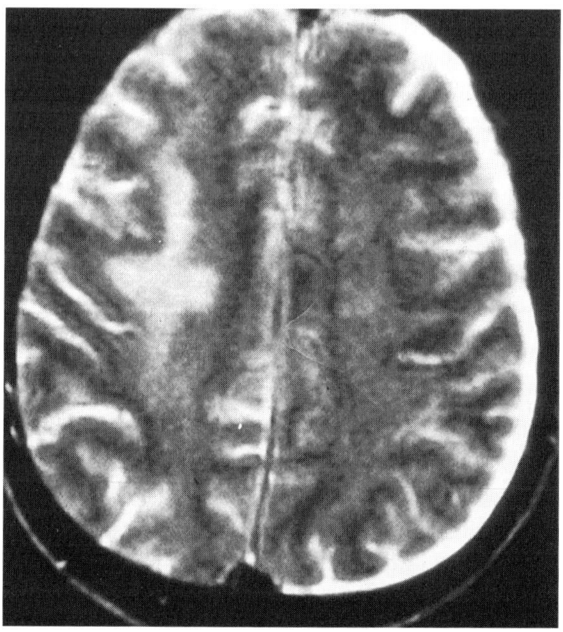

**Figure 2.1** $T_2$-weighted MRI of a patient with HIV-ADC showing asymmetric high-intensity signal in the white matter.

correlated with dementia (Dal Pan *et al.*, 1992; Kieburtz *et al.*, 1996). In a positron emission tomography study, relative subcortical hypermetabolism was present in early HIV-ADC and cortical and subcortical grey matter hypometabolism at later stages (Rottenberg *et al.*, 1987). There is no justification as yet for routine use of positron emission tomography in HIV-ADC.

## CSF abnormalities

CSF analysis is useful to exclude subacute opportunistic infections such as cryptococcosis or mycobacteria. Patients with HIV-ADC often show a mild mononuclear pleocytosis and increased protein content. Intrathecal synthesis of oligoclonal IgG bands is present in patients with HIV neurological abnormalities (Resnick *et al.*, 1985), but also in patients without AIDS or ARC (Goudsmit *et al.*, 1986). HIV has been isolated from the CSF of patients with HIV infection, both during seroconversion and in HIV-ADC (Ho *et al.*, 1985). Free HIV particles have been isolated in some patients at the early stage of infection and in most patients at the late stage (Chiodi *et al.*, 1988). Demonstration of HIV particles in the CSF could be a signal of virus replication in the brain. HIV has been cultured from the CSF in some patients (Ho *et al.*, 1985). HIV p24 antigen was detected more frequently in the CSF and blood of patients with HIV-ADC compared with non-demented patients; the concentration was higher in patients with low numbers of CD4 T cells (Brew, 1993; Royal *et al.*, 1994). Several reports have evaluated cytokine levels in the CSF: interleukin (IL)-1β, IL-1α and IL-6 were detected in the CSF of HIV patients with or without central nervous system involvement; levels of tumour necrosis factor α (TNF-α) were decreased (Gallo *et al.*, 1989); moderate elevation of IL-6 concentration was found (Perrella *et al.*, 1992); and increased levels of TNF-α were found (Grimaldi *et al.*, 1991; Perrella *et al.*, 1992; Wesselingh *et al.*, 1993). These observations support a possible intrathecal secretion of cytokines in some patients, but no correlation with the brain damage was possible (Grimaldi *et al.*, 1991) and contradictory results were obtained by others studies in which the authors were unable to detect TNF-α in the spinal fluid from HIV-infected patients (Shaskan and Thompson, 1992). However, in these different studies, the techniques used for the tests were different. CSF concentrations of neopterin, a marker of activated macrophages, were elevated in patients with HIV-ADC, brain lymphomas or opportunistic infections (Brew *et al.*, 1990). During the course of HIV-ADC, CSF neopterin levels correlated with the severity of the disease and decreased when the patients improved following treatment with zidovudine. This marker of activated macrophages is not specific but the results of this evaluation in 97 patients suggest a possible effect of zidovudine on macrophages (Brew *et al.*, 1990). Similar results were observed with CSF concentrations of quinolinic acid, with levels elevated over 20-fold in severe brain disorders and decreased when improvement occurred with administration of zidovudine or specific therapy for opportunistic infections (Heyes *et al.*, 1991).

### Electrophysiology

Electrophysiological abnormalities observed in HIV-ADC include non-specific alterations of the electroencephalogram, delayed somatosensory evoked potentials and long latency potentials, but such abnormalities lack specificity and reproducibility that would make them useful for screening or diagnostic purposes, or to evaluate the effect of any treatment.

## NEUROPATHOLOGY

An abundant literature has been published on CNS abnormalities in patients with HIV-ADC (Table 2.1) (Navia *et al.*, 1986b; Budka *et al.*, 1991). The large majority of the studies were done on autopsy samples and in many cases HIV-related lesions were concomitant to opportunistic infections or brain lymphomas (Kure *et al.*, 1991). Some stereotactic brain biopsies were performed in patients with focal brain lesions (Chappell *et al.*, 1992; Levy *et al.*, 1992). Only occasional cases of asymptomatic patients with HIV infection are available: mild chronic meningitis and gliosis in the white matter were present in the studies of Lenhardt *et al.* (1988) and McArthur *et al.* (1989).

Different morphological abnormalities have been observed in the CNS of patients with HIV-ADC and were classified into several morphological subtypes, which may be associated: multiple disseminated foci of microglia, necrosis, macrophages and multinucleated giant cells (MGCs) are usually associated with HIV antigens or nucleic acids; leucoencephalopathy characterized by diffuse damage to the white matter, myelin loss, reactive astrogliosis and MGCs (Gonzales and Davis, 1988); vacuolar leucoencephalopathy (de la Monte *et al.*, 1986); and diffuse poliodystrophy (Budka *et al.*, 1991).

**Table 2.1** Incidence of HIV-ADC in autopsy series

| Country | Reference | Number of patients | HIV-ADC (%) |
|---|---|---|---|
| USA | Petito et al. (1986) | 153 | 28 |
| Austria/Italy | Budka *et al.* (1987) | 100 | 38 |
| France | Hénin *et al.* (1987) | 31 | 30 |
| USA | de la Monte *et al.* (1987) | 30 | 90 |
| USA | Rhodes (1987) | 400 | 20 |
| USA | Kanzer *et al.* (1989) | 156 | 30 |
| Switzerland | Lang *et al.* (1989) | 135 | 18 |
| Germany | Stavrou *et al.* (1989) | 61 | 18 |
| France | Gray *et al.* (1991) | 135 | 38 |
| USA | Kure *et al.* (1991) | 268 | 26 |
| Brazil | Chimelli *et al.* (1992) | 252 | 10 |
| Canada | Cornford *et al.* (1992) | 39 | 43 |
| France | Matthiessen *et al.* (1992) | 174 | 19 |
| France | Lacroix, unpublished data* | 85 | 21 |

* Data taken from autopsies performed on patients with AIDS, in Bicêtre between 1986 and 1996.

The clinical dementia and abnormal neuropsychological tests were not associated with 'specific' brain changes at post-mortem examination in some series (Navia *et al.*, 1986b; Glass *et al.*, 1993). Long-term treatment with zidovudine might attenuate neuropathological changes (Glass *et al.*, 1993).

Low brain weight and cerebral atrophy are not always correlated with HIV-ADC, but the brains of most of our patients with HIV-ADC weighed less than 1000 g (normal brain weight 1500 g ± 100) (Gelman and Guinto, 1992; Kieburtz *et al.*, 1996).

Reports on neocortical damage are controversial, and furthermore any such changes are associated with subcortical damage (Ketzler *et al.*, 1990; Brew, 1991; Weis *et al.*, 1993a). Some authors have found qualitative and quantitative abnormalities (Everall *et al.*, 1991) and others denied any neuronal loss (Seilhean *et al.*, 1993; Weis *et al.*, 1993a). Vacuolar encephalopathy or spongiform changes have been observed (de la Monte *et al.*, 1986; Schwenk *et al.*, 1987), but a search for prions in brains from patients with AIDS was negative (Goldwater and Paton, 1989).

Progressive diffuse leucoencephalopathy, which is found in approximately 25% of patients with HIV-ADC, is characterized by diffuse loss of myelin, proliferation of astrocytes and infiltration by macrophages and giant cells (Budka *et al.*, 1987; Sharer, 1992). Diffuse or focal demyelination or pallor of the white matter are found in almost half of the patients with HIV-ADC (Figures 2.2 and 2.3) (Smith *et al.*, 1990; Glass *et al.*, 1993). In some cases, focal vacuolization and angiocentric areas of myelin pallor are present, suggesting alteration of the blood–brain barrier (Schmidbauer *et al.*, 1992; Power *et al.*, 1993).

White matter astrogliosis and fibrillary gliosis in the grey matter seem to be the more frequent findings in patients with HIV-ADC for some authors (de la Monte *et al.*, 1987). Other authors have found prominent gliosis in the subpial region, cortex–white matter junction and subcortical white matter associated with focal astrogliosis in the cortex, such as in most of our cases of HIV-ADC (von Einsiedel *et al.*, 1990; Weis *et al.*, 1993b). Immunocytochemistry with glial fibrillary acidic protein (GFAP) may be useful to determine the extension of the astrogliosis. In patients with HIV-ADC we observed a striking increase of GFAP-positive astrocytes in the white matter but no GFAP-positive astrocytes in the frontal cortex (Figure 2.4).

Microglial nodules made of macrophages, lymphocytes, a few giant cells, astrocytes and polymorphonuclear cells are found in the grey and white matter of the cerebral hemispheres, brainstem and cerebellum (Figure 2.5). Microglial nodules were believed to be directly and specifically due to HIV (Snider *et al.*, 1983; Anders *et al.*, 1986), but they can also be observed in association with cytomegalovirus (CMV), measles virus, *Cryptococcus* or *Toxoplasma gondii* infections (Kato *et al.*, 1987; Patsouris *et al.*, 1993).

The hallmark of HIV infection of the CNS is the presence of MGCs (Sharer *et al.*, 1985; Stavrou *et al.*, 1989). These giant cells, isolated or in microglial nodules (Figure 2.6), are usually found in the basal ganglia, brainstem and white matter, occasionally in the cortex (Budka, 1986). Some nuclear bridges may be observed, indicating probable division (Mizusawa *et al.*, 1987). HIV proteins can

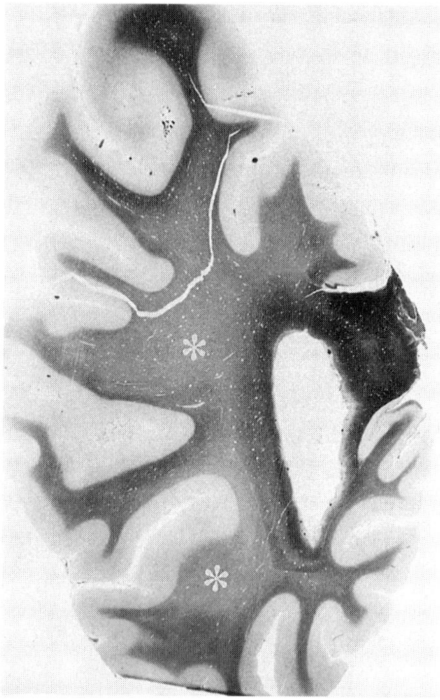

**Figure 2.2** Occipital lobe of a patient with HIV-ADC showing pallor of the myelin (*). (Vertical celloidin section; Woelcke's stain.)

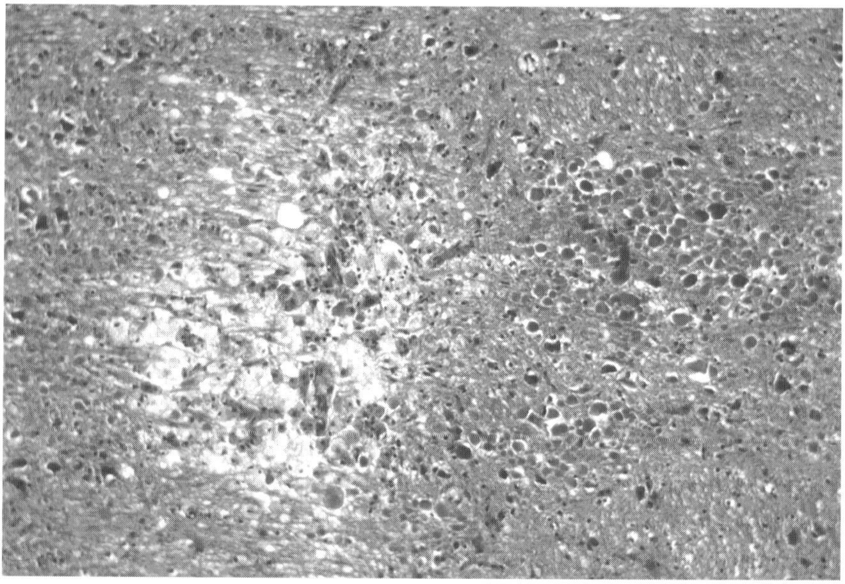

**Figure 2.3** Focal white matter necrosis in a patient with HIV-ADC. (Paraffin section; haematoxylin and eosin (H&E); ×710.)

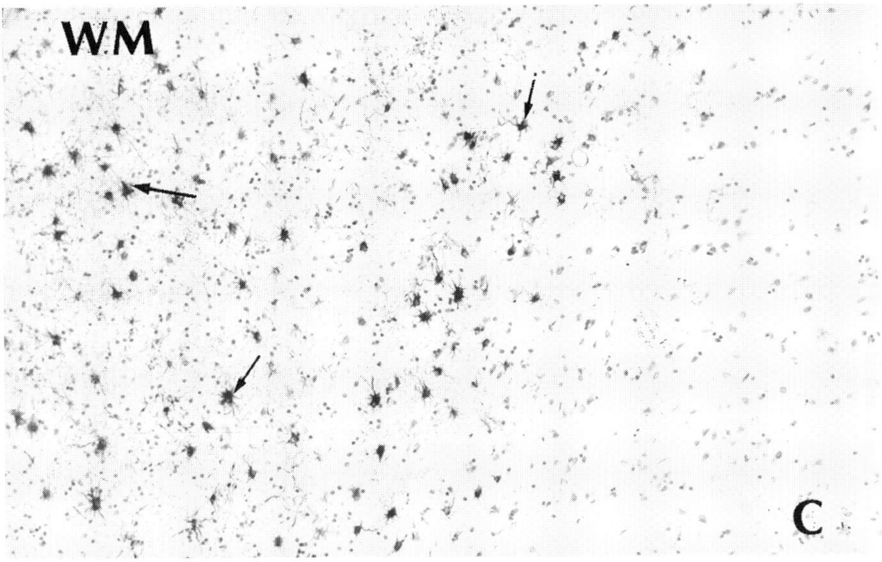


**Figure 2.4** Reactive astrogliosis (arrows) in the cortex (C)–white matter (WM) junction. (Paraffin section; glial fibrillary acidic protein (GFAP)/diamino benzidine (DAB); ×270.)

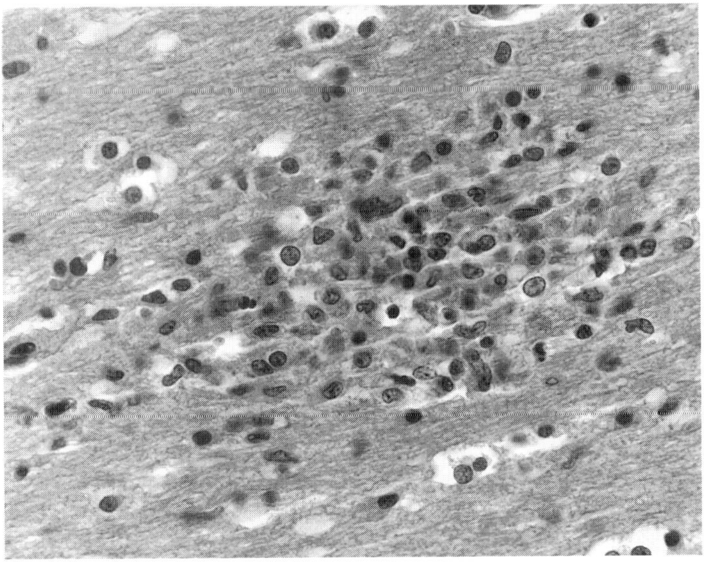

**Figure 2.5** Microglial nodule in the white matter of the cerebellum of an HIV-infected patient. (Paraffin section; H&E; ×1050.)

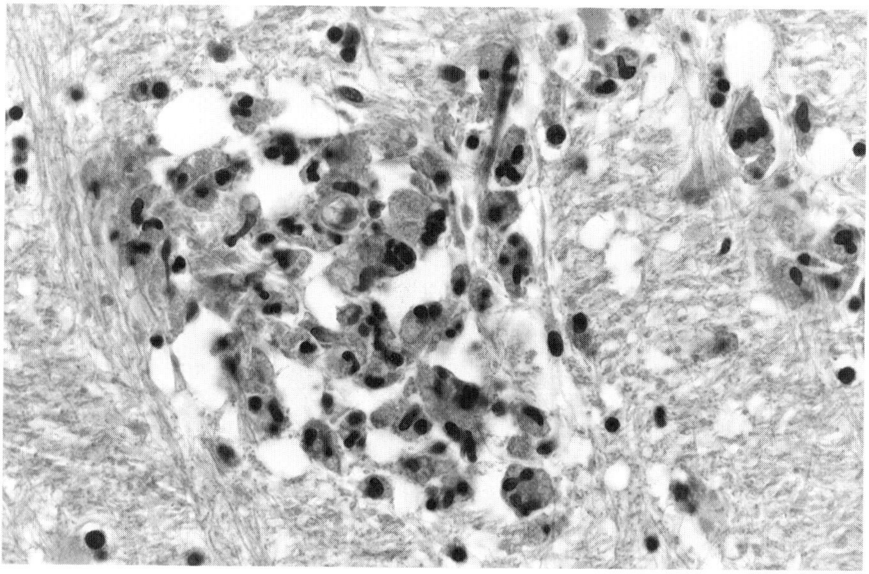

**Figure 2.6** A microglial nodule with many multinucleated giant cells in the basal ganglia of a patient with HIV-ADC. (Paraffin section; H&E; ×1050.)

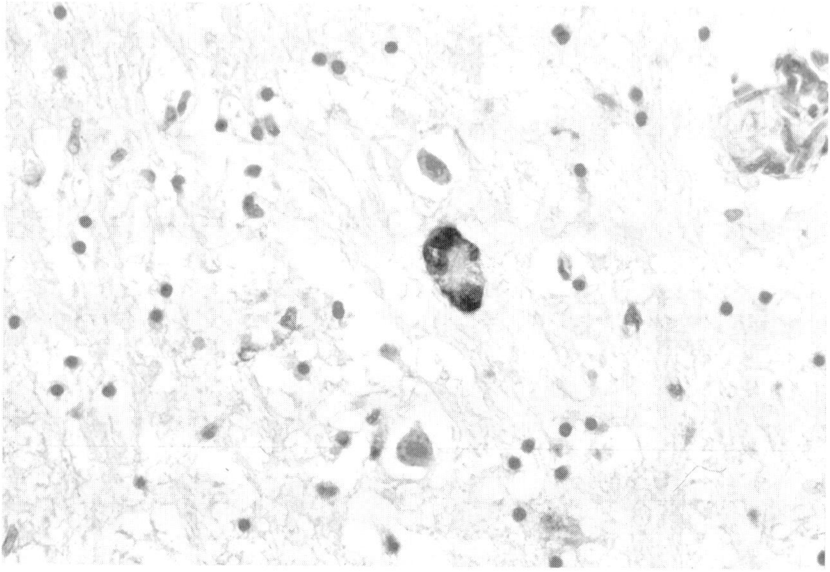

**Figure 2.7** HIV gp41 antibodies detected in the cytoplasm of a giant cell in the caudate nucleus of an HIV-demented patient. (Paraffin section; DAB; ×2740.)

be detected by immunocytochemistry in these MGCs (Figure 2.7) in agreement with electron microscopic observations (Mizusawa *et al.*, 1987). The presence of MGCs is essential for the diagnosis of HIV infection of the CNS if HIV antigens or nucleic acids are not detected with immunocytochemistry or *in situ* hybridization (Sharer and Kapila, 1985; Budka *et al.*, 1991). Identification of cells of the monocyte–macrophage lineage of MGCs has been performed using immunocytochemistry, *in situ* hybridization, electron microscopy and cultures from brain biopsies (Gartner *et al.*, 1986; Vazeux *et al.*, 1987; Hulette *et al.* 1992). A microglial origin for the giant cells is commonly accepted (Michaels *et al.*, 1988; Kure *et al.*, 1990a), but denied by some authors (Miles and Chou, 1988). Using a ferritin antibody, which is a marker for microglia, we have observed diffuse proliferation of microglial cells in the cerebral grey and white matter in most patients with HIV-ADC (Gelman, 1993).

Mild focal perivascular and leptomeningeal mononuclear cell infiltration is usually present, including monocyte–macrophages, T cells and rarely B cells (Weidenheim *et al.*, 1990). CD68-positive macrophages (Figure 2.8) containing p24 core protein are frequently detected in the thalamus and the external basal ganglia, but the cortical grey matter is usually spared (Neuen-Jacob *et al.*, 1993). In the basal ganglia, vascular mineralization is due to iron and aluminium deposition (Perl *et al.*, 1989). Abnormalities of vessel walls may be observed, such as thickening of capillary basal laminae (Budka, 1989) and increased reactivity of laminin in the basement membranes of capillary walls (Taruscio *et*

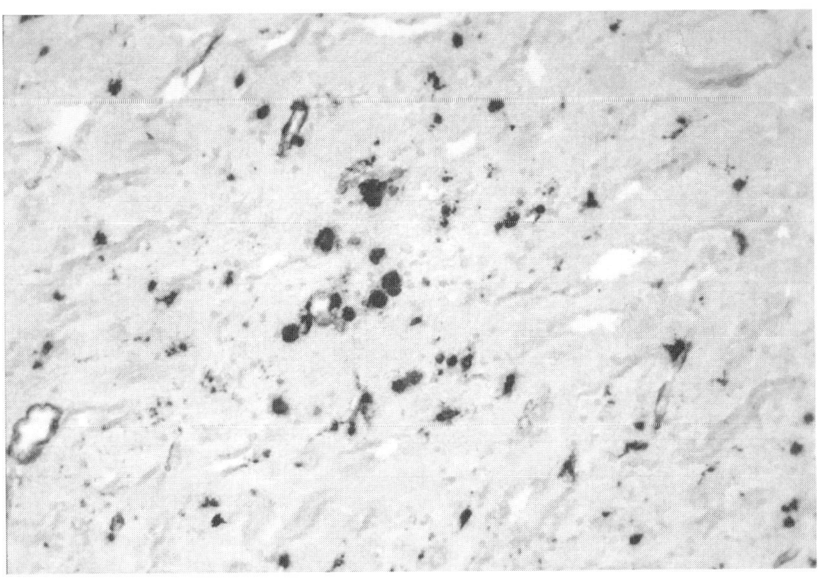

**Figure 2.8** Multiple macrophages stained by an anti-CD68 antibody in the white matter of a patient with severe HIV-ADC. (Frozen section; DAB; ×685.)

*al.*, 1991). Alterations of the blood–brain barrier have been proved by the presence of serum proteins in post-mortem brains of patients with AIDS, suggesting that the breakdown of the blood–brain barrier may facilitate entry of HIV into the brain and may be responsible for the gliosis and white matter pallor (Rhodes, 1991; Petito and Cash, 1992).

Ultrastructural examination of brain can show free viral particles of various shapes in the cytoplasm of macrophages and MGCs (Meyenhoffer *et al.*, 1987). High levels of HIV envelope proteins (gp41) and other viral proteins, including p17, p24 and p25, are present in perivascular and parenchymal macrophages, microglia and MGCs, endothelial cells (Gabuzda *et al.*, 1986; Wiley *et al.*, 1986; Budka, 1990; Kure *et al.*, 1990b) and, questionably, neurones (Pumarola-Sune *et al.*, 1987). Quantitation of gp41 antibodies did not demonstrate a correlation between abundant gp41 antibodies in the frontal cortex and basal ganglia and dementia: some non-demented patients had high levels of gp41 antibodies and some demented patients had little or no immunoreactivity (Glass *et al.*, 1995). In our experience, the higher levels of gp41 antigens compared with p24 and gp120 antigens in the deep grey matter of patients with HIV-ADC favour the use of gp41 antibody to detect HIV antigens in brain tissue. HIV RNA has been detected in brain macrophages and MGCs (Kure *et al.*, 1990a). Using *in situ* hybridization, HIV was found in capillary endothelial cells, macrophages and giant cells of both white and grey matter of the brain in patients with HIV-ADC (Wiley *et al.*, 1986; Walker *et al.*, 1989). Using the polymerase chain reaction (PCR), the presence of HIV DNA in brain tissue is well correlated with brain pathology for some authors (Weiser *et al.*, 1990; Wiley and Budka, 1991) but denied by others (Johnson *et al.*, 1996).

HIV-ADC may be associated with CMV encephalitis (Fuller *et al.*, 1989) or human T-lymphotropic virus type 1 (HTLV-1) infection (Berger *et al.*, 1991). Simultaneous infections, detected by immunocytochemistry in most cases, had led some authors to suggest an *in vivo* interaction between the two viruses in the pathogenesis of dementia (Wiley and Nelson, 1988). Infection with HTLV-1 does not seem to be important in the occurrence of higher function disorder, which is not common in patients infected with this virus alone. Severe brain encephalitis may occur in coinfection with HIV and JC viruses (Vazeux *et al.*, 1990). We have detected the virus antigens in different cells: HIV antigens in MGCs and microglia and JC antigens in oligodendrocytes (Figure 2.9).

## PATHOGENESIS

Studies on the pathogenesis of HIV-ADC have been the subject of several review articles (Achim *et al.*, 1991a; Geleziunas *et al.*, 1992; Epstein and Gendelman, 1993). Several key points must be considered in the pathogenesis.

(1) Although HIV penetrates the brain early in the course of HIV infection, HIV-ADC becomes symptomatic years later (except children, in whom the

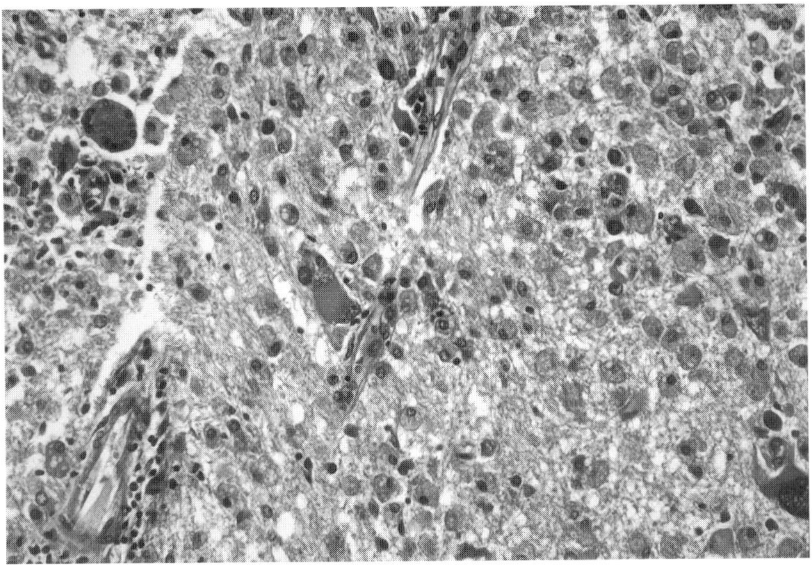

**Figure 2.9** Many macrophages, an HIV giant cell, bizarre astrocytes and dense inclusions in oligodendrocytes in the white matter of a patient with multifocal leucoencephalopathy and HIV-ADC. (Paraffin section; H&E; ×1369.) Immunocytochemistry demonstrated that different cells were infected by the two viruses: macrophages/multinucleated giant cells by HIV and oligodendrocytes exclusively by papovavirus.

dementia occurs earlier; see Chapter 6) when patients have already lost most of their CD4 T cells.

(2) Infection of neurones does not seem to be responsible for the dementia process, suggesting that other factors play a role in the brain pathology associated with HIV infection.

(3) Indirect factors induced by the presence of HIV are likely to be responsible for the pathological brain disorder. Such factors could include: astrocyte-mediated neuronal injury, microglia-mediated neuronal injury or both (Lipton, 1991); release of toxic substances in the brain in association with viral replication in macrophages/microglia, including viral proteins, cytokines, glutamate, quinolinic acid, *N*-methyl-D-aspartate (NMDA) receptor (Johnson *et al.*, 1988; Rosenberg and Fauci, 1990; Li *et al.*, 1991); and intercellular adhesion molecules such as integrins (Achim *et al.*, 1991a; Archelos *et al.*, 1993).

Unfortunately, experimental models have not yet cast much light on our understanding of HIV-ADC. Experimental simian immunodeficiency virus (SIV) infection and feline immunodeficiency virus infection, which induce similar brain lesions in monkeys and cats, have been proposed as possible models for HIV-ADC (Ringler *et al.*, 1988; Dean *et al.*, 1993; Gray *et al.*, 1993).

However, in a recent study, Rausch *et al.* (1994) found only minimal CNS lesions in SIV-infected rhesus monkeys with cognitive/motor abnormalities.

The virus might penetrate the CNS via pinocytic vesicles in endothelial cells, through choroid plexus epithelial cells or within circulating infected cells of the monocyte–macrophage lineage (Johnson *et al.*, 1988). Fibroblast-like cells of the human choroid plexus can be latently infected by HIV *in vitro*, indicating another possible route of entry for the virus into the brain (Harouse *et al.*, 1989). The virus penetrates the cells by binding its envelope gp120 protein to the CD4 antigen, which is present on brain macrophages and microglia (Kaiser *et al.*, 1990). Most studies suggest that HIV enters the CNS as a proviral form within infected macrophages, probably during the early stages of HIV infection (Achim *et al.*, 1991a). Comparison of isolates of HIV-1 from the CNS or blood showed that those from the brain represented a specific subgroup (Cheng-Mayer *et al.*, 1989). The three main forms of HIV DNA (linear, unintegrated circular and integrated) have been detected in the brains of demented patients, with a higher proportion of unintegrated viral DNA (Pang *et al.*, 1990). A segment of the envelope of the virus, the V3 loop, seems to be the stimulus for the replication of the virus in brain macrophages (Garry *et al.*, 1991; Chesebro *et al.*, 1992; Westervelt *et al.*, 1992). DNA sequencing of the *nef* gene, one of the regulatory genes of HIV, from brains of patients with HIV dementia showed a duplicated region in *nef*, suggesting selection for *nef* quasi-species in humans (Blumberg *et al.*, 1992). A variable interaction between the CD4 molecule and the viral envelope glycoprotein gp120 is also suspected (Lifson *et al.*, 1986; Vazeux *et al.*, 1987).

Since the recognition of HIV infection of the brain, macrophages have been suspected of playing a major role (Bowen *et al.*, 1985; Klatzmann and Gluckman, 1986). Macrophages and microglia, and astrocytes in the opinion of some authors (Shapshak *et al.*, 1990), are sites of replication for HIV *in vitro* (Gendelman *et al.*, 1990; Lyman *et al.*, 1992). The gp41 protein is the factor suspected of reducing chemotaxis. Brain macrophages and microglial cells are the major source of active HIV replication; peripheral blood macrophages located in the brain do not produce HIV antigen in early cultures (Brinkmann *et al.*, 1992). In primary human brain cultures astrocytes do not express HIV *gag* antigens, but in microglial cells the virus replicates actively, leading to cell fusion and death (Watkins *et al.*, 1990). Conversely, Peudenier *et al.* (1991), using other macrophage receptors, found that the HIV-infected cells in the brains of patients with HIV-ADC comprised peripheral monocytes that had crossed the blood–brain barrier and some resident macrophages (microglia) that had phagocytosed infected blood lymphocytes. Adults with the most severe dementia usually have the most critical lesions, together with, according to different authors, high levels of brain infection (Vazeux *et al.*, 1987) or low levels of brain infection (Johnson *et al.*, 1996). Children with severe dementia who have been infected at birth have low HIV replication in the brain (Vazeux *et al.*, 1992). Viral particles accumulate within Golgi-derived cytoplasmic vacuoles in brain macrophages and MGCs. Thus infection of brain macrophages and viral replication has been clearly demonstrated by numerous studies, but the absence of obvious neuronal and glial infection leads to a consideration of the pathogenic role of mediators released by infected macrophages (Giulian *et al.*, 1990; Merrill and Chen, 1991).

Expression of the major histocompatibility complex (MHC) has been studied in the brain of patients with HIV-ADC. MHC class I ($\beta_2$-microglobulin) has been detected at high levels on endothelial cells, macrophages and possibly on oligodendrocytes. MHC class II (HLA-DR), present only on macrophages, microglia and on occasional endothelial cells, and gp120 bind to the same ligand (CD4) on T cells and macrophages (Rosenberg and Fauci, 1990; Achim *et al.*, 1991b). Activated microglial cells express MHC and are involved in antigen presentation and lymphocyte activation in the CNS response of HIV-ADC (Thomas, 1992). Activation of microglia by HIV may thus disturb the normal homeostatic balance between microglia and astrocytes, oligodendrocytes, endothelial cells and neurones. Cytokines are suspected of playing a major role in this context (Dickson *et al.*, 1991). Activated peripheral macrophages and microglia may induce IL-1 and TNF-$\alpha$ production via signals mediated through the CD4 molecule on monocytes (Merrill and Chen, 1991). In brain tissue cultures, microglia and astrocytes produce IL-1 and TNF-$\alpha$ in the presence of infected T cells, whole virus or recombinant envelope proteins; antibodies against gp120 and gp41 block this production (Merrill *et al.*, 1992). In the brains of patients with HIV infection, there is a significant increase in MHC class II antigen, IL-1 and TNF-$\alpha$, but no correlation is present between levels of cytokines and the presence or absence of CNS pathology (Tyor *et al.*, 1992). The expression of TNF-$\alpha$ mRNA seems to be higher in the brains of patients with HIV-ADC compared with non-demented AIDS patients or seronegative controls (Glass *et al.*, 1993; Wesselingh *et al.*, 1993). Secretion of IL-1 and arachidonic acid metabolites is induced by the gp120 glycoprotein in cultures (Wahl *et al.*, 1989). In an *in vitro* study, HIV-infected macrophages, cocultivated with astroglia, produced elevated levels of TNF-$\alpha$ and arachidonic metabolites (Genis *et al.*, 1992). Interferon $\gamma$ produced by activated macrophages/microglia may lead to increased synthesis of neopterin and quinolinic acid, an agonist of the presumed neurotoxic NMDA receptor (Rabinoff, 1993) that could be involved in the CNS damage in AIDS patients. Neopterin levels are increased in the subcortical white matter but normal, compared with controls, in the cortex of patients with HIV-ADC and CMV pathology (Shaskan *et al.*, 1992). The neurotoxins produced by macrophages may act via NMDA receptors (Giulian *et al.*, 1990). The gp120 coat protein can increase the cellular concentration of $Ca^{2+}$ and induce neuronal damage and subsequently neuronal death (Lipton, 1992a). Suspecting the important role played by calcium channels in neuronal injuries, some authors have suggested the use of calcium channel antagonists, such as nimodipine, to prevent the *in vitro* neuronal damage induced by gp120 (Dreyer *et al.*, 1990; Lipton and Gendelman, 1995). The gp 120 coat protein could, in addition, induce excessive stimulation of excitatory amino acid binding at NMDA receptors and thus worsen neuronal damage. Memantine, which blocks NMDA receptors, can prevent gp120 neuronal damage *in vitro* (Lipton, 1992b; Lipton and Gendelman, 1995), but clinical use of this drug cannot be considered as yet.

If the role played by macrophages and microglial cells in the pathogenesis of HIV-ADC is established, the mechanisms of blood–brain barrier alteration are currently unknown. Some authors have suggested a role for activated B cells that may have crossed the blood–brain barrier; in our experience, however, the presence of B cells is very uncommon in the brains of patients who die with HIV-ADC (Houff, 1988). Some studies have focused on the role played by intercellular adhesion molecules (Sasseville *et al.*, 1992; Epstein and Gendelman, 1993; Mackay and Imhof, 1993). Two pairs of molecules seem to be frequently involved in immune processes: lymphocyte function associated antigen 1 and intercellular adhesion molecule 1 (ICAM-1); and very late antigen 4 and vascular cell adhesion molecule 1 (VCAM-1) (Mackay and Imhof, 1993). Primary cultures of human embryonic neurones and astrocytes are destroyed in the presence of HIV-infected macrophages, but not after direct infection; cell–cell adhesion of the neural cells with the infected macrophages is necessary to induce lesions (Tardieu *et al.*, 1992). In preliminary studies of HIV-ADC, the expression of VCAM-1 was increased but the expression of ICAM-1 was not significantly different from controls (McKelvie *et al.*, 1992).

The striking differences between the small numbers of infected cells, which contain potentially neurotoxic HIV proteins and factors such as cytokines, and the extent of CNS lesions has led some authors to suggest a role for astrocytes via abnormal cell–cell interaction (Epstein and Gendelman, 1993). Cultured human glial cells can be infected by HIV and some of them can express the CD4 molecule (Cheng-Mayer *et al.*, 1987; Brack-Werner *et al.*, 1992). Epstein and Gendelman (1993), convinced by the importance of the astrogliosis in HIV-ADC present in most of their cases, as in ours, think that cell–cell communication between astrocytes and infected monocytes induces and amplifies glial proliferation and production of neurotoxins.

Despite these multiple *in vivo*, post-mortem and *in vitro* studies, little is certain about the pathogenesis of HIV-ADC. Different indirect factors, such as cytokines, excitatory aminoacids receptors and intercellular adhesion molecules, are probably involved in addition to direct infection of the brain by different forms of HIV.

## TREATMENT

Since the outbreak of the epidemic of HIV infection, spectacular progress has been achieved in the treatment of opportunistic infections, especially cerebral toxoplasmosis and to some extent CMV infection of the nervous system. However, specific treatment of HIV infection with zidovudine is less than satisfactory as judged by daily clinical experience. Although some authors have reported promising results on the usefulness of zidovudine to prevent or treat HIV-ADC (Price *et al.*, 1988b), mainly on the basis of biological or pathological markers (Price *et al.*, 1988b; Royal *et al.*, 1994) and short-term controlled trials (Sidtis *et al.*, 1993), follow-up of larger series and over a longer period of time is needed to show significant clinical benefit. No significant reports on the use of dideoxyinosine, dideoxycytidine or antiproteases have been published.

## VASCULAR DISORDERS OF THE CNS IN AIDS

Children and adults may present with CNS vascular disorders (Mizusawa *et al.*, 1988; Park *et al.*, 1990). In some of them cerebrovascular lesions are symptomatic (Engstrom *et al.*, 1988; Kugler *et al.*, 1991), but more often vascular lesions are only found at autopsy, sometimes in association with lesions due to HIV, opportunistic infections or lymphoma (Gonzales and Davis, 1988; Rhodes, 1993).

A cerebral stroke is a rare event in patients with HIV infection and has been associated with hepatitis B and C antigenaemia (Atalaia *et al.*, 1992). Syphilitic arteritis may occur in patients with HIV infection and may improve on antibiotic therapy (Labauge *et al.*, 1991). In the presence of ischaemic or haemorrhagic stroke in a young patient without cardiovascular risk factors, syphilis and HIV must be searched for.

In some autopsy series, the frequency of cerebral infarcts was high, ranging from 10% (Kure *et al.*, 1991) to 29% (Mizusawa *et al.*, 1988). Ischaemic lesions were found in the cerebral hemispheres, the brainstem and sometimes the cerebellum or spinal cord (Budka *et al.*, 1987; Engstrom *et al.*, 1988; Fénelon *et al.*,

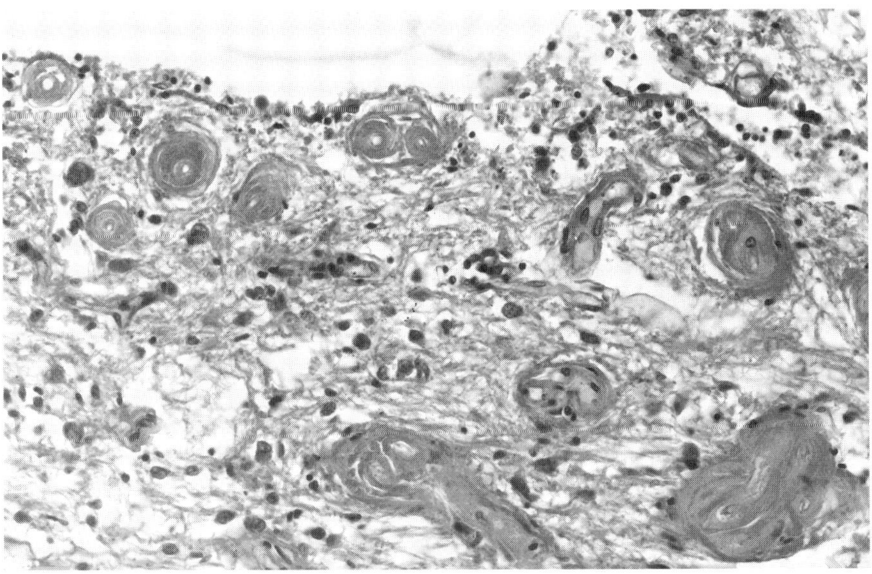

**Figure 2.10** Thickening of the small vessels and obstruction of their lumens in the pons of a patient with multiple small infarcts. (Paraffin section; H&E; ×500).

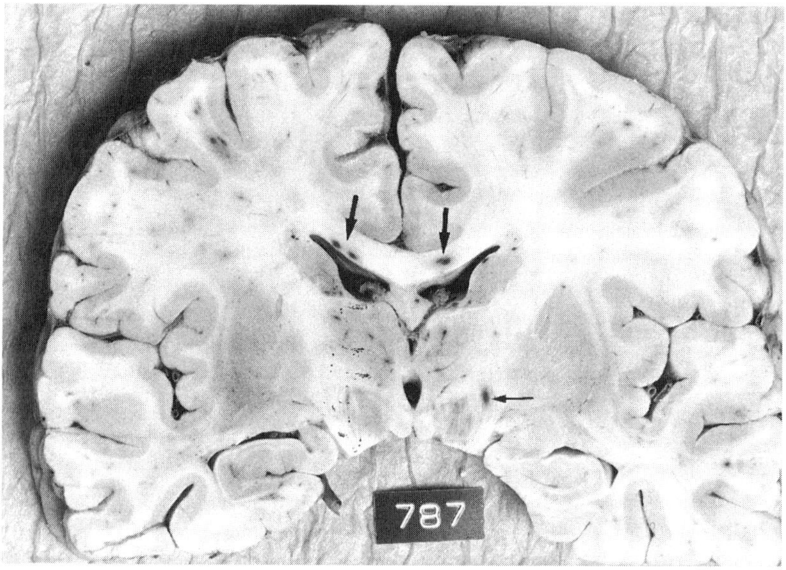


**(a)**

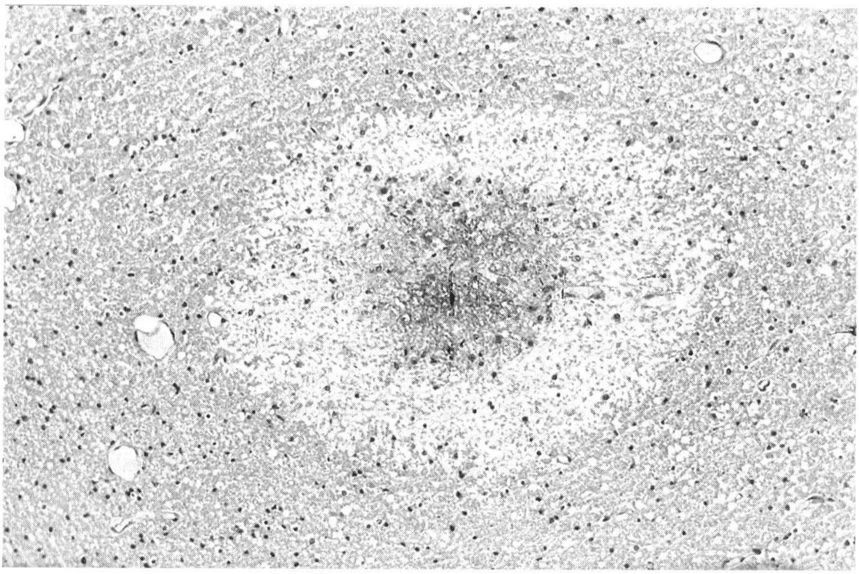

**(b)**

**Figure 2.11** (a) Frontal section of the brain showing multiple small haemorrhagic infarcts in the corpus callosum (thick arrows) and pyramidal tract (thin arrow). (b) One lesion of the white matter of the same patient showing a small round infarct with a haemorrhagic centre. (Paraffin section; H&E; ×270.)

1991). Occlusion of large vessels was observed in a few cases (Kato *et al.*, 1987; Atalaia *et al.*, 1992), but in most cases lesions of small arteries were present, involving the basal ganglia or brainstem (Mizusawa *et al.*, 1988). In two patients, we have observed ischaemic lesions in the thalamus and pons, resulting from occlusion of small vessels, thickening of the vessel walls and associated microthrombi (Figure 2.10) (Cho *et al.*, 1987). Disseminated thromboemboli have been detected (Anders *et al.*, 1986; Mizusawa *et al.*, 1988), secondary to endocarditis in some patients (Snider *et al.*, 1983). Ischaemic necrosis of the hippocampus may occur after preterminal hypoxia. Disseminated haemorrhagic small infarcts in the white matter were observed in one of our patients (Figure 2.11). Calcification of vessel wall and calcium deposits were frequent but occurred less often in adults than in children (Mizusawa *et al.*, 1988; Kure *et al.*, 1991).

In the absence of opportunistic infections or lymphomas, cerebral haemorrhages are uncommon. Large series have mentioned haemorrhagic lesions of the brain, epidural haematoma and subarachnoid haemorrhages secondary to disruption of a congenital aneurysm (Snider *et al.*, 1983; Moskowitz *et al.*, 1984; Anders *et al.*, 1986; Kato *et al.*, 1987).

Inflammatory vasculitis may affect both the central as well as the peripheral nervous system (Said *et al.*, 1988; Calabrese *et al.*, 1989). Multifocal necrotizing arteritis involving the brain and spinal cord was reported by Vinters *et al.* (1988); varicella-zoster virus was detected by immunocytochemistry in affected vessels. In several patients with CMV encephalitis, we have observed necrotizing arteritis of middle-sized arteries of the cerebral hemispheres or brainstem. One patient presented with a sudden stroke of the ventral peduncular region demonstrated on CT; the autopsy, performed 2 months after the initial symptoms, found ischaemia of the peduncles associated with CMV ventriculitis (Figure 2.12). Several cases of cerebral granulomatous angiitis have been reported (Yankner *et al.*, 1986; Anders *et al.*, 1989), associated with cerebral lymphoma in two cases (Anders *et al.*, 1989) and possibly in relation with a lymphoma in other reports (Colby, 1989; Labauge *et al.*, 1991).

Thus, most of the CNS ischaemic infarcts observed in the context of HIV infection are related to infection either by HIV itself, which can induce specific vasculitis, or to opportunistic infections including syphilis and CMV, which represent two potentially treatable causes of cerebral infarction.

## CONCLUSIONS

HIV-associated higher function disorders are common but often associated with opportunistic infections of the brain late in the course of the disease. The early penetration of the virus into the CNS, which contrasts with the clinical manifestations of HIV-ADC years later, suggests that HIV-associated brain lesions accumulate with time and become clinically detectable only when they have affected a critical number of sites or destroyed a large

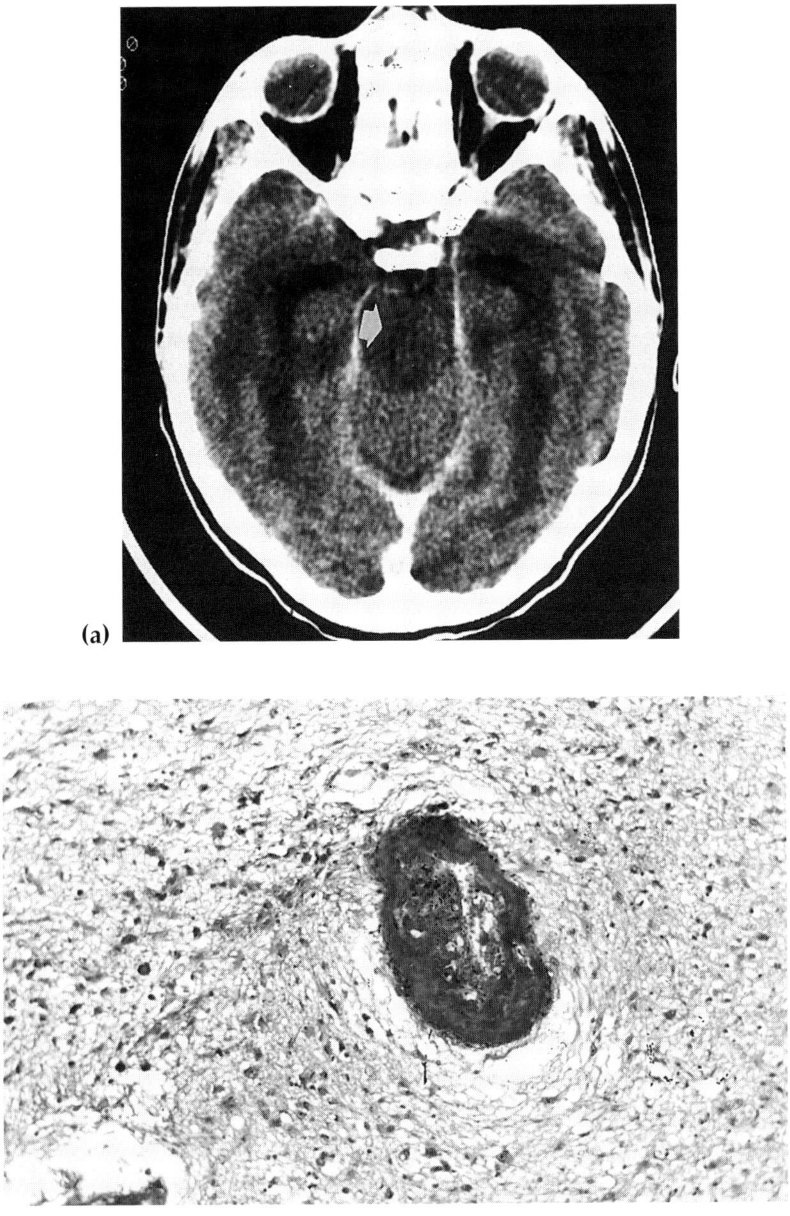

(a)

(b)

**Figure 2.12** (a) CT image of a patient with infarct of the mesencephalon (arrow) and cytomegalovirus (CMV) ventriculitis. This patient had an acute tetraparesis associated with profound coma; she improved progressively and presented with complex oculomotor paralysis; she died 2 months later and autopsy detected necrotizing arteritis and ischaemic lesions in the ventral mesencephalon and left caudate nucleus associated with CMV ventriculitis. (b) Mesencephalon of the same patient showing an artery with fibrinoid necrosis located in the parenchymal necrosis (Paraffin section; H&E; ×230.)

number of neurones. The mechanisms by which cerebral lesions occur are certainly complex and multiple. The role of macrophages in harbouring viruses and in releasing products of activation that can induce demyelination or neuronal death seems much more important than infection of neurones, which may lead to their death or interfere with their function. Another important issue to consider is the accessibility of the brain compartment to drugs used in the treatment of HIV infection. When more efficient treatment of HIV infection becomes available, it will be important to verify that the drugs cross the blood–brain barrier and control the replication of HIV in the brain. From a practical point of view, the occurrence of HIV-ADC in young people makes them totally dependent, often requiring long-term hospitalization, preferably in centres where doctors, nurses, physiotherapists and psychologists have some expertise in the field.

## REFERENCES

Achim CL, Schrier RD and Wiley CA (1991a) Immunopathogenesis of HIV encephalitis. *Brain Pathology* **1**: 177–184.

Achim CL, Morey MK and Wiley CA (1991b) Expression of major histocompatibility complex and HIV antigens within the brains of AIDS patients. *AIDS* **5**: 535–541.

Anders KH, Guerra WF, Tomiyasu U *et al.* (1986) The neuropathology of AIDS: UCLA experience and review. *American Journal of Pathology* **124**: 537–558.

Anders KH, Latta H, Chang BS *et al.* (1989) Lymphomatoid granulomatosis and malignant lymphoma of the central nervous system in the acquired immunodeficiency syndrome. *Human Pathology* **20**: 326–334.

Archelos JJ, Jung S, Mäurer M *et al.* (1993) Inhibition of experimental autoimmune encephalomyelitis by an antibody to the intercellular adhesion molecule ICAM-1. *Annals of Neurology* **34**: 145–154.

Atalaia A, Ferro J and Antunes F (1992) Stroke in an HIV-infected patient. *Journal of Neurology* **239**: 356–357.

Barohn RJ, Gronseth G, McVey A *et al.* (1990) Nervous system involvement in HIV infection is related to lymphocyte CD4 count. *Neurology* **40** (Suppl. 1): 237.

Berger JR, Sheremata WA, Resnick L *et al.* (1989) Multiple sclerosis-like illness occurring with human immunodeficiency virus infection. *Neurology* **39**: 324–329.

Berger JR, Raffanti S, Svenningsson A *et al.* (1991) The role of HTLV in HIV-1 neurologic disease. *Neurology* **41**: 197–202.

Berger JR, Tornatore C, Major EO *et al.* (1992) Relapsing and remitting human immunodeficiency virus-associated leukoencephalomyelopathy. *Annals of Neurology* **31**: 34–38.

Blumberg BM, Epstein LG, Saito Y *et al.* (1992) Human immunodeficiency virus type 1 *nef* quasispecies in pathological tissue. *Journal of Virology* **66**: 5256–5264.

Bornstein RA, Nasrallah HA, Para MF *et al.* (1993) Neuropsychological performance in symptomatic and asymptomatic HIV infection. *AIDS* **7**: 519–524.

Bowen DL, Lane HC and Fauci AS (1985) Immunopathogenesis of the acquired immunodeficiency syndrome. *Annals of Internal Medicine* **103**: 704–709.

Brack-Werner R, Kleinschmidt A, Ludvigsen A *et al.* (1992) Infection of human brain cells by HIV-1: restricted virus production in chronically infected human glial cell lines. *AIDS* **6**: 273–285.

Brew BJ (1991) Neuronal loss in frontal cortex in HIV infection. *Lancet* **338**: 129–130.

Brew BJ (1993) HIV-1-related neurological disease. *Journal of Acquired Immune Deficiency Syndromes* **6** (Suppl. 1): S10–S15.

Brew BJ and Perdices M (1992) HIV nomenclature. *Neurology* **42**: 265.

Brew BJ, Bhalla RB, Paul M *et al.* (1990) Cerebrospinal fluid neopterin in human immunodeficiency virus type 1 infection. *Annals of Neurology* **28**: 556–560.

Brinkmann R, Schwinn A, Narayan O *et al.* (1992) Human immunodeficiency virus infection in microglia: correlation between cells infected in the brain and cells cultured from infectious brain tissue. *Annals of Neurology* **31**: 361–365.

Budka H (1986) Multinucleated giant cells in brain: a hallmark of the acquired immune deficiency syndrome (AIDS). *Acta Neuropathologica* **69**: 253–258.

Budka H (1989) Human immunodeficiency virus (HIV)-induced disease of the central nervous system: pathology and implications for pathogenesis. *Acta Neuropathologica* **77**: 225–236.

Budka H (1990) Human immunodeficiency virus (HIV) envelope and core proteins in central nervous system tissues of patients with the acquired immune deficiency syndrome (AIDS). *Acta Neuropathologica* **79**: 611–619.

Budka H, Costanzi G, Cristina S *et al.* (1987) Brain pathology induced by infection with the human immunodeficiency virus (HIV): a histological, immunocytochemical, and electron microscopical study of 100 autopsy cases. *Acta Neuropathologica* **75**: 185–198.

Budka H, Wiley CA, Kleihues P *et al.* (1991) HIV-associated disease of the nervous system: review of nomenclature and proposal for neuropathology-based terminology. *Brain Pathology* **1**: 143–152.

Calabrese LH, Estes M, Yen-Lieberman B *et al.* (1989) Systemic vasculitis in association with human immunodeficiency virus infection. *Arthritis and Rheumatism* **32**: 569–576.

Carne CA, Tedder RS, Smith A *et al.* (1985) Acute encephalopathy coincident with seroconversion for anti-HTLV-III. *Lancet* **ii**: 1206–1208.

Chappell ET, Guthrie BL and Orenstein J (1992) The role of stereotactic biopsy in the management of HIV-related focal brain lesions. *Neurosurgery* **30**: 825–829.

Cheng-Mayer C, Rutka JT, Rosenblum ML *et al.* (1987) Human immunodeficiency virus can productively infect cultured human glial cells. *Proceedings of the National Academy of Sciences USA* **84**: 3526–3530.

Cheng-Mayer C, Weiss C, Seto D and Levy JA (1989) Isolates of human immunodeficiency virus type 1 from the brain may constitute a special group of the AIDS virus. *Proceedings of the National Academy of Sciences USA* **86**: 8575–8579.

Chesebro B, Wehrly K, Nishio J and Perryma, S (1992) Macrophage-tropic human immunodeficiency virus isolates from different patients exhibit unusual V3 envelope sequence homogeneity in comparison with T-cell-tropic isolates: definition of critical amino acids involved in cell tropism. *Journal of Virology* **66**: 6547–6554.

Chimelli L, Rosemberg S, Hahn MD *et al.* (1992) Pathology of the central nervous system in patients infected with the human immunodeficiency virus (HIV): a report of 252 autopsy cases from Brazil. *Neuropathology and Applied Neurobiology* **18**: 478–488.

Chiodi F and Fenyö EM (1991) Neurotropism of human immunodeficiency virus. *Brain Pathology* **1**: 185–191.

Chiodi F, Sönnerborg A and Albert J (1988) Human immunodeficiency virus infection of the brain. I: Virus isolation and detection of HIV specific antibodies in the cerebrospinal fluid of patients with varying clinical conditions. *Journal of the Neurological Sciences* **85**: 245–257.

Cho E-S, Sharer LR, Reress NS and Little B (1987) Intimal proliferation of leptomeningeal arteries and brain infarcts in subjects with AIDS. *Journal of Neuropathology and Experimental Neurology* **46**: 385.

Chrysikopoulos HS, Press GA, Grafe MR *et al.* (1990) Encephalitis caused by human immunodeficiency virus: CT and MR imaging manifestations with clinical and pathologic correlation. *Radiology* **175**: 185–191.

Clark SJ, Saag MS, Hahn BH *et al.* (1991) Primary HIV-1 infection. *New England Journal of Medicine* **325**: 734–735.

Coffin J, Haase A, Levy JA *et al.* (1986) Human immunodeficiency viruses (letter). *Science* **232**: 697.

Colby TV (1989) Central nervous system lymphoid granulomatosis in AIDS. *Human Pathology* **20**: 301–302.

Cooper DA, Gold J, Maclean P *et al.* (1985) Acute AIDS retrovirus infection. Definition of a clinical illness associated with seroconversion. *Lancet* **i**: 537–540.

Cornford ME, Holden JK, Boyd MC *et al.* (1992) Neuropathology of the acquired immune deficiency syndrome (AIDS): report of 39 autopsies from Vancouver, British Columbia. *Canadian Journal of Neurological Sciences* **19**: 442–452.

Dal Pan GJ, McArthur JH, Aylward E *et al.* (1992) Patterns of cerebral atrophy in HIV-1 infected individuals. Results of a quantitative MRI analysis. *Neurology* **42**: 2125–2130.

Dean AF, Montgomery M, Baskerville A *et al.* (1993) Different patterns of neuropathological disease in rhesus monkeys infected by simian immunodeficiency virus, and their relation to the humoral immune response. *Neuropathology and Applied Neurobiology* **19**: 336–345.

de la Monte SM, Moore T and Hedley-Whyte ET (1986) Vacuolar encephalopathy of AIDS. *New England Journal of Medicine* **315**: 1549–1550.
de la Monte SM, Ho DD, Schooley RT *et al.* (1987). Subacute encephalomyelitis of AIDS and its relation to HTLV-III infection. *Neurology* **37**: 562–569.
de Martini R, Turner RR, Formenti SC *et al.* (1988) Peripheral blood mononuclear cell abnormalities and their relationship to clinical course in homosexual men with HIV infection. *Clinical Immunology and Immunopathology* **46**: 258–271.
Dickson DW, Matteace LA, Kure K *et al.* (1991) Microglia in human disease, with emphasis on acquired immune deficiency syndrome. *Laboratory Investigation* **64**: 135–156
Dreyer EB, Kaiser PK, Offerman JT and Lipton SA (1990) HIV-1 coat protein neurotoxicity prevented by calcium channel antagonists. *Science* **248**: 364–367.
Engstrom J, Lowenstein DH and Bredesen D (1988) Cerebral infarctions and transient neurologic deficits associated with AIDS. *Neurology* **38**: 241.
Epstein LG and Gendelman HE (1993) Human immunodeficiency virus type 1 infection of the nervous system: pathogenic mechanisms. *Annals of Neurology* **33**: 429–436.
Everall IP, Luthert PJ and Lantos PL (1991) Neuronal loss in the frontal cortex in HIV infection. *Lancet* **337**: 1119–1121.
Fénelon G, Gray F, Scaravilli F *et al.* (1991) Ischemic myelopathy secondary to disseminated intravascular coagulation in AIDS. *Journal of Neurology* **238**: 51–54.
Fuller GN, Guiloff RJ, Scaravilli F *et al.* (1989) combined HIV–CMV encephalitis presenting with brainstem signs. *Journal of Neurology, Neurosurgery and Psychiatry* **52**: 975–979.
Gabuzda DH and Hirsch MS (1987) Neurologic manifestations of infection with human immunodeficiency virus. *Annals of Internal Medicine* **107**: 383–391.
Gabuzda DH, Ho DD, de la Monte SM *et al.* (1986). Immunohistochemical identification of HTLV-III antigen in brains of patients with AIDS. *Annals of Neurology* **20**: 289–295.
Gallo P, Frei K, Rordorf C *et al.* (1989) Human immunodeficiency virus type 1 (HIV-1) infection of the central nervous system: an evaluation of cytokines in cerebro-spinal fluid. *Journal of Neuroimmunology* **23**: 109–116.
Garry RF, Kort JJ, Koch-Nolte F and Koch G (1991) Similarities of viral proteins to toxins that interact with monovalent cation channels. *AIDS* **5**: 1381–1384.
Gartner S, Markovits P, Markovits D *et al.* (1986) Virus isolation from and identification of HTLV-III/LAV producing cells in brain tissue from a patient with AIDS. *Journal of the American Medical Association* **256**: 2365–2371.
Geleziunas R, Schipper HM and Wainberg MA (1992) Pathogenesis and therapy of HIV-1 infection of the central nervous system. *AIDS* **6**: 1411–1426
Gelman BB (1993) Diffuse microgliosis associated with cerebral atrophy in the acquired immunodeficiency syndrome. *Annals of Neurology* **34**. 65–70.
Gelman BB and Guinto FC (1992) Morphometry, histopathology, and tomography of cerebral atrophy in the acquired immunodeficiency syndrome. *Annals of Neurology* **32**: 31–40.
Gendelman HE, Baca LM, Husayni H *et al.* (1990) Macrophage–HIV interaction: viral isolation and target cell tropism. *AIDS* **4**: 221–228.
Genis P, Jett M, Bernton EW *et al.* (1992) Cytokines and arachidonic metabolites produced during human immunodeficiency virus (HIV)-infected macrophage–astroglia interactions: implications for the neuropathogenesis of HIV disease. *Journal of Experimental Medicine* **176**: 1703–1718.
Giulian D, Vaca K and Noonan CA (1990) Secretion of neurotoxins by mononuclear phagocytes infected with HIV-1. *Science* **250**: 1593–1596.
Glass JD, Wesselingh SL, Selnes OA and McArthur JC (1993) Clinical–neuropathologic correlation in HIV-associated dementia. *Neurology* **43**: 2230–2237.
Glass JD, Fedor H, Wesselingh SL and McArthur JC (1995) Immunocytochemical quantitation of human immunodeficiency virus in the brain: correlations with dementia. *Annals of Neurology* **38**: 755–762.
Goldwater PN and Paton JC (1989) Apparunt0non-ynvo l vement of prions in the pathogenesis of spongiform change in HIV-infected brain. *Journal of Neuropathology and Experimental Neurology* **48**: 184–186.
Gonzales MF and Davis RL (1988) Neuropathology of acquired immunodeficiency syndrome. *Neuropathology and Applied Neurobiology* **14**: 345–363.
Goudsmit J, Wolters EC, Bakker M *et al.* (1986) Intrathecal synthesis of antibodies to HTLV-III in patients without AIDS or AIDS related complex. *British Medical Journal* **292**: 1231–1234.
Gray F, Geny C, Lionnet F *et al.* (1991) Etude neuropathologique de 135 cas adultes de syndrome d'immuno-deficience acquise (SIDA). *Annales de Pathologie* **11**: 236–247.

Gray F, Hurtrel M and Hurtrel B (1993) Early central nervous system changes in human immunodeficiency virus (HIV) infection. *Neuropathology and Applied Neurobiology* **19**: 3–9.

Grimaldi LME, Martino GV, Franciotta DM *et al.* (1991) Elevated alpha-tumor necrosis factor levels in spinal fluid from HIV-1-infected patients with central nervous system involvement. *Annals of Neurology* **29**: 21–25.

Hardy WD, Daar ES, Sokolov Jr, RT and Ho DD (1991) Acute neurologic deterioration in a young man. *Reviews of Infectious Diseases* **13**: 745–750.

Harouse JM, Wroblewska Z, Laughlin MA *et al.* (1989) Human choroid plexus cells can be latently infected with human immunodeficiency virus. *Annals of Neurology* **25**: 406–411.

Harter DH (1989) Neuropsychological status of asymptomatic individuals seropositive to HIV-1. *Annals of Neurology* **26**: 589–591.

Hénin D, Duyckaerts C, Chaunu MP *et al.* (1987) Etude neuropathologique de 31 cas de syndrome d'immuno-dépression acquise. *Revue Neurologique* **143**: 631–642.

Heyes MP, Brew BJ, Martin A *et al.* (1991) Quinolinic acid in cerebrospinal fluid and serum in HIV-1 infection: relationship to clinical and neurological status. *Annals of Neurology* **29**: 202–209.

Ho DD, Rota TR, Schooley RT *et al.* (1985) Isolation of HTLV-III from cerebrospinal fluid and neural tissues of patients with neurologic syndromes related to the acquired immunodeficiency syndrome. *New England Journal of Medicine* **313**: 1493–1497.

Ho DD, Bredesen DE, Vinters HV and Daar ES (1989). Acquired immunodeficiency syndrome dementia complex. *Annals of Internal Medicine* **111**: 400–410.

Houff SA (1988) Neuroimmunology of human immunodeficiency virus infection. In: *AIDS and the Nervous System* (ed Rosenblum ML), pp. 347–375. New York: Raven Press.

Hulette CM, Downey BT and Burger PC (1992) Macrophage markers in diagnostic neuropathology. *American Journal of Surgical Pathology* **16**: 493–499.

Jansen RS, Saykin AJ, Kaplan JE *et al.* (1988) Neurological complications of human immunodeficiency virus infection in patients with lymphadenopathy syndrome. *Annals of Neurology* **23**: 49–55.

Janssen RS, Saykin AJ, Cannon L *et al.* (1989) Neurological and neuropsychological manifestations of HIV-1 infection: association with AIDS-related complex but not asymptomatic HIV-1 infection. *Annals of Neurology* **26**: 592–600.

Janssen RS, Nwanyanwu OC, Selik RM and Stehr-Green JK (1992) Epidemiology of human immunodeficiency virus encephalopathy in the United States. *Neurology* **42**: 1472–1476.

Jarvik JG, Hesselink JR, Kennedy C *et al.* (1988) Acquired immunodeficiency syndrome: magnetic resonance patterns of brain involvement with pathologic correlation. *Archives of Neurology* **45**: 731–736.

Johnson R, McArthur JC and Narayan O (1988) The neurobiology of human immunodeficiency virus infections. *FASEB Journal* **2**: 2970–2981.

Johnson RT, Glass JD, McArthur JC and Chesebro BW (1996) Quantitation of human immunodeficiency virus in brains of demented and nondemented patients with acquired immunodeficiency syndrome. *Annals of Neurology* **39**: 392–395.

Jones HR, Ho DD, Forgacs P *et al.* (1988) Acute fulminating fatal leukoencephalopathy as the only manifestation of human immunodeficiency virus infection. *Annals of Neurology* **23**: 519–522.

Kaiser PK, Offermann JT and Lipton SA (1990) Neuronal injury due to HIV-1 envelope protein is blocked by anti-gp 120 antibodies but not by anti-CD4 antibodies. *Neurology* **40**: 1757–1761.

Kanzer MD, Parisi JE, Tuur SM and Lo SC (1989) The autopsy neuropathology of AIDS (abstract) *Journal of Neuropathology and Experimental Neurology* **48**: 314.

Kato T, Hirano A, Llena JF and Dembitzer HM (1987) Neuropathology of the acquired immune deficiency syndrome (AIDS) in 53 autopsy cases with particular emphasis on microglial nodules and multinucleated giant cells. *Acta Neuropathologica* **73**: 287–294.

Ketzler S, Weis S, Haug H and Budka H (1990) Loss of neurons in the frontal cortex in AIDS brains. *Acta Neuropathologica* **80**: 92–94.

Kieburtz K, Ketonen L, Cox C *et al.* (1996) Cognitive performance and regional brain volume in human immunodeficiency virus type 1 infection. *Archives of Neurology* **53**: 155–158.

Klatzmann D and Gluckman (1986) HIV infection: facts and hypothesis. *Immunology Today* **7**: 291–296.

Kugler SL, Barzilai A, Hodes DS *et al.* (1991) Acute hemiplegia associated with HIV infection. *Pediatric Neurology* **7**: 207–210.

Kure K, Weidenheim KM, Lyman WD and Dickson DW (1990a) Morphology and distribution of HIV-1 gp41-positive microglia in subacute AIDS encaphalitis. Pattern of involvement resembling a multisystem degeneration. *Acta Neuropathologica* **80**: 393–400.

Kure K, Lyman WD, Weidenheim KM and Dickson DW (1990b) Cellular localisation of an HIV-1 antigen in subacute AIDS encephalitis using an improved double-labelling immunohistochemical method. *American Journal of Pathology* **136**: 1085–1092.

Kure K, Llena JF, Lyman WD *et al.* (1991) Human immunodeficiency virus-1 infection of the nervous system: an autopsy study of 268 adult, pediatric, and fetal brains. *Human Pathology* **22**: 700–710.

Labauge R, Pagès M, Tourniaire D and Blard JM (1991) Infarctus pontique, syphilis nerveuse et infection par le VIH. *Revue Neurologique* **147**: 406–408.

Lang W, Miklossy J, Dernaz JP *et al.* (1989) Neuropathology of the acquired immune deficiency syndrome (AIDS): a report of 135 consecutive autopsy cases from Switzerland. *Acta Neuropathologica* **77**: 379–390.

Lenhardt TM, Super MA and Wiley CA (1988) Neuropathological changes in an asymptomatic HIV seropositive man. *Annals of Neurology* **23**: 209–210.

Levy RM, Bredesen DE and Rosenblum ML (1985) Neurological manifestations of the acquired immune deficiency syndrome (AIDS): experience at UCSF and review of the literature. *Journal of Neurosurgery* **62**: 465–495.

Levy RM, Rosenblum S and Perrett LV (1986) Neuroradiologic findings in AIDS: a review of 200 cases. *American Journal of Roentgenology* **147**: 977–983.

Levy RM, Russell E, Yungbluth M *et al.* (1992) The efficacy of image-guided stereotactic brain biopsy in neurologically symptomatic acquired immunodeficiency syndrome patients. *Neurosurgery* **30**: 186–189; discussion 189–190.

Li Y, Kappes JC, Conway JA *et al.* (1991) Molecular characterisation of human immunodeficiency virus type 1 cloned directly from uncultured human brain tissue: identification of replication-competent and -defective viral genomes. *Journal of Virology* **65**: 3973–3985.

Lie JT (1992) Primary (granulomatous) angiitis of the central nervous system: a clinicopathologic analysis of 15 cases and review of the literature. *Human Pathology* **23**: 164–171.

Lifson JD, Reyes GR, McGrath S *et al.* (1986) AIDS retrovirus induced cytopathology: giant cell formation and involvement of CD4 antigen. *Science* **232**: 1123–1127.

Lipton SA (1991) HIV-related neurotoxicity. *Brain Pathology* **1**: 193–200.

Lipton SA (1992a) Models of neuronal injury in AIDS: another role for the NMDA receptor? *Trends in Neuroscience* **15**: 75–79.

Lipton SA (1992b) Memantine presents HIV coat protein-induced neuronal injury *in vitro*. *Neurology* **42**: 1403–1405.

Lipton SA and Gendelman HE (1995) Dementia associated with the acquired immunodeficiency syndrome. *New England Journal of Medicine* **332**: 934–940.

Lyman WD, Hatch WC and Rashbaum WK (1992) HIV-1 infection of human microglia and astrocytes *in vitro*. *Journal of Neuropathology and Experimental Neurology* **51**: 354.

McArthur JC, Becker PS, Parisi JE *et al.* (1989) Neuropathological changes in early HIV-1 dementia. *Annals of Neurology* **26**: 681–684.

McArthur JC, Hoover DR, Bacellar H *et al.* (1993) Dementia in AIDS patients: incidence and risk factors. *Neurology* **43**: 2245–2252.

Mackay CR and Imhof BA (1993) Cell adhesion in the immune system. *Immunology Today* **14**: 99–102.

McKelvie PA, De Girolami U and Nasser I (1992) Expression of endothelial adhesion molecules in HIV encephalopathy. *Journal of Neuropathology and Experimental Neurology* **51**: 354.

Masliah E, Achim CL, Ge N *et al.* (1992) Spectrum of human immunodeficiency virus-associated neocortical damage. *Annals of Neurology* **32**: 321–329.

Matthiessen L, Marche C, Labrousse F *et al.* (1992) Etude neuropathologique de l'encéphale de 174 patients morts du SIDA dans un hôpital parisien, de 1982 à 1988. *Annales de Medecine Interne* **143**: 43–49.

Merrill JE and Chen ISY (1991) HIV-1, macrophages, glial cells, and cytokines in AIDS nervous system disease. *FASEB Journal* **5**: 2391–2397.

Merrill JE, Koyanagi Y, Zack J *et al.* (1992) Induction of interleukin-1 and tumor necrosis factor alpha in brain cultures by human immunodeficiency virus type 1. *Journal of Virology* **66**: 2217–2225.

Meyenhoffer MMF, Epstein LG, Cho ES and Sharer LR (1987) Ultrastructural morphology and intracellular production of human immunodeficiency virus (HIV) in brain. *Journal of Neuropathology and Experimental Neurology* **46**: 474–484.

Michaels J, Price RW and Rosenblum MK (1988) Microglia in the giant cell encephalitis of acquired immunodeficiency syndrome: proliferation, infection, and fusion. *Acta Neuropathologica* **76**: 373–379.

Miles JM and Chou SM (1988) Multinucleated giant cells in AIDS encephalopathy are not derived from microglia. *Journal of Neuropathology and Experimental Neurology* **47**: 302.
Mizusawa H, Hirano A, Llena JF and Kato T (1987) Nuclear bridges in multinucleated giant cells associated with primary lymphoma of the brain in acquired immune deficiency syndrome (AIDS). *Acta Neuropathologica* **75**: 23–26.
Mizusawa H, Hirano A, Llena JF and Shintaku M (1988) Cerebrovascular lesions in acquired immune deficiency syndrome (AIDS). *Acta Neuropathologica* **76**: 451–457.
Moskowitz LB, Hensley GT, Chan JC *et al.* (1984) The neuropathology of acquired immune deficiency syndrome. *Archives of Pathology and Laboratory Medicine* **108**: 867–872.
Navia BA and Price RW (1987) The acquired immunodeficiency syndrome dementia complex as the presenting or sole manifestation of human immunodeficiency virus infection. *Archives of Neurology* **44**: 65–69.
Navia BA, Jordan BD and Price RW (1986a) The AIDS dementia complex: I. Clinical features. *Annals of Neurology* **19**: 517–524.
Navia BA, Cho E-S, Petito CK and Price RW (1986b) The AIDS dementia complex: II. Neuropathology. *Annals of Neurology* **19**: 525–535.
Neuen-Jacob E, Arendt G, Wendtland B *et al.* (1993) Frequency and topographical distribution of CD68-positive macrophages and HIV-1 core proteins in HIV-associated brain lesions. *Clinical Neuropathology* **12**: 315–324.
Pang S, Koyanagi Y, Miles S *et al.* (1990) High levels of unintegrated HIV-1 DNA in brain tissue of AIDS dementia patients. *Nature* **343**: 85–89.
Park YD, Belman AL, Kim T-S *et al.* (1990) Stroke in pediatric acquired immunodeficiency syndrome. *Annals of Neurology* **28**: 303–311.
Patsouris E, Kretzschmar HA, Stavrou D and Mehraein P (1993) Cellular composition and distribution of gliomesenchymal nodules in the central nervous system of AIDS patients. *Clinical Neuropathology* **12**: 130–137.
Perl DP, Good PE and Jabbar G (1989) Basal ganglia vascular mineralization in AIDS: evidence of massive aluminium deposition. *Journal of Neuropathology and Experimental Neurology* **48**: 384.
Perrella O, Carrieri PB, Guarnaccia D and Soscia M (1992) Cerebrospinal fluid cytokines in AIDS dementia complex. *Journal of Neurology* **239**: 387–388.
Petito CK and Cash KS (1992) Blood–brain barrier abnormalities in the acquired immunodeficiency syndrome: immunohistochemical localisation of serum proteins in post-mortem brains. *Annals of Neurology* **32**: 658–666.
Petito C, Cho E, Leman W *et al.* (1986) Neuropathology of acquired immunodeficiency syndrome (AIDS). An autopsy review. *Journal of Neuropathology and Experimental Neurology* **45**: 635–646.
Peudenier S, Hery C, Montagnier L and Tardieu M (1991) Human microglial cells: characterization in cerebral tissue and in primary culture, and study of their susceptibility to HIV-1 infection. *Annals of Neurology* **29**: 152–161.
Post J, Tate L, Quencer R *et al.* (1988) CT, MR, and pathology in HIV encephalitis and meningitis. *American Journal of Radiology* **151**: 373–380.
Power C, Kong P-A, Crawford TO *et al.* (1993) Cerebral white matter changes in acquired immunodeficiency syndrome dementia: alterations of the blood–brain barrier. *Annals of Neurology* **34**: 339–350.
Price RW and Brew B (1988) The AIDS dementia complex. *Journal of Infectious Diseases* **158**: 1079–1083.
Price RW, Brew B, Sidtis JJ *et al.* (1988a) The brain in AIDS: central nervous system HIV-1 infection and the AIDS dementia complex. *Science* **239**: 586–592.
Price RW, Sidtis JJ and Rosenblum M (1988b) AIDS dementia complex: some current questions. *Annals of Neurology* **23** (Suppl.): S27–S33.
Price RW, Sidtis JJ and Brew BJ (1991) AIDS dementia complex and HIV-1 infection: a view from the clinic. *Brain Pathology* **1**: 155–162.
Pumarola-Sune T, Navia BA, Cordon-Cardo C *et al.* (1987) HIV antigen in the brain of patients with the AIDS-dementia complex. *Annals of Neurology* **21**: 490–496.
Rabinoff M (1993) Mononuclear metabolic products and human immunodeficiency virus-associated neurological damage. *Annals of Neurology* **34**: 240.
Rausch DM, Heyes MP, Murray EA *et al.* (1994) Cytopathologic and neurochemical correlates of progression to motor/cognitive impairment in SIV-infected rhesus monkeys. *Journal of Neuropathology and Experimental Neurology* **53**: 165–175.
Resnick L, diMarzo-Veronese F and Schupbach J (1985) Intra-blood–brain-barrier synthesis of

HTLV-III-specific IgG in patients with neurologic symptoms associated with AIDS-related complex. *New England Journal of Medicine* **313**: 1498–1504.

Rhodes RH (1987) Histopathology of the central nervous system in the acquired immunodeficiency syndrome. *Human Pathology* **18**: 636–643.

Rhodes RH (1991) Evidence of serum-protein leakage across the blood–brain barrier in the acquired immunodeficiency syndrome. *Journal of Neuropathology and Experimental Neurology* **50**: 171–183.

Rhodes RH (1993) Histopathologic features in the central nervous system of 400 acquired immunodeficiency syndrome cases: implications of rates of occurrence. *Human Pathology* **24**: 1189–1198.

Ringler DJ, Hunt RD, Desrosiers RC *et al.* (1988) Simian immunodeficiency virus-induced meningoencephalitis: natural history and retrospective study. *Annals of Neurology* **23** (Suppl.): S101–S107.

Rosenberg ZF and Fauci AS (1990) Immunopathogenic mechanisms of HIV infection: cytokine induction of HIV expression. *Immunology Today* **11**: 176–180.

Rottenberg DA, Moeller JR, Strother SC *et al.* (1987) The metabolic pathology of the AIDS dementia complex. *Annals of Neurology* **22**: 700–706.

Royal III W, Selnes OA, Concha M *et al.* (1994) Cerebrospinal fluid human immunodeficiency virus type 1 (HIV-1) 24 antigen in HIV-1-related dementia. *Annals of Neurology* **36**: 32–39.

Said G, Lacroix-Ciaudo C, Fujimura H, Blas C and Faux N. (1988) The peripheral neuropathy of necrotizing arteritis: a clinicopathological study. *Annals of Neurology* **23**: 461–465.

Sasseville VG, Newman WA, Lackner AA *et al.* (1992) Elevated vascular cell adhesion molecule-1 in AIDS encephalitis induced by simian immunodeficiency virus. *American Journal of Pathology* **141**: 1021–1030.

Schmidbauer M, Huemer M, Cristina S *et al.* (1992) Morphological spectrum, distribution and clinical correlation of white matter lesions in AIDS brains. *Neuropathology and Applied Neurobiology* **18**: 489–501.

Schwenk J, Cruz-Sànchez F, Gosztonyi G, Cervos-Navarro J (1987) Spongiform encephalopathy in a patient with acquired immune deficiency syndrome (AIDS). *Acta Neuropathologie* (Berlin) **74**: 389–392.

Seilhean D, Duyckaerts C, Vazeux R *et al.* (1993) HIV-1-associated cognitive/motor complex: absence of neuronal loss in the cerebral neocortex. *Neurology* **43**: 1492–1499.

Shapshak P, Yoshioka M, Svenningsson A *et al.* (1990) Combined immunocytochemistry and *in situ* hybridization to detect HIV in AIDS brain cells. *Journal of Neuropathology and Experimental Neurology* **49**: 351.

Sharer LR (1992) Pathology of HIV-1 infection of the central nervous system. *Journal of Neuropathology and Experimental Neurology* **51**: 3 11.

Sharer LR and Kapila R (1985) Neuropathologic observations in the acquired immunodeficiency syndrome. *Acta Neuropathologica* **66**: 188–198.

Sharer LR, Cho ES and Epstein LG (1985) Multinucleated giant cells and HTLV-III in AIDS encephalopathy. *Human Pathology* **16**: 760.

Shaskan EG and Thompson RM (1992) Undetectable tumor necrosis factor-alpha in spinal fluid from HIV-1 infected patients. *Annals of Neurology* **31**: 687–689.

Shaskan EG, Brew BJ, Rosenblum M *et al.* (1992) Increased neopterin levels in brains of patients with human immunodeficiency virus type 1 infection. *Journal of Neurochemistry* **59**: 1541–1546.

Sidtis JJ, Gatsonis C, Price RW *et al.* (1993) Zidovudine treatment of the AIDS dementia complex: results of a placebo-controlled trial. *Annals of Neurology* **33**: 434–439.

Smith TW, DeGirolami U, Hénin D *et al.* (1990) Human immunodeficiency virus (HIV) leukoencephalopathy and the microcirculation. *Journal of Neuropathology and Experimental Neurology* **49**: 357–370.

Snider WD, Simpson DM, Nielsen S *et al.* (1983) Neurological complications of acquired immune deficiency syndrome: analysis of 50 patients. *Annals of Neurology* **14**: 403–418.

Stavrou D, Mehraein P, Mellert W *et al.* (1989) Evaluation of intracerebral lesions in patients with acquired immunodeficiency syndrome: neuropathological findings and experimental data. *Neuropathology and Applied Neurobiology* **15**: 207–222.

Tardieu M, Hery C, Peudenier S *et al.* (1992) Human immunodeficiency virus type 1-infected monocytic cells can destroy human neural cells after cell-to-cell adhesion. *Annals of Neurology* **32**: 11–17.

Taruscio D, Malchiodi Albedi F, Bagnato R *et al.* (1991) Increased reactivity of laminin in the basement membranes of capillary walls in AIDS brain cortex. *Acta Neuropathologica* **81**: 552–556.

Thomas WE (1992) Brain macrophages: evaluation of microglia and their functions. *Brain Research Reviews* **17**: 61–74.

Tyor WR, Glass JD, Griffin JW *et al.* (1992) Cytokine expression in the brain during the acquired immunodeficiency syndrome. *Annals of Neurology* **31**: 349–360.

Vazeux R, Brousse N, Jarry A *et al.* (1987) AIDS subacute encephalitis: identification of HIV-infected cells. *American Journal of Pathology* **126**: 403–410.

Vazeux R, Cumont M, Girard PM *et al.* (1990) Severe encephalitis resulting from coinfection with HIV and JC virus. *Neurology* **40**: 944–948.

Vazeux R, Lacroix-Ciaudo C, Blanche S *et al.* (1992) Low levels of human immunodeficiency virus replication in the brain tissue of children with severe acquired immunodeficiency syndrome encephalitis. *American Journal of Pathology* **140**: 137–144.

Vinters HV, Guerra WF, Eppolito L and Reith PE (1988) Necrotizing vasculitis of the nervous system in a patient with AIDS-related complex. *Neuropathology and Applied Neurobiology* **14**: 417–424.

von Einsiedel RW, Minami E, Secor DL *et al.* (1990) Structural components of the AIDS dementia complex: correlation of brain parenchymal astrogliosis with HIV-1 DNA in cerebral tissues. *Journal of Neuropathology and Experimental Neurology* **49**: 351.

Wahl LM, Corcoran ML, Pyle SW *et al.* (1989) Human immunodeficiency virus glycoprotein (gp 120) induction of monocyte arachidonic acid metabolites and interleukin 1. *Proceedings of the National Academy of Sciences USA* **86**: 621–625.

Wahl SM, Allen JB, McCartney FN *et al.* (1991) Macrophage- and astrocyte-derived transforming growth factor beta as a mediator of central nervous system dysfunction in acquired immune deficiency syndrome. *Journal of Experimental Medicine* **173**: 981–991.

Walker DG, Itagaki S, Berry K and McGeer PL (1989) Examination of brains of AIDS cases for human immunodeficiency virus and human cytomegalovirus nucleic acids. *Journal of Neurology, Neurosurgery and Psychiatry* **52**: 583–590.

Watkins BA, Dorn HH, Kelly WB *et al.* (1990) Specific tropism of HIV-1 for microglial cells in primary human brain cultures. *Science* **249**: 549–553.

Weidenheim KM, Dickson DW, Kure K and Lyman (1990) Identification of T-lymphocytes in adult AIDS patients with and without subacute giant cell encephalitis. *Journal of Neuropathology and Experimental Neurology* **49**: 323.

Weis S, Haug H and Budka H (1993a) Neuronal damage of the cerebral cortex of AIDS brains: a morphometric study. *Acta Neuropathologica* **85**: 185–189.

Weis S, Haug H and Budka H (1993b) Astroglial changes in the cerebral cortex of AIDS brains: a morphometric and immunohistochemical investigation. *Neuropathology and Applied Neurobiology* **19**: 329–335.

Weiser B, Peress, La Neve *et al.* (1990) Human immunodeficiency virus type 1 expression in the central nervous system correlates directly with extent of disease. *Proceedings of the National Academy of Sciences USA* **87**: 3997–4001.

Wesselingh SL, Power C, Glass JD *et al.* (1993) Intracerebral cytokine messenger RNA expression in acquired immunodeficiency syndrome dementia. *Annals of Neurology* **33**: 576–582.

Westervelt P, Trowbridge DB, Epstein LG *et al.* (1992) Macrophage tropism determinants of human immunodeficiency virus type 1 *in vivo*. *Journal of Virology* **66**: 2577–2582.

Wiley CA and Budka H (1991) HIV-induced central nervous system lesions. *Brain Pathology* **1**: 153–154.

Wiley CA and Nelson JA (1988) Role of human immunodeficiency virus and cytomegalovirus in AIDS encephalitis. *American Journal of Pathology* **133**: 73–81.

Wiley CA, Schier RD, Nelson JA *et al.* (1986) Cellular localization of human immunodeficiency virus infection within the brains of acquired immunodeficiency syndrome patients. *Proceedings of the National Academy of Sciences USA* **83**: 7089–7093.

Yankner BA, Skolnik PR, Shoukimas GM *et al.* (1986) Cerebral granulomatous angiitis associated with isolation of human T-lymphotropic virus type III from the central nervous system. *Annals of Neurology* **20**: 362–364.

# 3

# *Neoplasms of the Nervous System*

## PRIMARY LYMPHOMA OF THE CNS

### Epidemiology

Since the outbreak of HIV infection, a number of studies have shown the high frequency of primary non-Hodgkin's lymphomas in the CNS of patients with AIDS. The incidence of primary lymphoma of this type is estimated at 2% of patients with AIDS, and the risk for an HIV-infected patient to develop this type of brain tumour is 10-fold that observed in non-HIV-infected subjects (Rosenblum *et al.*, 1988). The occurrence of primary lymphoma of the CNS characterizes stage IV(d) of AIDS (Centers for Disease Control, 1985). In patients with AIDS, 5–10% of neurological disorders are due to CNS lymphomas (Snider *et al.*, 1983; Amberson *et al.*, 1985). Primary brain lymphomas are the most frequent site of extranodal lymphomas in AIDS (Knowles *et al.*, 1988). In European autopsy series, CNS lymphomas are observed in 6–18% of AIDS patients (Budka *et al.* 1987; Gray *et al.*, 1991; Matthiessen *et al.*, 1992), with the exception of one study (Lang *et al.*, 1989). In our own series of 85 autopsies of patients with HIV infection (unpublished data, but see Table 4.7), 11 adults (13%) had a brain lymphoma. In a series from the USA the percentage of primary brain lymphoma is around 6% (Petito *et al.*, 1986; Kure *et al.*, 1991; Rhodes, 1993) and in Brazil 4% (Chimelli *et al.*, 1992). A role has been suggested for treatment with zidovudine (azidothymidine, AZT) in the development of lymphoma in patients with AIDS (Pluda *et al.*, 1990). Within a cohort of 55 patients treated with zidovudine for up to 3 years, eight patients developed an extranodal lymphoma, including five primary CNS localizations. In the USA, primary CNS lymphomas have also been reported in nine children (Epstein *et al.*, 1988), in which age group it seems more frequent than opportunistic infections of the nervous system (Kozlowski *et al.*, 1990). In contrast, brain lymphoma is virtually unknown in children with AIDS in Europe (Lacroix *et al.*, 1993). From a radiological standpoint, lymphomas of the CNS represent the most common enhancing lesion on brain CT after toxoplasmic abscesses.

**Clinical presentation**

The clinical presentation of primary brain lymphoma is that of a brain tumour with a rapidly progressive course. Usually, rapid alteration of intellectual performance occurs with apathy, confusion, behavioural changes, memory loss, walking difficulty, hemiparesis, cranial nerve involvement and lethargy (Gill *et al.*, 1986; Carbone *et al.*, 1991; Marelle *et al.*, 1994). Headache is present in 30–40% of patients and focal deficits in 30–50% (Rosenblum *et al.*, 1988). Fever and seizures are less common than in cerebral toxoplasmosis (Scully *et al.*, 1983; Freeman *et al.*, 1986). Intramedullary or epidural lymphomas may occur (Loureiro *et al.*, 1988; Herida *et al.*, 1993).

**Imaging and biological investigations**

CT shows single or, more often, multiple mass lesions (Orron *et al.*, 1989; Poon *et al.*, 1989). Without contrast, CT shows isodense or slightly hypodense or hyperdense lesion(s) (Figure 3.1a) and variable oedema (Gill *et al.*, 1986; Levy *et al.*, 1986; Remick *et al.*, 1990). CT may be normal or show only cerebral atrophy (Amberson *et al.*, 1985; So *et al.*, 1988). Contrast injection produces a nodular, ring or patchy enhancement of the mass, sometimes with preferential involvement of the subependymal area (Figure 3.2a) (Rosenblum *et al.*, 1988; So *et al.*, 1988). MRI may detect smaller lesions; the signal is hypointense on $T_1$-weighted sequences and hyperintense on $T_2$-weighted sequences, with gadolinium enhancement (Gill *et al.*, 1986; Marelle *et al.*, 1994). MIR is by far the most efficient method for spinal cord lesions.

The CSF examination may be normal in some patients; others may have a pleocytosis associated with high protein levels and low glucose content (So *et al.*, 1988). In cases of pleocytosis the lymphocytes are usually normal; tumoral lymphocytes are rarely found (So *et al.*, 1988). Levels of $\beta_2$-microglobulin in CSF were higher in patients with AIDS-related brain lymphoma than in those with opportunistic infections (Brew *et al.*, 1989). By means of PCR, Epstein–Barr virus (EBV) DNA was detected in patients with HIV-related brain lymphoma and the titres were higher when the meninges were infiltrated by the lymphoma (Clifford *et al.*, 1994). Most patients with AIDS-related lymphoma have profound immunodepression, demonstrated by a $CD4^+$ T-cell count under 100/ml, and polyclonal secretion of immunoglobulins in the blood.

**Neuropathology**

In the absence of regression of a mass in the brain after 3 weeks of empirical antitoxoplasmic treatment, a lymphoma becomes the first diagnostic possibility, but histological confirmation is theoretically required (Knowles *et al.*, 1988; So *et al.*, 1988). In some patients stereotactic biopsy or open brain biopsy of the lesion has even been performed (Scully *et al.*, 1983; Feiden *et al.*, 1993). The high risk of cerebral haemorrhage during the biopsy (Pichenik *et al.*, 1983; Feiden *et al.*, 1993) has led us to avoid cerebral biopsy in the majority of cases. The prognosis is so poor in most patients, even after treatment, that a brain biopsy should be considered only for those in good general condition. The frequently necrotic

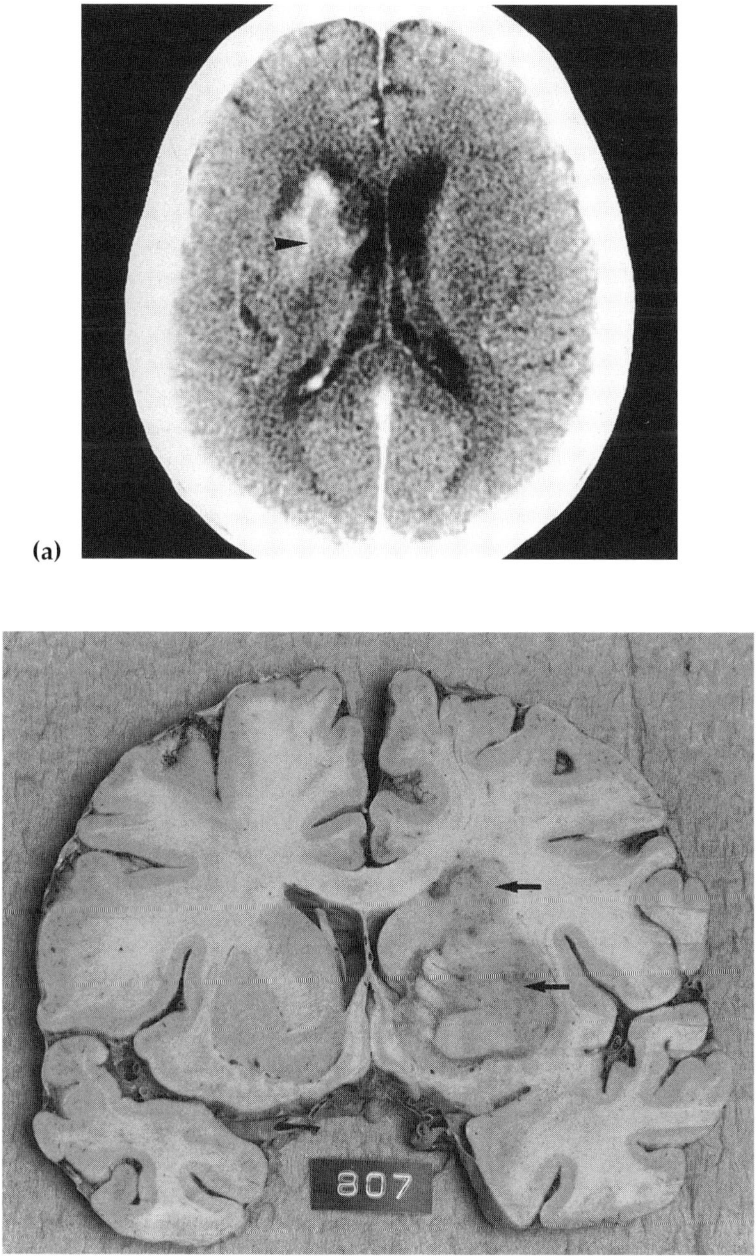


**(a)**

**(b)**

**Figure 3.1** (a) CT image with contrast showing a heterogeneous enhancing lesion of the right basal ganglia and the periependymal region (arrowhead) in an HIV-infected patient with brain lymphoma. (b) Frontal section of the brain of the same patient: the right caudate nucleus and the lenticular nucleus are invaded by the lymphoma (arrows).

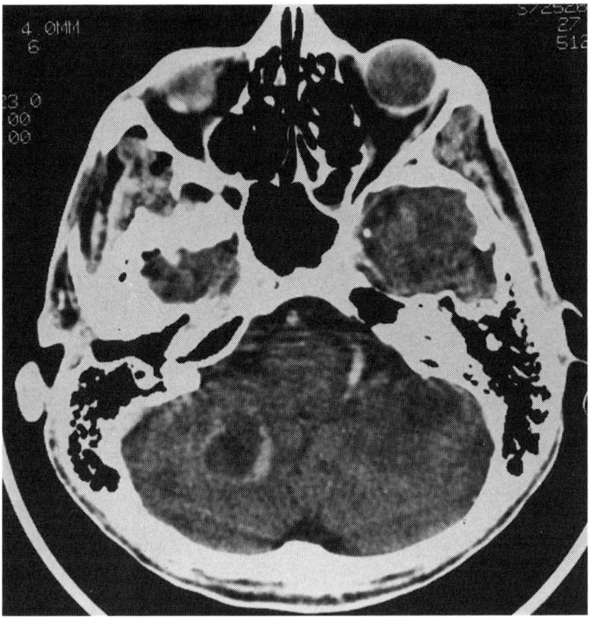

(a)

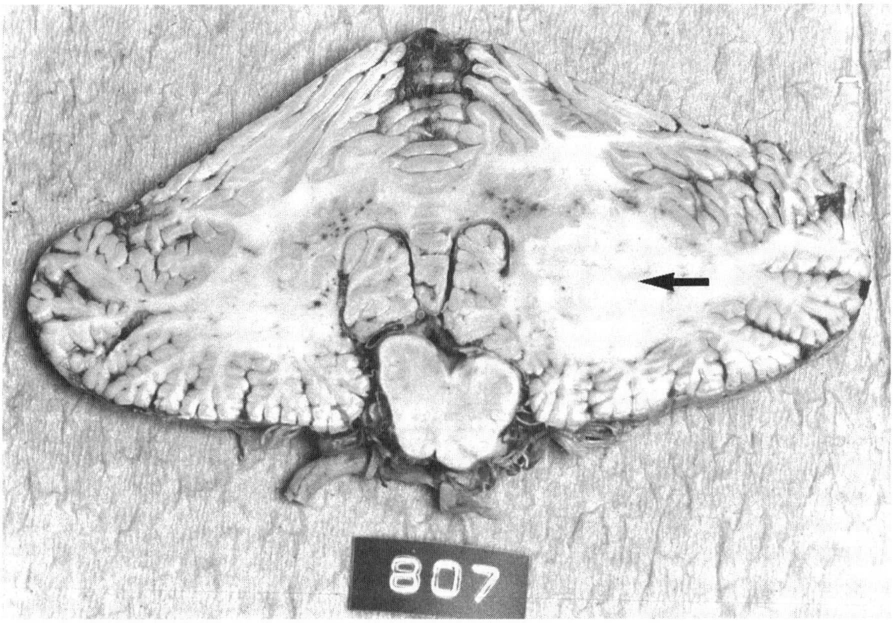



(b)

**Figure 3.2** (a) CT image with contrast showing ring enhancement in the right hemisphere of an HIV-infected patient with cerebellar lymphoma. (b) Section of the cerebellum of the same patient: the lymphoma of the right hemisphere is necrotic (arrow).

aspect of tumour samples taken by biopsy can make histological diagnosis more difficult. In many patients the clinical deficit increases so rapidly that the brain lymphoma is found only at autopsy (Loureiro *et al.*, 1988; Marelle *et al.*, 1994).

Primary brain lymphomas are multicentric and located in the periependymal area (see Figure 3.1b) (Rosenblum *et al.*, 1988). Usually, a large hemispheric mass is present, associated with several other smaller disseminated lesions in the brainstem and cerebellum (see Figure 3.2b). Spinal cord localization is uncommon (Snider *et al.*, 1983; Stavrou *et al.*, 1989; Herida *et al.*, 1993). Primary brain lymphomas are high- or intermediate-grade pathological types (Freeman *et al.*, 1986; Ioachim *et al.*; 1991; Marelle *et al.*, 1994), including a large majority of large-cell immunoblastic or small-cell non-cleaved types (So *et al.*, 1986; Rosenblum *et al.*, 1988); low-grade lymphomas are rare (Kaplan *et al.*, 1989). Nuclear abnormalities and atypical mitosis are frequent (Figure 3.3). In the CNS, tumoral lymphocytes have a perivascular arrangement (Figure 3.4). Tumoral necrosis is frequent; macrophages and some glial cells are mixed with tumour cells (Figure 3.5). The large majority of primary brain lymphomas are of the B-cell type, including the anaplastic variety (Figure 3.6), exceptionally of the T-cell type (Rao *et al.*, 1989; Ruff *et al.*, 1989). CNS localization of Burkitt-like lymphoma occurs (Ziegler *et al.*, 1982). Both monoclonal and polyclonal secretion of immunoglobulins has been observed (Loureiro *et al.*, 1988; Hamilton-Dutoit *et al.*, 1991; Meeker *et al.*, 1991). In five of our patients with

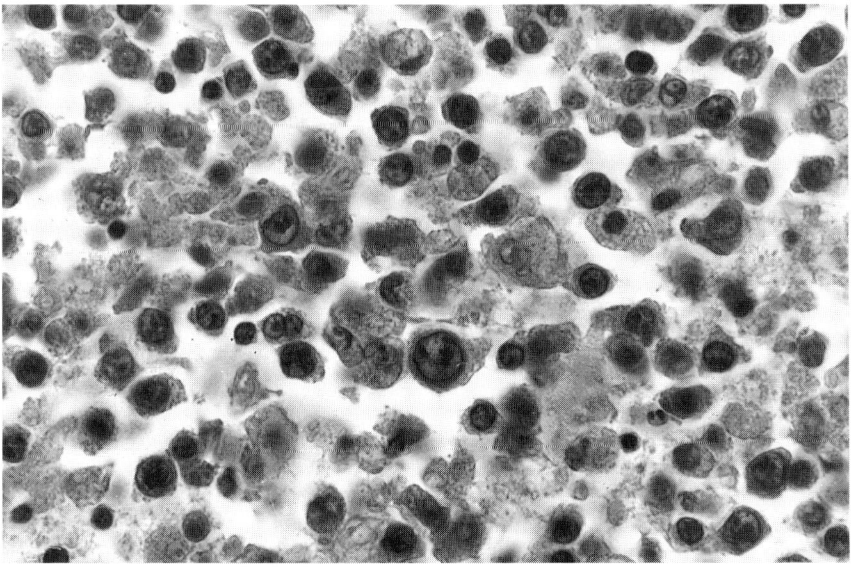

**Figure 3.3** Large immunoblastic lymphocytes and nuclear abnormalities in a brain lymphoma of an HIV-infected patient. (Paraffin section; H&E; ×1640.)

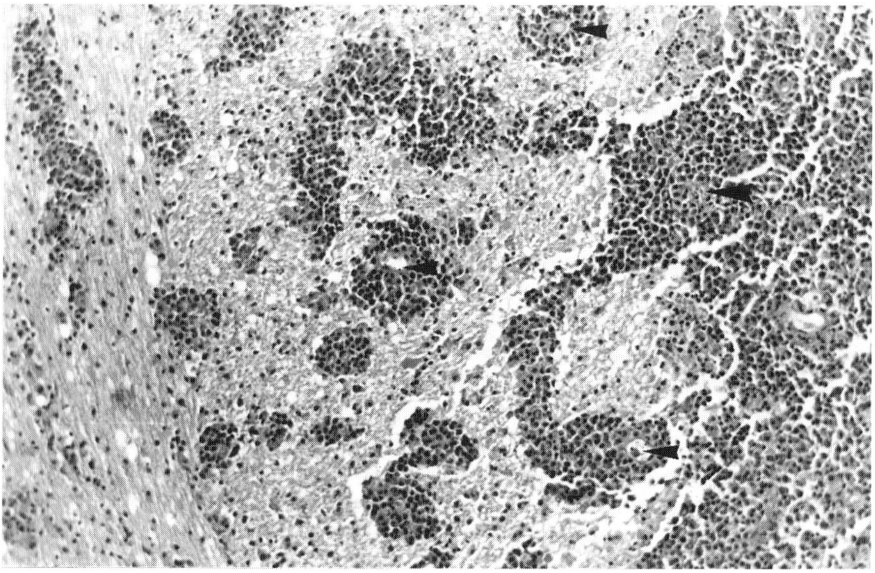

**Figure 3.4** Tumoral lymphocytes are located around the vessels (arrowheads) in a brain lymphoma of an HIV-infected patient. (Paraffin section; H&E; ×30.)

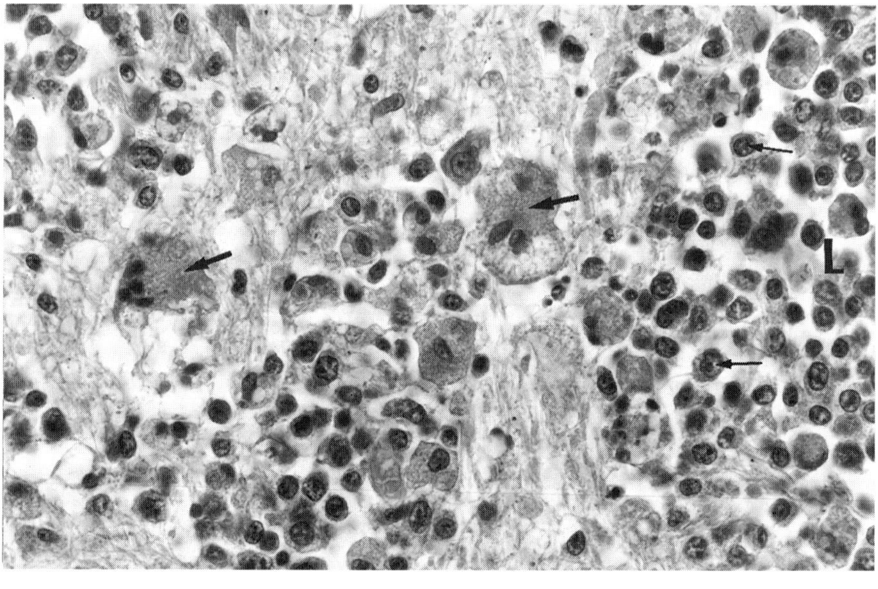


**Figure 3.5** Lymphoid cells (thin arrows) are associated with macrophages and giant cells (thick arrows) in a brain lymphoma (L) of an HIV-infected patient. (Paraffin section; H&E; ×1330.)

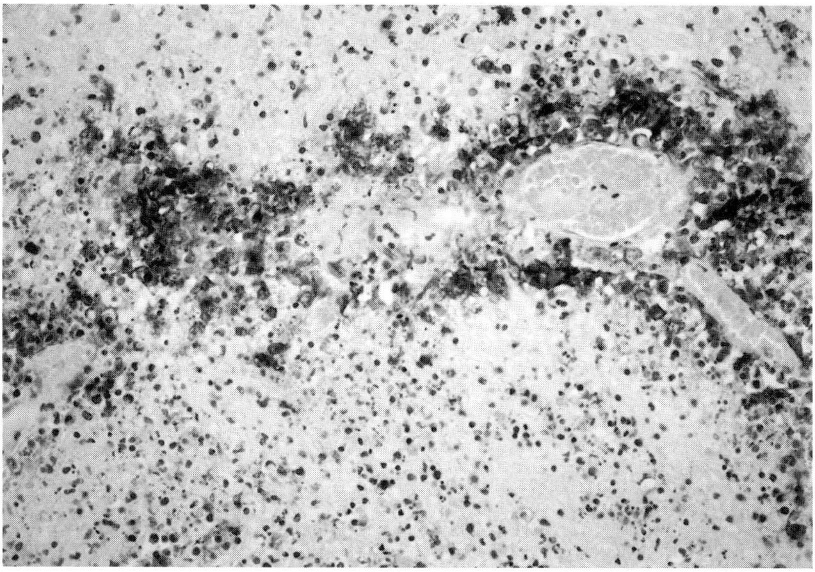

**Figure 3.6** Immunocytochemistry with a CD20 (L26, Dako) antibody showing B cells around vessels in a brain lymphoma of an HIV-infected patient. (Paraffin section; avidin–biotin/DAB; ×60.)

AIDS, brain lymphoma was associated with HIV encephalitis and cerebral toxoplasmosis and CMV encephalitis. Cerebral toxoplasmosis is the most important differential diagnosis of cerebral lymphomas, and antitoxoplasmic challenge therapy for a few weeks is the best way to approach the diagnosis (see Chapter 4).

### Pathogenesis

The similarities between primary CNS lymphoma in AIDS patients and Burkitt's lymphoma have led to study of the expression of EBV in these lymphomas (Ziegler *et al.*, 1982). Patients with AIDS or AIDS-related complex have a high number of EBV-infected B cells in the peripheral blood and a profound defect of T-cell immunity to EBV (Birx *et al.*, 1986). EBV DNA was found in frozen samples of a lymphoma using Southern hybridization with a fragment of EBV as the probe (Rosenberg *et al.*, 1986). Further studies using *in situ* hybridization were able to demonstrate EBV RNA in 100% of primary CNS lymphomas but only 30–50% of systemic lymphomas in AIDS patients (Hamilton-Dutoit *et al.*, 1991; MacMahon *et al.*, 1991). In a large proportion of primary CNS lymphomas in HIV-infected patients, the surface proteins of EBV were expressed in greater amounts than in lymphomas of non-AIDS patients (Meeker *et al.*, 1991; Auperin *et al.*, 1993; Bashir *et al.*, 1993). In our experience, EBV surface proteins are expressed in all brain lymphomas obtained at autopsy or biopsy of AIDS patients (Figure 3.7). EBV might induce abnormalities of the c-*myc* oncogene and then multiplication of one or several clones of B lymphocytes (Rosenblum *et al.*, 1988). A direct role for HIV in the induction of primary cerebral lymphomas is possible, even though the virus has not yet been detected in tumoral cells. In primary brain lymphoma with anaplastic large-type cells (CD30 positive) (Chadburn *et al.*, 1993), a few tumoral cells were positive for the p24 antigen but this needs confirmation. Coinfection by HIV and EBV may induce differences between primary CNS lymphomas and systemic lymphomas: rearrangements in the c-*myc* oncogene in brain lymphomas have not been detected, but have been found in 50% of systemic lymphomas (Meeker *et al.*, 1991; Ballerini *et al.*, 1993). These results could indicate that primary and secondary brain lymphomas might have different genetic patterns (Baumgartner *et al.*, 1989; Meeker *et al.*, 1991).

**Treatment and evolution**

The prognosis of brain lymphoma in HIV-infected patients is extremely poor and in the first reports the average survival time was less than 2 months with or without treatment (Gill *et al.*, 1986; So *et al.*, 1986). In many patients, the diagnosis of primary CNS lymphoma is made only at autopsy (Snider *et al.*, 1983; Loureiro *et al.*, 1988; Stavrou *et al.*, 1989; Matthiessen *et al.*, 1992). The evolution is more rapid compared with primary lymphomas affecting non-AIDS patients (Rosenblum *et al.* 1988). In systemic AIDS-related

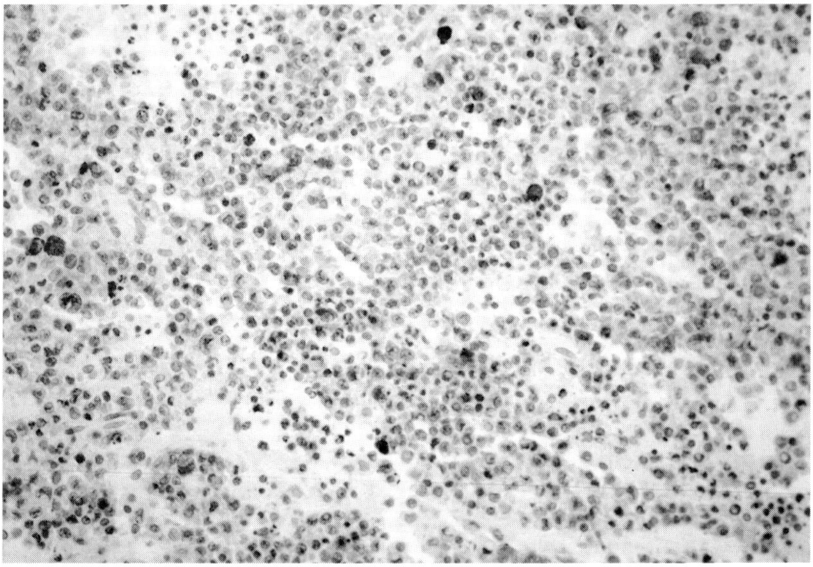

**Figure 3.7** Immunocytochemistry with a capsid Epstein–Barr virus antibody (EBV-LMP, Dako) of a brain lymphoma in an HIV-infected patient. Numerous tumoral lymphocytes are stained in brown. (Paraffin section; avidin–biotin/DAB; ×60.)

lymphomas, patients with a $CD4^+$ T-cell count over 400/ml have a longer survival time than those with a $CD4^+$ T-cell count under 100/ml, regardless of the histological type of the lymphoma (Andrieu et al., 1988; Knowles *et al.*, 1988; Marelle *et al.*, 1994). However, CNS brain lymphomas usually occur in severely immunosuppressed patients (Levine *et al.*, 1991a). The median survival time of patients with treated (surgery, radiotherapy and chemotherapy) primary brain lymphoma is 2.5 months compared with 6 months for AIDS-related systemic lymphoma. Death results from opportunistic infections in most patients (Lowenthal *et al.*, 1988; Levine *et al.*, 1991a). Because nearly all patients have multifocal localization that cannot be removed, surgery is useful only for performing a biopsy to histologically characterize the mass lesion (So *et al.*, 1988; Marelle *et al.*, 1994). In one series, only 2/21 patients with primary brain lymphoma were still alive 22 months after radiation and chemotherapy (Ziegler *et al.*, 1982). Some patients received oral steroids but cerebral lymphomas in AIDS patients do not respond as well as they do in non-immunosuppressed patients. Cranial radiotherapy has also been proposed by different authors (Formenti *et al.*, 1989; Baumgartner *et al.*, 1990). In a series of 10 patients who received 2200–5000 cGy, six had complete response of brain masses on CT and one had partial response but median survival time of the group was 5.5 months (Formenti *et al.*, 1989). The median survival time was less than 3 months after radiation therapy in another series (Rosenblum *et al.*, 1988). Chemotherapy has seldom been given in AIDS patients because of the immunological depression already present in these patients (Bermudez *et al.*, 1989; Levine *et al.*, 1991b).

## CNS LOCALIZATION OF SYSTEMIC LYMPHOMAS

Systemic non-Hodgkin's lymphomas occur in 5% of HIV-infected patients (Knowles *et al.*, 1988) and 19% of patients with systemic lymphoma have CNS localization (Ziegler *et al.*, 1984). In addition to brain metastasis, lymphomatous infiltration of the meninges, cranial nerves and epidural spaces has been observed (Snider *et al.*, 1983; Loureiro *et al.*, 1988). The lymphomas are usually of the large-cell immunoblastic type, but great cellular polymorphism is observed. A few Burkitt's lymphomas have been described in patients with AIDS (Ziegler *et al.*, 1982; Snider *et al.*, 1983; So *et al.*, 1988), but to our knowledge no Hodgkin's lymphomas of the CNS have been found. Treatment of systemic lymphomas consists of chemotherapy associated with radiotherapy, but in patients with AIDS the median survival time is only 5–6 months (Lowenthal *et al.*, 1988; Kaplan *et al.*, 1989). A multi-institutional trial in patients with systemic lymphomas without CNS localization used low-dose chemotherapy with CNS prophylaxis (intrathecal cytosine arabinoside) together with cranial irradiation and zidovudine in some patients; 45% of the patients had a complete response and their median survival time was 15 months (Levine *et al.*, 1991b).

## LYMPHOMATOID GRANULOMATOSIS

Lymphomatoid granulomatosis was observed by Anders *et al.* (1989) in the CNS of three patients with AIDS in association with malignant lymphoma that affected other parts of the brain. These authors suggested that lymphomatoid granulomatosis could progress to malignant lymphomas. Colby (1989) suggested that the different patterns of lymphomas actually represented varieties of malignant lymphomas. In our autopsy series, disseminated brain and extraneural lesions of lymphomatoid granulomatosis were present in an HIV-infected child (see Table 4.7) (Lacroix *et al.*, 1993).

## KAPOSI'S SARCOMA

Cutaneous and visceral localization of Kaposi's sarcoma are extremely common in AIDS, but the nervous system is seldom involved. Isolated reports have mentioned Kaposi's sarcoma of the dura mater (Ariza and Kim, 1988) or brain metastasis (Gorin *et al.*, 1985; So *et al.*, 1988). A spontaneous haemorrhagic aspect on CT may be a marker for diagnosis (Gorin *et al.*, 1985). Treatment is based on radiotherapy, chemotherapy and zidovudine, but the prognosis is poor (Bachelez and Revuz, 1989).

## OTHER TUMOURS

Other tumours (probably coincidental), including astrocytomas, cerebral metastasis and leiomyosarcoma, have been occasionally encountered (Gasnault *et al.*, 1988; Anders *et al.*, 1989; Kozlowski *et al.*, 1990).

## REFERENCES

Amberson JB, di Carlo EF, Metroka CE *et al.* (1985) Diagnostic pathology in the acquired immunodeficiency syndrome. *Archives of Pathology and Laboratory Medicine* **109**: 345–351.

Anders KH, Latta H, Chang BS *et al.* (1989) Lymphomatoid granulomatosis and malignant lymphoma of the central nervous system in the acquired immunodeficiency syndrome. *Human Pathology* **20**: 326–334.

Andrieu JM, Toledano M, Raphael M *et al.* (1988) HIV-related haematological neoplasias in France. *Recent Results in Cancer Research* **112**: 46–53.

Ariza A and Kim JH (1988) Kaposi's sarcoma of the dura mater. *Human Pathology* **19**: 1461–1463.

Auperin I, Morinet F, Oksenhendler E and Mikol J (1993) Primary B-cell lymphoma of the central nervous system from HIV infected and non-infected patients: expression of cellular surface proteins and Epstein–Barr viral markers. *Neuropathology and Applied Neurobiology* **19**: 191.

Bachelez H and Revuz J (1989) Traitement de la maladie de Kaposi. *Presse Medicale* **18**: 484–487.

Ballerini P, Gaidano G, Gong JZ *et al.* (1993) Multiple genetic lesions in AIDS-related non-Hodgkin's lymphoma. *Blood* **81**: 166–176.

Bashir R, Luka J, Cheloha K *et al.* (1993) Expression of Epstein–Barr virus proteins in primary CNS lymphoma in AIDS patients. *Neurology* **43**: 2358–2362.

Baumgartner JE, Meeker TK, Garibaldi C *et al.* (1989) Patterns of gene rearrangement in AIDS-associated primary central nervous system lymphoma. Satellite conference to the V International Conference on AIDS, Québec, Canada, Abstract BS9.

Baumgartner JE, Rachlin JR, Beckstead JH *et al.* (1990) Primary central nervous system lymphomas: natural history and response to radiation in 55 patients with acquired immunodeficiency syndrome. *Journal of Neurosurgery* **73**: 206–211.

Bermudez M, Grant KM, Rodvien R and Mendes F (1989) Non-Hodgkin's lymphoma in a population with or at risk for acquired immunodeficiency syndrome: indications for intensive chemotherapy. *American Journal of Medicine* **86**: 71–76.

Birx D, Redfield RR and Tosato G (1986) Defective regulation of Epstein–Barr virus infection in patients with acquired immunodeficiency syndrome (AIDS) or AIDS-related disorders. *New England Journal of Medicine* **314**: 874–879.

Brew BJ, Bhalla RB, Fleisher M *et al.* (1989) Cerebrospinal fluid $\beta_2$ microglobulin in patients infected with human immunodeficiency virus. *Neurology* **39**: 830–834.

Budka H, Costanzi G, Cristina S *et al.* (1987) Brain pathology induced by infection with the human immunodeficiency virus (HIV): a 100 autopsy cases. *Acta Neuropathologica* **75**: 185–198.

Carbone A, Tirelli U, Vaccher E *et al.* (1991) A clinicopathologic study of lymphoid neoplasias associated with human immunodeficiency virus infection in Italy. *Cancer* **68**: 842–852.

Centers for Disease Control (CDC) (1985) Revision of the case definition of acquired immunodeficiency syndrome for national reporting – United States. *Annals of Internal Medicine* **103**: 402–403.

Chadburn A, Cesarman E, Jagirdar J *et al.* (1993) CD30 (Ki-1) positive anaplastic large cell lymphomas in individuals infected with the human immunodeficiency virus. *Cancer* **72**: 3078–3090.

Chimelli L, Rosemberg S, Hahn MD *et al.* (1992) Pathology of the central nervous system in patients infected with the human immunodeficiency virus (HIV): a report of 252 autopsy cases from Brazil. *Neuropathology and Applied Neurobiology* **18**: 478–488.

Clifford DB, Arribas JR, Fichtenbaum CJ and Storch GA (1994) Detection of Epstein–Barr virus DNA in cerebrospinal fluid of patients with HIV-related central nervous system lymphoma. *Annals of Neurology* **36**: 329.

Colby TV (1989) Central nervous system lymphomatoid granulomatosis in AIDS? *Human Pathology* **20**: 301–302.

Epstein LG, di Carlo FJ, Joshi VV *et al.* (1988) Primary lymphoma of the central nervous system in children with acquired immuno-deficiency syndrome. *Pediatrics* **82**: 355–363.

Feiden W, Bise K, Steude U *et al.* (1993) The stereotactic biopsy diagnosis of focal intracerebral lesions in AIDS patients. *Acta Neurologica Scandinavica* **87**: 228–233.

Formenti SC, Gill PS, Lean E *et al.* (1989) Primary central nervous system lymphoma in AIDS. Results of radiation therapy. *Cancer* **63**: 1101–1107.

Freeman CR, Shastik C, Brisson M-L, Meagher-Villemure K and Dylewski I (1986) Primary malignant lymphoma of the central nervous system. *Cancer* **58**: 1106–1111.

Gasnault J, Roux FX and Vedrenne C (1988) Cerebral astrocytoma in association with HIV infection. *Journal of Neurology, Neurosurgery and Psychiatry* **51**: 422–424.

Gill PS, Graham RA, Boswell W *et al.* (1986) A comparison of imaging, clinical, and pathologic aspects of space-occupying lesions within the brain in patients with acquired immune deficiency syndrome. *American Journal of Physiologic Imaging* **1**: 134–141.

Gorin FA, Bale JF, Hack S *et al.* (1985) Kaposi's sarcoma metastatic to the CNS. *Archives of Neurology* **42**: 162–165.

Gray F, Geny C, Lionnet F *et al.* (1991) Etude neuropathologique de 135 cas adultes de syndrome d'immuno-deficience acquise (SIDA). *Annales de Pathologie* **11**: 236–247.

Hamilton-Dutoit SJ, Pallesen G, Franzmann MB *et al.* (1991) AIDS-related lymphoma: histopathology, immunophenotype and association with Epstein–Barr virus as demonstrated by *in situ* nucleic acid hybridization. *American Journal of Pathology* **138**: 149–163.

Herida M, Khuong MA, De Broucker T *et al.* (1993) Lymphome primitif du système nerveux central à localisation médullaire révélatrice chez un patient infecté par le virus de l'immunodéficience humaine. *Annales de Medecine Interne* **144**: 64–66.

Ioachim HL, Dorsett B, Cronin W *et al.* (1991) Acquired immunodeficiency syndrome-associated lymphomas: clinical, pathologic, immunologic, and viral characteristics of 111 cases. *Human Pathology* **22**: 659–673.

Kaplan LD, Abrams DI, Feigal E *et al.* (1989) AIDS-associated non-Hodgkin lymphomas in San Francisco. *Journal of the American Medical Association* **261**: 719–724.

Knowles DM, Chamulak GA, Subar M J *et al.* (1988) Clinicopathologic, immunophenotypic, and molecular genetic analysis of AIDS-associated lymphoid neoplasia. Clinical and biologic implications. *Pathology Annual* **23**: 33–67.

Kozlowski PB, Sher JH, Dickson DW *et al.* (1990) Central nervous system in pediatric HIV infection: a multicenter study. In: *Brain in Pediatric AIDS* (eds PB Kozlowski, DA Snider, PM Vietze and HM Wisniewski), pp. 132–146. Basel: Karger.

Kure K, Llena JF, Lyman WD *et al.* (1991). Human immunodeficiency virus-1 infection of the nervous system: an autopsy study of 268 adult, pediatric, and foetal brains. *Human Pathology* **22**: 700–710.

Lacroix C, Vazeux R, Brousse N *et al.* (1993) Etude neuropathologique de 10 enfants infectés par le VIH. *Revue Neurologique* **149**: 37–45.

Lang W, Miklossy J, Dernaz JP *et al.* (1989) Neuropathology of the acquired immune deficiency syndrome (AIDS): a report of 135 consecutive autopsy cases from Switzerland. *Acta Neuropathologica* **77**: 379–390.

Levine AM, Sullivan-Halley J, Pike MC *et al.* (1991a) Human immunodeficiency virus-related lymphoma: prognostic factors predictive of survival. *Cancer* **68**: 2466–2472.

Levine AM, Wernz JC, Kaplan L *et al.* (1991b) Low dose chemotherapy with central nervous system prophylaxis and azidothymidine maintenance in AIDS related lymphoma. *Journal of the American Medical Association* **266**: 84–88.

Levy RM, Rosenblum S and Perrett LV (1986) Neuroradiologic findings in AIDS: a review of Chimelli *et al.* 19920 cases. *American Journal of Roentgenology* **147**: 977–983.

Loureiro C, Gill PS, Meyer PR, Rhodes R, Rarick MU and Levine AM (1988) Autopsy findings in AIDS-related lymphoma. *Cancer* **62**: 735–739.

Lowenthal DA, Straus DJ, Wise Campbell S *et al.* (1988) AIDS-related lymphoid neoplasia. The memorial hospital experience. *Cancer* **61**: 2325–2327.

MacMahon EME, Glass JD, Hayward SD *et al.* (1991) Epstein–Barr virus in AIDS-related primary central nervous system lymphoma. *Lancet* **338**: 969–980.

Marelle L, Raphael M, Hénin D *et al.* (1994) Les lymphomes cérébraux du SIDA: étude clinique et corrélations clinico-pathologiques. *Revue Neurologique* **150**: 123–132.

Matthiessen L, Marche C, Labrousse F *et al.* (1992) Etude neuropathologique de l'encéphale de 174 patients morts du SIDA dans un hôpital parisien, de 1982 à 1988. *Annales de Medecine Interne* **143**: 43–49.

Meeker TC, Shiramizu B, Kaplan L *et al.* (1991) Evidence for molecular subtypes of HIV-associated lymphomas: division into peripheral monoclonal, polyclonal and central nervous system lymphoma. *AIDS* **5**: 669–674.

Orron DE, Kuhn MJ, Malholtra V, Mildvan D and Leeds N (1989) Primary cerebral lymphoma in acquired immunodeficiency syndrome (AIDS) – CT manifestations. *Computerized Medical Imaging and Graphics* **13**: 207–214.

Petito C, Cho E, Leman W *et al.* (1986) Neuropathology of acquired immunodeficiency syndrome (AIDS). An autopsy review. *Journal of Neuropathology and Experimental Neurology* **45**: 635–646.

Pichenik AE, Fischl MA and Walls KW (1983) Evaluation of cerebral mass lesions in acquired immunodeficiency syndrome. *New England Journal of Medicine* **308**: 1099–1100.

Pluda JM, Yarchoan R, Jaffe ES *et al.* (1990) Development of non-Hodgkin lymphoma in a cohort of patients with severe human immunodeficiency virus (HIV) infection on long-term antiretroviral therapy. *Annals of Internal Medicine* **113**: 276–282.

Poon T, Matoso I, Tchertkoff V *et al.* (1989) CT features of primary cerebral lymphoma in AIDS and non-AIDS patients. *Journal of Computer Assisted Tomography* **13**: 6–9.

Rao C, Wrzolek M, Kozlowski PB *et al.* (1989) Primary T cell central lymphoma in AIDS. *Journal of Neuropathology and Experimental Neurology* **48**: 302.

Remick SC, Diamond C, Migliozzi JA *et al.* (1990) Primary central nervous system lymphoma in patients with and without the acquired immune deficiency syndrome: a retrospective analysis and a review of the literature. *Medicine* **69**: 345–360.

Rhodes RH (1993) Histopathologic features in the central nervous system of 400 acquired immunodeficiency syndrome cases: implications of rates of occurrence. *Human Pathology* **24**: 1189–1198.

Rosenberg NL, Hochberg FH, Miller G, Kleinschmidt-De Masters BK (1986) Primary central nervous system lymphoma related to Epstein–Barr virus in a patient with acquired immune deficiency syndrome. *Annals of Neurology* **20**: 98–102.

Rosenblum ML, Levy RM, Bredesen DE *et al.* (1988) Primary central nervous system lymphomas in patients with AIDS. *Annals of Neurology* **23**: S13–16.

Ruff P, Bagg A and Papadopoulos K (1989) Precursor T-cell lymphoma associated with human immunodeficiency virus type 1 (HIV-1) infection. *Cancer* **64**: 39–42.
Scully RE, Mark EJ and McNeely BU (1983) Case records of the Massachusetts General Hospital. *New England Journal of Medicine* **309**: 359–369.
Snider WD, Simpson DM, Nielsen S *et al.* (1983) Neurological complications of acquired immune deficiency syndrome: analysis of 50 patients. *Annals of Neurology* **14**: 403–418.
So YT, Beckstead JH and Davis RL (1986) Primary central nervous system lymphoma in acquired immune deficiency syndrome: a clinical and pathological study. *Annals of Neurology* **20**: 566–572.
So YT, Choucair A, Davis RL *et al.* (1988) Neoplasms of the central nervous system in acquired immunodeficiency syndrome. In: *AIDS and the Nervous System* (ed, Rosenblum ML), pp. 285–300. New York: Raven Press.
Stavrou D, Mehraein P, Mellert W *et al.* (1989) Evaluation of intracerebral lesions in patients with acquired immunodeficiency syndrome. Neuropathological findings and experimental data. *Neuropathology and Applied Neurobiology* **15**: 207–222.
Ziegler JL, Miner RC, Rosenbaum E *et al.* (1982) Outbreak of Burkitt's like lymphoma in homosexual men. *Lancet* **18ii**: 631–633.

# 4

# *Opportunistic Infections of the Central Nervous System*

## PROTOZOAL INFECTION: CEREBRAL TOXOPLASMOSIS

More than 40% of all AIDS patients develop neurological manifestations, and in 10% of them the neurological manifestations represent the first symptoms of AIDS. At autopsy, 75% or more have CNS lesions, mostly opportunistic infections (Table 4.1 lists infections detected in two composite autopsy series of 791 and 309 patients from the USA and Europe respectively).

Before the 1980s, opportunistic infections of the CNS were uncommon (Table 4.2). They affected immunocompromised patients with reticuloendothelial malignancies, collagen vascular disease or transplanted organs; despite profound immunosuppression, the incidence of toxoplasmosis in these patients was low, ranging from 2 to 5% (Vietzke *et al.*, 1968; Israelski and Remington, 1993). Since the advent of AIDS, some of these infections (*Toxoplasma gondii*

**Table 4.1** Opportunistic infections of the CNS (%) at autopsy in AIDS

| | USA (791 patients)* | France/Switzerland (309 patients)[†] |
|---|---|---|
| Toxoplasmosis | 11.1 | 31.6 |
| Cryptococcosis | 8.4 | 4.4 |
| Cytomegalovirus | 16.9 | 12.3 |
| Progressive multifocal leucoencephalopathy | 3.5 | 4.7 |
| Mycobacteria | <0.5 | <0.5 |
| Varicella-zoster virus encephalitis | 0.6 | — |
| Candidiasis | 1.3 | <0.5 |
| Other fungi | <0.5 | <0.5 |

* Sources: Levy *et al.* (1985), Anders *et al.* (1986), Navia *et al.* (1986b), Petito *et al.* (1986), Rhodes (1987), Kure *et al.* (1991).
[†] Sources: Lang *et al.* (1989), Matthiessen *et al.* (1992).

**Table 4.2** CNS pathogens associated with disorders of cell-mediated immunity known before 1980 compared with after 1980 (the AIDS era)

| | Before 1980 | | AIDS (after 1980) | |
|---|---|---|---|---|
| | Common | Rare | Common | Rare |
| Bacterial | *Listeria monocytogenes*<br>*Nocardia* sp. | *Mycobacterium tuberculosis* | | *Listeria monocytogenes*<br>*Mycobacterium tuberculosis*<br>*Nocardia* sp. |
| Viral | Herpes simplex virus | Papovavirus | Papovavirus | Herpes simplex virus type 1 |
| | Varicella-zoster virus | Cytomegalovirus (extremely infrequent) | Cytomegalovirus | Herpes simplex virus type 2 |
| Fungi | *Cryptococcus neoformans* | *Aspergillus fumigatus* | *Cryptococcus neoformans* | *Aspergillus fumigatus*<br>*Histoplasma capsulatum* |
| Parasites | | *Toxoplasma gondii* | *Toxoplasma gondii* | |

encephalitis, CMV encephalitis, progressive multifocal leucoencephalitis) occur at an unusually high rate in this chronically immunodeficient population (Levy *et al.*, 1985; Matthiessen *et al.*, 1992).

*Toxoplasma gondii* encephalitis (toxoplasmic encephalitis), once rare, even in the immunocompromised patient, now accounts for about 40% of CNS infections and more than one-third of intracerebral mass lesions (Whelan *et al.*, 1983; Levy RM *et al.*, 1986; Luft & Remington, 1992; Strittmatter *et al.*, 1992) and is a major cause of neurological morbidity and mortality among patients at an advanced stage of HIV infection. It is one of the most significant neurological complications in HIV-infected patients as it is both preventable and treatable (Handler *et al.*, 1983; Whelan *et al.*, 1983; Levy *et al.*, 1985; Navia *et al.*, 1986a; Luft and Remington, 1988, 1992). *Toxoplasma gondii*, like *Pneumocystis carinii*, is a typical example of a major AIDS-related opportunistic infection: primary infection (acute, newly acquired infection) is asymptomatic or mildly symptomatic and self-limited in at least 90% of normal children and adults, while *T. gondii* encephalitis is a cause of rapidly progressive and fatal disease in AIDS patients if left untreated.

In an immunocompetent host, infection with *Toxoplasma* remains asymptomatic. The advent of AIDS and accompanying progressive impairment of immune function, especially of cell-mediated immunity, reactivates latent infection, thus placing individuals at high risk for *T. gondii* encephalitis (Luft and Remington, 1988).

**The organism (Luft, 1989; Pfefferkorn, 1990; Wong and Remington, 1993)**

*Toxoplasma gondii*, a ubiquitous, obligate, intracellular protozoan parasite widely distributed in human populations, is the agent most often responsible for latent infection of the CNS. Its natural reservoirs include cats, birds and a variety of animals in which it can proliferate, but its only definitive hosts are members of the cat family (i.e. felines), while humans and other mammals are incidental hosts. *Toxoplasma gondii* has a complex life cycle with three separate forms potentially infectious for humans: the oocyst (containing sporozoites), which is the product of the sexual cycle; the tachyzoite (containing trophozoites), which is the asexual invasive form; and the tissue cyst (containing bradyzoites), which persists in the latent phase of infection. The complete cycle, which only occurs in the cat, includes both an enteroepithelial sexual cycle and an extraintestinal asexual cycle. In humans and other incidental hosts, the organism has only an extraintestinal phase of development. The principal forms by which *T. gondii* is transmitted are the tissue cyst and the oocyst. Cats are the only animals that pass oocysts in their faeces. Sporulated oocysts can survive for more than 12 months in warm and humid soils. Oocysts are a cause of infection in humans who have contact with cat faeces or objects contaminated with cat faeces. The tachyzoite form is the obligate intracellular form found during acute infection; it can invade virtually all mammalian cell types, where it multiplies through an asexual cycle. When the host cell ruptures, released organisms may infect nearby cells, pursuing the replicative process. Tachyzoites also form cysts.

Tissue cysts contain viable organisms that persist for the lifespan of the host and are responsible for the chronic latent phase of infection. Any tissue previously infected, but mainly brain, skeletal and heart muscle cells, may harbour these cysts, allowing reactivation in the context of impaired cell-mediated immunity with the unwelcome release of invasive tachyzoites (Remington and Cavanaugh, 1965).

Humans are infected either through ingestion of oocysts (after handling cat faeces or soil contaminated with cat faeces) or tissue cysts (after eating infected food), or transplacentally. Nevertheless, pet cats are probably seldom the direct source of infection (Wallace *et al.*, 1993; Glaser *et al.*, 1994). Animals raised for human consumption become infected when they eat soil contaminated with cat faeces. Thus, ingestion of undercooked meats, mainly pork and mutton that contain tissue cysts, and vegetables or other food products contaminated with oocysts is the major means of transmission and the most common source of human toxoplasmosis (Dubey, 1986; Jackson and Hutchison, 1989). In countries with a high standard of living the infection is mainly linked to the consumption of raw meat. The role of undercooked meat as a source of toxoplasmosis in humans is well established: in France (where meat is often eaten rare, whereas it is well cooked in Anglo-Saxon and Asian countries), 84% of pregnant women in Paris were found to have antibodies to *T. gondii* compared with only 22% in London (Dubey and Beattie, 1988). In France, differences in dietary habits are probably responsible for differences in prevalence between pregnant women from different geographic origins (71% among French women, 61% among those from North Africa, 41% among those from black Africa, and 13% among women from Asia). The fall in seroprevalence observed over recent years in women of child-bearing age is apparently due to the more frequent consumption of frozen meat (Jeannel *et al.*, 1988).

### Seroprevalence of infection with *T. gondii* and incidence of toxoplasmic encephalitis

The incidence of toxoplasmic encephalitis is correlated with the seroprevalence of antibodies against *T. gondii* and with the clinical status or the $CD4^+$ cell counts of HIV-infected patients in a given population. The prevalence of seropositivity for *T. gondii* among HIV-infected individuals is similar to that in the general population (Renold *et al.*, 1992). However, this prevalence varies considerably from one geographic area to the next and with environmental conditions, past exposure and culinary habits that favour ingestion of raw or undercooked meat. These variations account for the differences in the incidence of toxoplasmic encephalitis between regional locales and countries on both sides of the Atlantic Ocean (see below).

#### *Seroprevalence of* Toxoplasma

The prevalence of toxoplasmosis in the general population varies from one country to another (Feldman, 1982; Dubey and Beattie, 1988; Dumas *et al.*, 1991).

In Africa, the prevalence of toxoplasmosis is higher in the humid and relatively humid areas of North, Central and West Africa (40–60%). The prevalence becomes very low (less than 25%) in desert areas, the Sahel (Senegal, Niger, etc.) and zones with a large Anglo-Saxon population (e.g. South Africa).

In general, the prevalence is very low in South-East Asia and Japan (4–14%). It appears to be higher in the Middle East, India, Indonesia and Malaysia (20–30%).

In the Pacific region, data are only partial but suggest prevalences below 30% in Australia and 25–60% in New Zealand. The prevalence in the Pacific atolls can be quite high (30–70%).

There is a strong contrast between the high prevalence sometimes observed in South America (30–80%) and the very low prevalence in North America. Rates vary from one part of North America to another: for example, the prevalence in pregnant women is 41% in Quebec, 30% in New York, 8% in Oregon and 5% in Manitoba (Feldman, 1965; Jeannel *et al.*, 1988; McCabe and Remington, 1990; Chatterton, 1992).

Three geographic areas emerge in Europe: Scandinavia and the UK have a prevalence below 25%, France and Germany have a high prevalence (40–70%) and countries around the Mediterranean Sea have a moderate prevalence (20–50%). The difference between the first two zones is explained by different culinary habits.

In HIV-infected patients in the USA, 4–45% have been found seropositive for *Toxoplasma* antibodies: 9.7% among the 723 patients in the Naval Health Research Center at San Diego (Wallace *et al.*, 1993); 4% among the HIV-positive participants in the Chicago Multicenter AIDS Cohort (Israelski *et al.*, 1993); 8–16% of adults in major urban areas, with a higher prevalence (25%) among undetailed ethnic groups (Wong *et al.*, 1995); in other studies, the range of prevalence for *Toxoplasma* antibodies was 15–45% (Wong and Remington, 1994).

In HIV-infected adults from Europe, Africa, Haiti and Latin America, and for identical epidemiological factors, the prevalence of *Toxoplasma* infection is correspondingly higher than in the USA. The incidence increases with age, and in all populations there are no differences in prevalence between the sexes. In Switzerland, prevalence of positive serology for *T. gondii* among 163 patients with AIDS registered between November 1989 and May 1991 was 50% (Renold *et al.*, 1992). Among 1499 HIV-seropositive Parisian patients the seroprevalence was 75% (Derouin *et al.*, 1991). In tropical areas (Central America and Equatorial Africa) the range of prevalence in HIV-infected adults is 50–78% (Remington *et al.*, 1970; Clumeck *et al.*, 1984; Ndumbe *et al.*, 1992; Sinibaldi and De Ramirez, 1992) and may exceed 90% (Beaman *et al.*, 1994).

*Incidence of toxoplasmic encephalitis*

Toxoplasmic encephalitis was recognized early in the AIDS epidemic (Hauser *et al.*, 1982; Luft *et al.*, 1983) and all HIV-infected patients who have antibody to *T. gondii*, with or without AIDS, must be considered at risk for toxoplasmic encephalitis. The incidence of toxoplasmic encephalitis is proportional to the prevalence of antibodies to *T. gondii* in a given population: among HIV-infected patients, up to 97% of toxoplasmic encephalitis develops in those infected with the parasite (Luft and Remington, 1988, 1992; Beaman *et al.*, 1994). Toxoplasmic encephalitis is extremely rare in patients seronegative for *Toxoplasma*. Only 1–3% of patients with neurotoxoplasmosis lack specific serological markers against *T. gondii* (Israelski and Remington, 1988; Suzuki *et al.*, 1988; Pedrol *et al.*, 1990; Derouin *et al.*, 1991). In a prospective prophylaxis study, all but one of 51 patients in whom toxoplasmosis developed had serological evidence of past exposure to *T. gondii* at the time of inclusion in the study (Girard *et al.*, 1993). More recently, none of the 183 participants in the Chicago Multicenter AIDS Cohort Study (MACS) who developed AIDS and who were seronegative for *Toxoplasma* antibodies developed toxoplasmic encephalitis (Israelski *et al.*, 1993). Available data from Europe, the USA, Equatorial Africa, Central and South America show that 25–50% of HIV-infected patients seropositive for *T. gondii* could develop toxoplasmic encephalitis (Aspock and Hassl, 1990; Grant *et al.*, 1990; Matheron *et al.*, 1990; Zangerle *et al.*, 1991; Luft and Remington, 1992).

In countries with a relatively low prevalence for *T. gondii* the percentage of patients with AIDS who develop toxoplasmic encephalitis is lower than in geographic areas that have populations with a higher seroprevalence. In the USA, toxoplasmic encephalitis has been reported in only 1–5% of patients with AIDS (Levy *et al.*, 1988; Porter and Sande, 1992) and, among the patients with an AIDS-defining disease reported to the Centers for Disease Control (CDC) in 1989, 5% had toxoplasmic encephalitis (Centers for Disease Control, 1990). Using the AIDS surveillance data from the USA, it was shown that among 203 470 persons with AIDS 11 058 (5.4%) had a diagnosis of toxoplasmosis (Hu *et al.*, 1995). Toxoplasmic encephalitis was the index diagnosis in 44–58% of HIV-infected patients with toxoplasmic encephalitis (Wong and Remington, 1994). These data obviously underestimate the prevalence of toxoplasmic encephalitis as the majority of HIV-infected patients who develop toxoplasmic encephalitis do so after the diagnosis of AIDS and are not reported to the CDC (Luft *et al.*, 1983; Wong *et al.*, 1984; Navia *et al.*, 1986a; Selik *et al.*, 1990).

In the USA, depending on regional seroprevalence of toxoplasmic infection, toxoplasmic encephalitis has been reported in 5–40% of patients with AIDS (review in Wong *et al.*, 1995). A retrospective study has suggested that 28–30% of HIV-infected patients seropositive for *Toxoplasma* will develop CNS toxoplasmosis (Grant *et al.*, 1990). In a recent prospective study (Israelski *et al.*, 1993), the risk of toxoplasmic encephalitis in HIV-infected patients with previous exposure to *Toxoplasma* was higher than that previously reported (Porter and Sande, 1992), with 5 of 13 patients (38%) developing toxoplasmic encephalitis.

Among the 203 470 individuals with AIDS in the USA, multivariate analysis showed that toxoplasmosis was more common among Hispanics compared with whites and among foreign-born compared with US-born subjects, but was less common among men having sex with men (risk ratio 0.8) compared with drug users (Hu *et al.*, 1995). The highest incidence of toxoplasmic encephalitis in patients with AIDS has been reported in Europe (Clumeck, 1991). Up to 47% of patients with AIDS in Austria could eventually develop toxoplasmic encephalitis (Zangerle *et al.*, 1991) and 37% in France (Matheron *et al.*, 1990; Matthiessen *et al.*, 1992). Also in France, toxoplasmic encephalitis was the AIDS-defining diagnosis in 12% of patients reported with AIDS in 1994 (European Centre for the Epidemiological Monitoring of AIDS 1994, 1995). In summary, in areas with a high seroprevalence for *Toxoplasma*, up to 50% of all AIDS patients will develop toxoplasmic encephalitis (Luft and Remington, 1992).

The majority of AIDS patients developing toxoplasmic encephalitis are at a very advanced stage of immunodeficiency and their $CD4^+$ T-cell counts are extremely low (Redfield *et al.*, 1986; Crowe *et al.*, 1991). The risk of toxoplasmic encephalitis in patients who have antibodies against both HIV and *T. gondii* increases markedly as the $CD4^+$ T-cell count falls. In patients with toxoplasmic encephalitis, the median $CD4^+$ T-cell count is approximately 50 $ml^{-1}$ (Eliaszewicz *et al.*, 1990; Matheron *et al.*, 1990; Dannemann *et al.*, 1992; Hu *et al.*, 1995), 90% have a $CD4^+$ T-cell count $< 200$ $ml^{-1}$ and about 80% have a $CD4^+$ T-cell count $< 100$ $ml^{-1}$ (Eliaszewicz *et al.*, 1990; Matheron *et al.*, 1990; Dannemann *et al.*, 1992). A study by the AIDS Mission (Direction des Hôpitaux-Ministère de la Santé-Paris; F. Bourdillon, personal communication), which examined 903 cases of toxoplasmosis and the $CD4^+$ T-cell count at onset, showed that the $CD4^+$ T-cell count was $< 50$ $ml^{-1}$ in 75% of cases, $< 20$ $ml^{-1}$ in 50% and $< 7$ $ml^{-1}$ in 26%. Interestingly, of the 903 cases analysed 8.9% of patients had $CD4^+$ T-cell counts $> 100$ $ml^{-1}$, 2.5% had $CD4^+$ T-cell counts $> 200$ $ml^{-1}$ and 1.4% had $CD4^+$ T-cell counts $> 300$ $ml^{-1}$. These data have important implications for primary prophylaxis.

### Clinical presentation

In countries or geographic locales with a high seroprevalence of *T. gondii* infection, toxoplasmic encephalitis is frequently the first AIDS-indicating disease. Moreover, toxoplasmic encephalitis can occur in a subject whose HIV serostatus is unknown. For example, in a recent French series, toxoplasmic encephalitis revealed HIV infection in 19% of cases (Ragnaud *et al.*, 1993). When seroprevalence is lower, as in the USA, patients generally develop toxoplasmic encephalitis when they already have AIDS (Luft *et al.*, 1983; Wong *et al.*, 1984; Luft and Remington, 1985; Navia *et al.*, 1986a; Selik *et al.* 1990).

Since toxoplasmic encephalitis is a multifocal necrotizing encephalitis, a wide spectrum of neurological manifestations can be observed, varying between focal and non-focal signs and symptoms (Luft *et al.*, 1984; Luft and Remington, 1985; Cohn *et al.*, 1989) (Tables 4.3 and 4.4). Constitutional symptoms such as fever occurs in a variable proportion of cases (40–74% in the main series). Similarly, the reported frequency of headache ranges from 38 to 73%. Neurological manifestations include mental disturbances and neuropsychiatric disorders, motor and sensory abnormalities, seizures, cerebellar dysfunction and movement disorders or even coma, which can be present at first presentation (Levy *et al.*, 1985; Navia, 1986a; Haverkos, 1987; Leport *et al.*, 1988; Dannemann *et al.*, 1992; Porter, 1992; Renold *et al.*, 1992).

**Table 4.3** Initial findings in patients with toxoplasmic encephalitis (%)

| Signs/symptoms | USA (115 patients)* | Switzerland (86 patients)† |
|---|---|---|
| Headache | 55 | 49 |
| Abnormal consciousness | 42 | 31.4 |
| Fever | 47 | 40.7 |
| Seizures | 29 | 24.4 |
| Meningismus | 10 | 16.3 |
| Focal signs | 69 | 75.6 |

* Source: Porter *et al.* (1992).
† Source: Renold *et al.* (1992).

**Table 4.4** Focal neurological signs in patients with toxoplasmic encephalitis (%)

| Signs | USA (115 patients)* | Switzerland (86 patients)† |
|---|---|---|
| Hemiparesia/hemiplegia | 39 | 48.8 |
| Ataxia | 30 | 2.3 |
| Cranial nerve palsies | 28 | 17.4 |
| Aphasia | 8 | 5.8 |
| Visual field defect | 7 | 8.1 |

* Source: Porter *et al.* (1992).
† Source: Renold *et al.* (1992).

The typical presentation is one of subacute onset, over a matter of days or even weeks, with focal manifestations in more than 60% of patients (Navia *et al.*, 1986a; Haverkos, 1987; Cohn *et al.*, 1989; Pedrol *et al.*, 1990; Renold *et al.*, 1992) but the different clinical signs can develop abruptly, within days or hours. Mental disturbances such as confusion, disorientation, agitation or cognitive impairment are present in 50–65% of patients. Seizures reveal toxoplasmic encephalitis in 15–25% of patients (Whelan *et al.*, 1983; Leport, 1988; Pedrol, 1990; Levy and Bredesen, 1992); focal deficits are present in 49–85% of cases (approximately 60%) (Haveikos, 1987; Leport, 1988; Pedrol *et al.*, 1990; Dannemann *et al.*, 1992; Luft and Remington, 1992).

Hemiparesis or hemiplegia, cranial nerve palsies and speech disorders are common findings but ataxia, visual disturbances, cerebellar tremor and dysmetria are also observed. Uncommon manifestations including hemiballismus (Navia *et al.*, 1986a; Sanchez-Ramos *et al.*, 1989; Said *et al.*, 1996), involuntary movements such as focal dystonia (Tolge and Factor, 1991; Mattos *et al.*, 1993; Manji *et al.*, 1995), panhypopituitarism (Milligan *et al.*, 1984; Luft and Remington, 1992), diabetes insipidus and Schwartz–Bartter syndrome (Luft *et al.*, 1984; Farkash *et al.*, 1986; Wijdicks *et al.*, 1991) have also been described. Clinical meningeal syndrome (meningismus) is rare because infection causes encephalitis with few or no meningeal involvement. Other neurological manifestations include diffuse toxoplasmic encephalitis and spinal cord toxoplasmosis.

Diffuse toxoplasmic encephalitis is a panencephalitis that was initially discovered only at autopsy because it presented clinically as global brain dysfunction without focal neurological manifestations and normal findings on CT (Gray *et al.*, 1989; Khuong *et al.*, 1990). If untreated, the clinical course of diffuse toxoplasmic encephalitis results in death within a few days or weeks.

Spinal cord involvement with *T. gondii* is probably more frequent than previously reported. It includes diverse types of spinal cord manifestations including myelitis and conus medullaris syndrome (Mehren *et al.*, 1988; Herskovitz *et al.*, 1989; Harris *et al.*, 1990; Kayser *et al.*, 1990; Overhage *et al.*, 1990). Each of the above manifestations can be associated with extra neurological involvement due to *T. gondii*, e.g. chorioretinitis, pneumonia, myocarditis, gastrointestinal involvement or septic shock (Morlat *et al.*, 1993). Concurrent toxoplasmic encephalitis and chorioretinitis is found in 29–63% of patients (Holland *et al.*, 1988; Friedman, 1991; Cochereau-Massin *et al.*, 1992). Ocular toxoplasmosis rarely presents as a harbinger of toxoplasmic encephalitis (Parke and Font, 1986; Weiss *et al.*, 1986; Holland *et al.*, 1988; Friedman, 1991).

Overall, the neurological manifestations of toxoplasmic encephalitis pose a problem of differential diagnosis with other major CNS diseases in AIDS, such as cerebral lymphoma, progressive multifocal leucoencephalopathy (PML), CMV, herpes simplex virus (HSV), varicella-zoster virus (VZV), HIV encephalitis, and neuromeningeal cryptococcosis. Other fungal or bacteriological pathogens can, at times, be discussed (*Aspergillus* sp., *Coccidioides immitis*, mycobacteria). In addition, these conditions can coexist in patients with AIDS. In all cases, HIV-infected patients with CNS involvement must undergo brain imaging.

**Neuroimaging**

Toxoplasmic encephalitis is the most common cause of focal or multifocal lesions in HIV-infected patients (Table 4.4). On CT, the characteristic pattern is one of focal, often multiple (57–85% of cases), bilateral, rounded lesions that are isodense or hypodense before contrast enhancement. A mass effect is frequent. Contrast enhancement is ring shaped in 44–91% of cases and associated with peripheral oedema that together generate a target-like image (Figures 4.1 and 4.2). These lesions are multifocal in 40% of patients and 50% are ring enhancing (Weisberg *et al.*, 1988). A delayed double-dose contrast can improve ring enhancement. However, single lesions may be present and CT can underestimate the number of lesions found at autopsy (Navia, 1986a; Petito *et al.*, 1986). The lesions are most commonly located in the basal ganglia and corticomedullary junction (Post, 1983; Whelan *et al.*, 1983; Post, 1985; Levy *et al.*, 1986; De La Paz, 1988; Beaman *et al.*, 1994) but are found occasionally in the subtentorial space (Morlat *et al.*, 1993). Diffuse encephalitic forms may show diffuse hypodensity of the periventricular white matter, cortical/subcortical atrophy and even normal images (Khuong *et al.*, 1990).

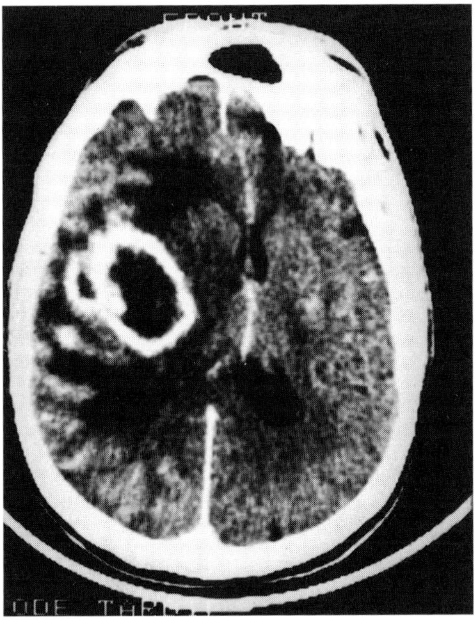

**Figure 4.1** CT image with contrast enhancement showing the typical appearance of a toxoplasmic abscess, with ring enhancement and conspicuous brain oedema.

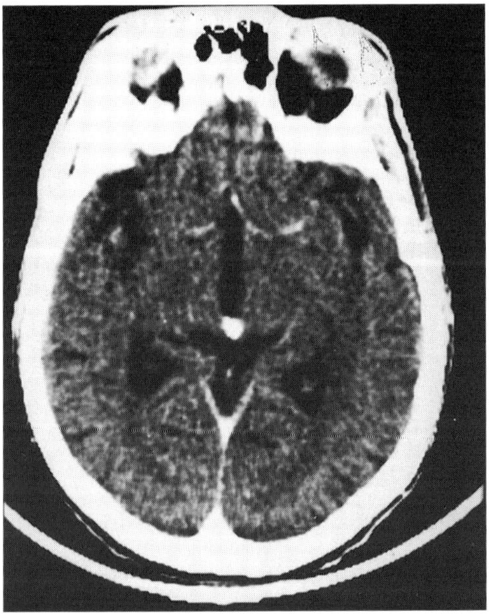

**Figure 4.2** The same patient as in Figure 4.1, 2 months later.

The sensitivity of MRI for toxoplasmic encephalitis appears to be far better than that of CT (Jarvik *et al.*, 1988a). MRI can be carried out first or when CT is normal or doubtful despite suggestive clinical signs. In particular, MRI can reveal lesions smaller than 1 cm diameter, as well as those located at the corticomedullary junction or lacking a mass effect (Blas and Meary, 1991) (Figure 4.3). MRI usually reveals multiple lesions when CT is unrevealing or shows only one lesion (Ciricillo and Rosenblum, 1990; Kupfer *et al.*, 1990; Levy *et al.*, 1990). In addition, diffuse encephalitic forms are often better identified, appearing as diffuse involvement of the white matter generating hyperintense areas on $T_2$-weighted images (usually periventricular). The lesions shown on MRI are typically high-signal abnormalities on $T_2$-weighted images. Deep lesions are 1–3 cm in diameter, but peripheral ones are smaller (1 cm or less). The higher sensitivity of MRI is also useful since it can show small lesions at the corticomedullary junction or multiple lesions not demonstrated on CT (Ciricillo and Rosenblum, 1990; Kupfer *et al.*, 1990; Levy *et al.*, 1990). Also, gadolinium-enhanced MRI may show focal lesions in patients with normal CT (Jarvik *et al.*, 1988a). It has been shown that a solitary lesion on MRI is suggestive of a diagnosis of lymphoma (Gill *et al.*, 1986; Ostertun *et al.*, 1988). It is thus wiser to perform an MRI in patients seropositive for *T. gondii*, who have neurological symptoms and normal CT.

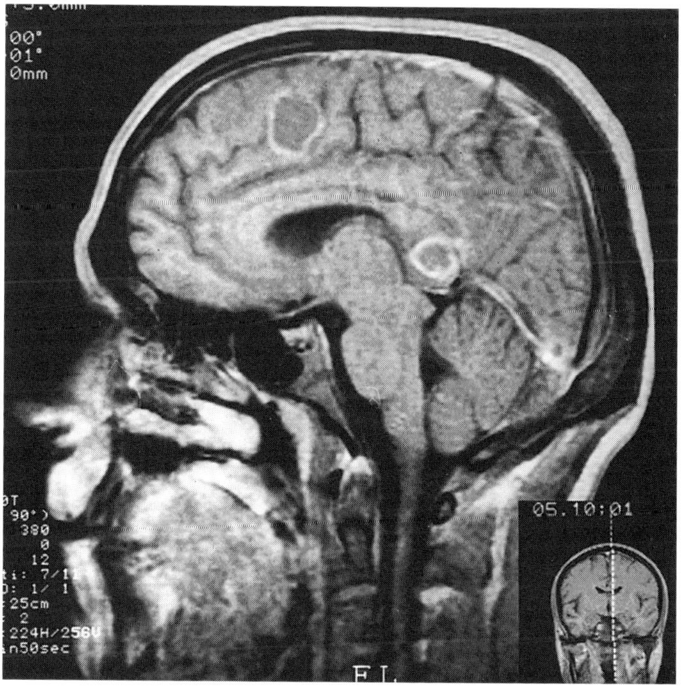


**Figure 4.3** $T_1$-weighted MRI showing two toxoplasmic abscesses, in the frontal lobe and the corpus callosum. Both abscesses disappeared after therapy.

None of the clinical and radiological signs described above are pathognomonic for toxoplasmic encephalitis, even in the presence of typical lesions on CT or MRI; for example, multifocal lesions with ring enhancement may be observed on CT in as many as 40% of patients with lymphoma. None the less, even if a firm initial diagnosis cannot be made on the sole basis of the history, physical examination and imaging findings, the rule to be applied is to begin presumptive treatment (Toxoplasmose et Infection HIV, 1993).

## Laboratory diagnosis

### *Serology*

The serological criteria generally used for the diagnosis of primary *Toxoplasma* infection in immunocompetent subjects are of little value for the diagnosis of toxoplasmic encephalitis in HIV-infected subjects. Serology is of clinical interest for the identification of HIV-infected patients at risk for toxoplasmic encephalitis, and in patients with brain lesions possibly due to *T. gondii* living in areas with low prevalence for toxoplasmic infection. Specific IgM antibodies are generally absent since they persist at low titres after primary infection (Remington and Desmonts, 1990) and are rarely found in AIDS patients (Luft *et al.*, 1984; Wong *et al.*, 1984; Haverkos, 1987). The specific IgG titre rises little in most cases (Grant *et al.*, 1990; Derouin *et al.*, 1991); if such a rise is observed its significance remains to be determined. Other serological methods have been developed to identify a characteristic response to clinical reactivation but none are sufficiently reliable for the firm diagnosis of cerebral toxoplasmosis (Derouin *et al.*, 1991).

Almost all patients have serological markers before the onset of cerebral toxoplasmosis, and at the time of diagnosis fewer than 3% of subjects do not have specific antibodies. Documented cases are rare but two have been proven histologically: one patient with cerebral toxoplasmosis (Luft *et al.*, 1984) and one with acute generalized toxoplasmosis (Oksenhendler *et al.*, 1990; Derouin *et al.*, 1991) were seronegative at the time of death with all serological methods available. In a recent series of 115 cases of cerebral toxoplasmosis, 13 (16%) of the 80 patients studied by means of immunofluorescence had no detectable antibodies (Porter and Sande, 1992); the diagnosis was confirmed histologically in four of these cases, but the results are very controversial. The poor sensitivity of certain commercial reagents for low antibody titres must be taken into account when negative results are obtained. Serological reactivation, i.e. increase in the antibody titre, can be observed in immunocompetent subjects but appears to be more frequent in immunodeficient patients. The yearly incidence of reactivation has been estimated at 12% in 177 HIV-infected patients; in only 24% of these cases (five patients) did reactivation engender immediate clinical manifestations (Derouin *et al.*, 1991). In a Swiss study, elevations of the anti-toxoplasma antibody later correlated with the diagnosis of TE with a sensitivity of only 44% (Renold *et al.*, 1992), serological reactivation is therefore not a convincing diagnostic argument but calls for closer clinical and radiological monitoring.

*Other laboratory methods*

Tests for anti-*Toxoplasma* antibodies in blood and CSF are of little value for the diagnosis of toxoplasmic encephalitis in HIV-infected subjects, and tests for specific antigens are no better. Histological features and genomic amplification of brain biopsy material are difficult to interpret. Other methods for detecting *T. gondii* in peripheral or CNS samples must thus be developed. Inoculation of blood into mice or cell culture can be used to detect *T. gondii* in patients with AIDS. However, the predictive value of these tests (parasitaemia revealing toxoplasmic encephalitis) remains to be established. Experience with PCR amplification is too limited, even if it has given some positive results in body fluids and tissues, such as brain (Holliman *et al.*, 1990), CSF (Lavrard *et al.*, 1992; Lebech, 1992; Parmley *et al.*, 1992), bronchoalveolar lavage (Schoondemark *et al.*, 1993) and blood samples (Dupouy-Camet *et al.*, 1993). Some authors have reported positive results in 68% of buffy coat studies (Wong *et al.*, 1995).

Identification of the parasite in other tissue specimens (liver, pleural fluid, muscle, eye, various biopsies, etc.) reflects parasite dissemination, but its predictive value for cerebral involvement remains to be determined. Techniques for detecting *T. gondii* can thus be useful in some cases, but are of no diagnostic or prognostic value in terms of TE.

Conventional studies of CSF are disappointing for the diagnosis of toxoplasmic encephalitis. In addition, performance of a spinal tap may be harmful in a patient with toxoplasmic brain abscess and intracranial hypertension. Changes in cellularity and protein content are inconsistent and non-specific (Parmley *et al.*, 1992). Specific IgG is detectable in the CSF of 70–80% of patients. Intrathecal synthesis of specific antibodies, interpreted in the light of total immunoglobulin concentrations in CSF and serum, has been proposed as an indirect specific diagnostic method (Potasman *et al.*, 1988). However, its sensitivity (63%) and specificity (68%) are of little value (Bougnoux *et al.*, 1990), and not confirmed in this setting. *Toxoplasma gondii* can be detected directly in CSF after staining the cell pellet (Dement *et al.*, 1987), by cell culture or after inoculation into mice (Grob *et al.*, 1992). However, direct visualization of the parasite is too unreliable to be used routinely and inoculation into mice is too lengthy to have any real diagnostic value. In contrast, direct detection of toxoplasmic DNA by hybridization to a specific probe (Anger *et al.*, 1992) or PCR amplification might be of value, but these methods need further evaluation; 6 of 11 cases of cerebral toxoplasmosis were identified by PCR of CSF (amplification of gene B1), with a specificity of 100% (Potasman *et al.*, 1988; Lebech *et al.*, 1992). Overall, laboratory studies of CSF have proved disappointing for the diagnosis of toxoplasmic encephalitis. Only DNA detection methods have been validated by teams other than those that developed the techniques. For the time being, lumbar puncture is not indicated for the diagnosis of toxoplasmic encephalitis.

## Pathology

### *Brain biopsy*

At present, AIDS patients with focal brain lesions generally receive challenge therapy for toxoplasmic encephalitis (Cohn *et al.*, 1989; Luft and Remington, 1992). However, toxoplasmic encephalitis does not always respond rapidly to this treatment, and the possibility of other causes of focal brain lesions raises the issue of the usefulness of brain biopsy. In theory, brain biopsy has the advantage of diagnosing toxoplasmosis in cases where no convincing response to challenge treatment is obtained after 14 days, an incomplete clinical or radiological response has been obtained, or treatment has to be interrupted because of side-effects (Cimino *et al.*, 1991; Luft *et al.*, 1993), but also when radiological signs are atypical, especially if serological tests for toxoplasmosis are negative, or the neurological condition deteriorates during the first 15 days of antitoxoplasmic therapy (Raffi, 1993). Sampling of the brain lesion by biopsy could also detect a treatable lesion of another origin, especially a malignant lymphoma or a non-toxoplasmic brain abscess.

The frequency of the different causes of focal CNS lesions is based on autopsy studies (Levy *et al.*, 1985; Anders *et al.*, 1986; Navia *et al.*, 1986b; Petito *et al.*, 1986; Rhodes, 1987; Lang *et al.*, 1989; Kure *et al.*, 1991; Matthiessen *et al.*, 1992) and the results of brain biopsy series (De La Paz and Enzmann, 1988; Cimino *et al.*, 1991; Chappell *et al.*, 1992) (Table 4.5). All these studies suffer from marked biases in recruitment, therapy and evaluation. However, toxoplasmic encephalitis is by far the most frequent cause of such lesions, followed by lymphoma and PML; the other causes are far less frequent (cryptococcosis, mycobacteriosis and candidosis) and can generally be diagnosed by other means (cryptococcal antigenaemia, blood culture, lumbar puncture). PML often shows characteristic neuroradiological signs (Ciricillo and Rosenblum, 1990). In addition, most published studies have been carried out in areas (e.g. the USA) where the prevalence of toxoplasmosis is much lower than in Europe.

**Table 4.5** Frequency of the different causes of focal brain lesions during AIDS

| CNS lesion | Frequency (%) | | |
|---|---|---|---|
| | De La Paz & Enzmann, 1988 | Cimino *et al.*, 1991 | Chappell *et al.*, 1992 |
| Toxoplasmosis | 50–70 | 53 | 34 |
| Lymphoma | 10–25 | 9 | 34 |
| PML | 10–22 | 9 | 20 |
| No diagnosis | 10 | 29 | 8 |
| Candida abscess | 3 | NA | 0 |
| Cryptococcoma | 2 | NA | 1.5 |
| Tumours | 2 | NA | 1.5 |
| Other | 2 | NA | 1.5 |

It is currently accepted that neither PML nor cerebral lymphoma can be effectively treated in AIDS patients. Taking into account toxoplasmosis, other treatable infectious lesions and lymphomas, the frequency of useful diagnoses obtained by brain biopsy in five studies was between 44 and 84% (Ciricillo and Rosenblum, 1990; Cimino *et al.*, 1991; Chappell *et al.*, 1992; Levy and Bredesen 1992; Zimmer *et al.*, 1992; Moulignier *et al.*, 1993) (Table 4.6). All the patients biopsied in these studies did not respond to antitoxoplasmic therapy for atypical brain lesions or severe neurological manifestations at onset. Brain biopsy confirmed the diagnosis of toxoplasmosis in 8–44% of the cases. In three of these studies, half the diagnoses made by brain biopsy were of toxoplasmic encephalitis.

**Table 4.6** Frequency of useful diagnosis obtained with brain biopsy

| Reference | Country | Year | Biopsies (*n*) | Useful diagnosis (%) | Toxo-plasmosis (%) | Toxo-plasmosis among useful diagnosis (%) |
|---|---|---|---|---|---|---|
| Cimino *et al.* (1991) | USA | 1991 | 58 | 52 | 26 | 54 |
| Chappell *et al.* (1992) | USA | 1992 | 25 | 44 | 8 | 18 |
| Levy *et al.* (1992) | USA | 1992 | 50 | 56 | 28 | 46 |
| Zimmer *et al.* (1992) | Germany | 1992 | 25 | 84 | 44 | 52 |
| Moulignier *et al.* (1993) | France | 1992 | 68 | 53 | 16 | 26 |

Adapted from Raffi (1993).

Not all lesions are accessible and, in the case of multiple lesions, biopsy of a single lesion may miss a second aetiology. Biopsy at some sites carries a risk of sequelae. The morbidity (mainly haemorrhagic) of stereotactic biopsy is estimated at 2–5%, but actually depends on the type of lesion and its location. Thrombocytopenia < 100 000 $ml^{-1}$ is a strict contraindication (Raffi, 1993). The diagnostic yield of biopsy depends on the conditions in which it is done and how the specimens are examined. It is important to sample both the centre and edges of the lesion, taking several fragments if possible (for microbiological and pathological studies, and a frozen sample for immunohistochemistry). The biopsy specimens must be examined in rigorous conditions, although 20–30% of biopsies remain negative despite thorough testing. In cases of toxoplasmic encephalitis, the frequency of false-negatives is also high when histology is used alone (Luft et al., 1984) instead of being combined with the immunoperoxidase method (Zimmer *et al.*, 1991). Note that toxoplasmosis can engender necrotic pseudolymphomatous lesions. A negative biopsy does not rule out any diagnoses. The indications and timing for a brain biopsy remain a matter of discussion.

In the case of typical lesions with contrast enhancement, challenge therapy for toxoplasmosis should be started and first assessed on day 7. As the absence of response does not rule out toxoplasmosis, we recommend continuing treatment for a further 8–15 days if possible because late improvement of toxoplasmic brain lesions is relatively common. The choice of approach will also depend on the site of the lesion and whether it is isolated or multiple. A single lesion that does not respond rapidly to antitoxoplasmic treatment is suggestive of lymphoma (Dina, 1991). Challenge therapy for toxoplasmic encephalitis should also be undertaken in the case of a hypodense lesion not showing contrast enhancement. Failure of a white-matter lesion to respond by day 15, together with confirmation of the lack of contrast uptake or a mass effect on brain imaging, is suggestive of PML, in which case brain biopsy is not useful. However, if a lymphoma is suspected and treatment becomes available, brain biopsy should be considered. In the absence of a biopsy-based diagnosis, it seems best to continue antitoxoplasmic treatment for at least 6–8 weeks. The chosen approach should take into account the time since the onset of AIDS (first neurological complication or onset during the terminal phase), the patient's overall condition, and the short-term and mid-term prognosis. The most difficult decision is whether to perform a biopsy in a patient with 'early AIDS' and a Karnofsky index > 50%. For some authors, the view that diagnosis of another CNS aetiology by means of biopsy is valueless should be weighed against the potential danger of challenge cerebral radiation therapy or palliative corticotherapy for suspected lymphoma; conversely, biopsy-based diagnosis has several advantages, including the possibility for withdrawal of unnecessary treatments (e.g. antitoxoplasmic drugs), determining the prognosis, trying a new therapeutic approach (for PML and lymphoma) and identifying another, curable, infectious cause (cryptococcosis, herpes, tuberculosis, nocardiosis, etc.). In patients with advanced HIV disease (long-standing AIDS, low Karnofsky index, $CD4^+$ T-cell count $< 50\ ml^{-1}$), the indications for brain biopsy must be considered in view of the possible therapies for lesions that do not respond to challenge treatment for toxoplasmosis (Edwards and Pendlebury, 1987). However, this choice has never been assessed in terms of morbidity, cost and survival. The only value of brain biopsy is to diagnose lymphoma or atypical toxoplasmosis and, occasionally, another disease. In all cases, the decision should be made by a multidisciplinary team consisting of clinicians, radiologists, neurosurgeons and pathologists.

To summarize the indications for brain biopsy of AIDS patients with intracranial lesions (Said, 1993), stereotactic brain biopsy with MRI guidance can be considered the least aggressive method and also the best way of obtaining high-quality specimens. In patients with AIDS, the most frequent cause of focal and diffuse lesions (and virtually the only cause for which an effective treatment is available) is toxoplasmic encephalitis. Clinical manifestations are highly varied, ranging from focal signs with intracranial hypertension to rapid mental deterioration with no focal signs or symptoms. High-quality neuroimaging (CT and MRI) before and after contrast enhancement generally provides good diagnostic evidence. However, in some cases the images are atypical and can be suggestive of another cause, especially cerebral lymphoma. The approach is identical in such cases, i.e. antitoxoplasmic treatment for 15 days (or more, according to the patient's condition), followed by a new comparative scan. If the lesion has remained stable or increased in size, a stereotactic biopsy with MRI guidance can be considered in order to provide histological evidence of lymphoma. Here again the potential risks and benefits must be weighed up carefully. The location of the target lesion is a crucial element, as is the risk of life-threatening bleeding. Another factor to take into account is the poor prognosis of cerebral lymphoma in patients who have AIDS and who are in very poor overall condition; in one series the mean survival time was only 6 weeks (Chappell *et al.*, 1992). In such cases, corticotherapy and radiotherapy can be considered. Since there is no non-invasive diagnostic method for toxoplasmic encephalitis, biopsy of intracerebral lesions is indicated for HIV-infected patients in good overall condition after failed antitoxoplasmic therapy, although biopsy is the exception rather than the rule in AIDS. However, recent advances in tests based on PCR amplification of CSF for the diagnosis of lymphoma (Cinque *et al.*, 1993), multifocal leucoencephalopathy (Tornatore *et al.*, 1992; Moret *et al.*, 1993) and CMV encephalitis, as well as more refined scan technology (Heald *et al.*, 1991), may well further limit the place of brain biopsy.

*Autopsy findings*

Currently, most patients with cerebral toxoplasmosis are treated and in recent autopsy series the percentage of acute or subacute toxoplasmosis has decreased to 3% (Table 4.7), in agreement with our own experience. Cerebral toxoplasmosis is most frequently found in the frontal and parietal lobes (Figure 4.4) (Lantos *et al.*, 1989; Porter and Sande, 1992) and the basal ganglia (Gastaut *et al.*, 1992), is usually multiple but may be diffuse (Gray *et al.*, 1989), is rarely unique (Alonso *et al.*, 1984) or restricted to the periventricular area (Figure 4.5). Spinal cord (Horowitz, *et al.*, 1983; Mehren *et al.*, 1988; Harris *et al.*, 1990) and conus medullaris (Kayser *et al.*, 1990; Overhage *et al.*, 1990) toxoplasmosis have been observed in a few patients.

Three histological types of lesion are identified: acute or necrotizing, organizing and chronic. Necrotic abscesses are usually found in untreated patients or after a few days of treatment. They contain lipid-laden macrophages, polymorphonuclear cells and vascular proliferation associated with surrounding oedema and haemorrhagic lesions (Navia *et al.*, 1986a; Vinters and Anders, 1990). The haemorrhages are occasionally multiple and massive (Wijdicks *et al.*, 1991). *Toxoplasma gondii* cysts with bradyzoites and free tachyzoites are found at the periphery of the abscesses (Figure 4.6) (Horowitz *et al.*, 1983). Occlusive hypertrophied arteritis has been observed in some cases (Huang and Chou, 1988). In patients treated for a few weeks, organizing abscesses are observed with large areas of central coagulation necrosis surrounded by foamy macrophages (Figure 4.7); scattered tachyzoites or

**Table 4.7** Autopsy series of HIV-infected patients from different countries

| Reference | Country (city) | Total cases | HIV (%) | Cytomegalo-virus (%) | Toxo-plasmosis (%) | Lymphoma (%) | Crypto-coccosis | Progressive multifocal leucoencep halopathy (%) | Others (%) |
|---|---|---|---|---|---|---|---|---|---|
| Moskowitz *et al.* (1984) | USA (Miami) | 52 | 10 | 4 | 30 | 2 | 0 | 4 | 8 |
| Anders *et al.* (1986) | USA (Los Angeles, UCLA | 89 | 47 | 16 | 7 | 5 | 14 | 7 | 4 |
| Petito *et al.* (1986) | USA (New York) | 153 | 28 | 26 | 10 | 6 | 2 | 3 | 6 |
| Budka *et al.* (1987) | Austria, Italy | 100 | 38 | 18 | 17 | 6 | 9 | 5 | 2 |
| Lang *et al.* (1989) | Switzerland | 206 | 18 | 7 | 24 | 0 | 4 | 7 | ? |
| Lantos *et al.* (1989) | UK (London) | 26 | 23 | 7 | 7 | 12 | 0 | 0 | 4 |
| Stavrou *et al.* (1989) | Germany | 61 | 18 | 20 | 11 | 6 | 6 | 0 | 1 |
| Burns *et al.* (1991) | USA (Dallas) | 141 | 38 | 20 | 3 | 6 | 9 | 3 | 8 |
| Gray *et al.* (1991) | France (Créteil) | 135 | 38 | 15 | 41 | 11 | 4 | <1 | 4 |
| Kure *et al.* (1991) | USA (New York; A. Einstein) | 268 | 26 | 13 | 13 | 7 | 9 | 5 | 7 |
| Chimelli *et al.* (1992) | Brazil | 252 | 10 | 8 | 34 | 4 | 13 | 1 | 14 |
| Matthiessen *et al.* (1992) | France (Paris; Bichat) | 174 | 19 | 14 | 37 | 18 | 6 | 3 | 1 |
| Rhodes (1993) | USA (Los Angeles, SCMC) | 400 | 20 | 8 | 8 | 6 | 6 | ? | ? |
| Lacroix, unpublished data | France (Kremlin Bicêtre) | 85 | 21 | 19 | 8 | 13 | 3.5 | 10.5 | 25 |

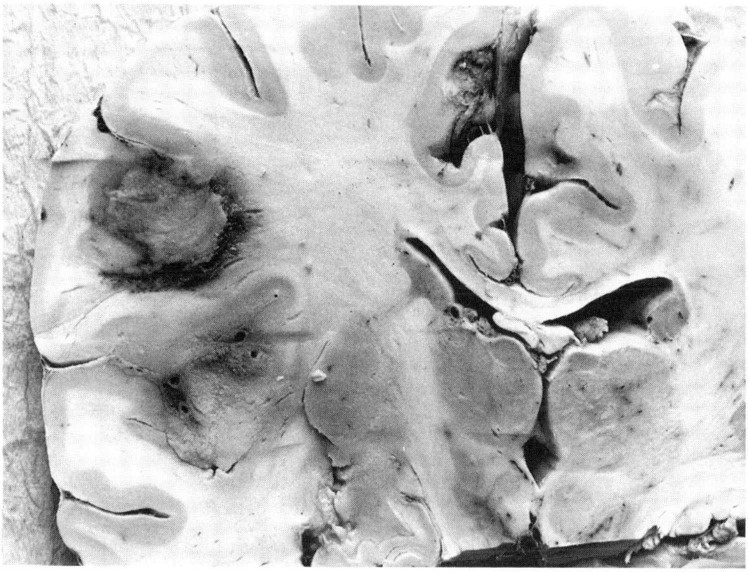

**Figure 4.4** Toxoplasmic abscess in the frontal cortex of a patient with haemophilia.

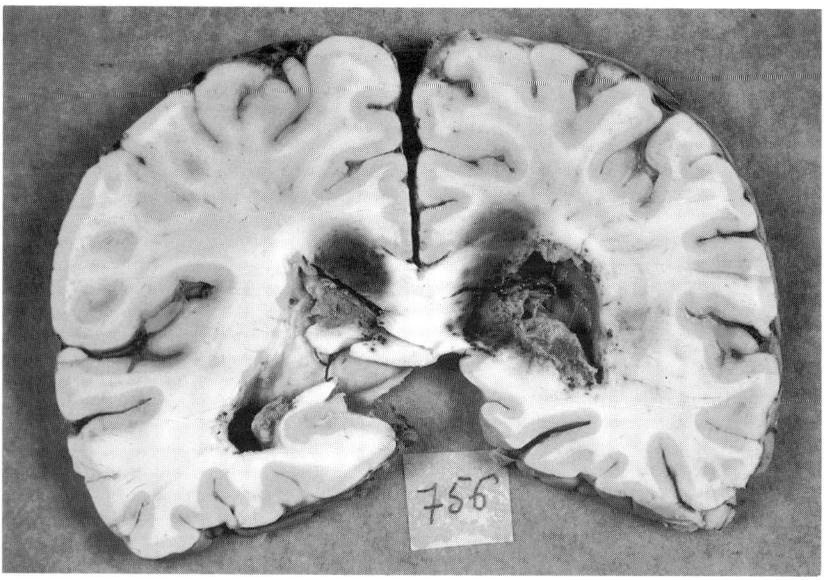


**Figure 4.5** Haemorrhagic toxoplasmic ventriculitis.

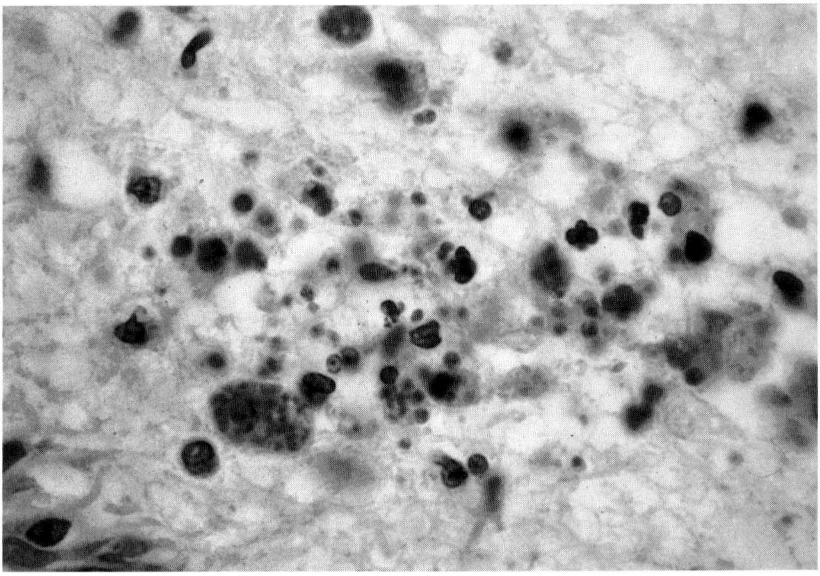

**Figure 4.6** Toxoplasmic abscess of the frontal lobe showing cyst and free tachyzoites. (Paraffin section; Nissl; ×1550.)

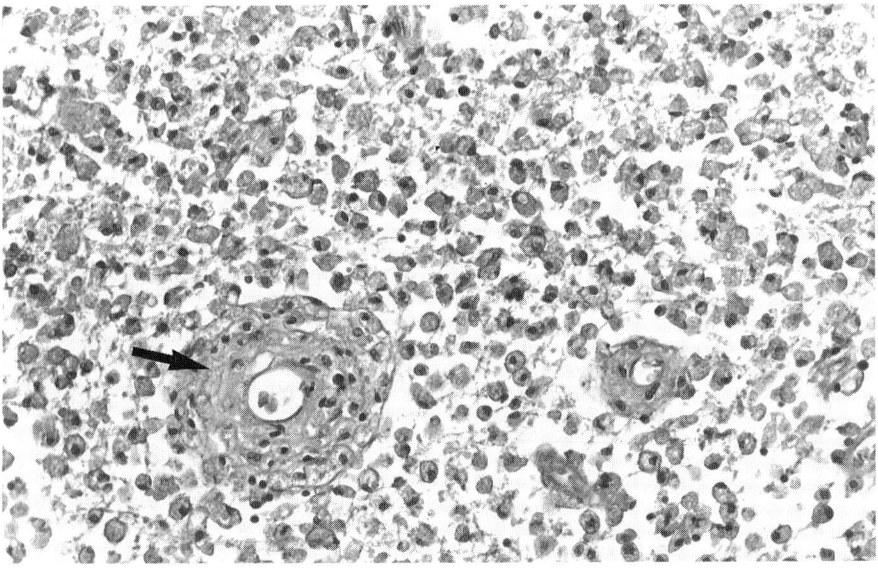

**Figure 4.7** Toxoplasmic abscess of the parietal lobe treated for a few weeks. Note the presence of necrosis, foamy macrophages and necrotizing vasculitis (arrow). (Paraffin section; H&E; ×550.)

isolated cysts may be observed at the periphery of the abscess. Chronic abscesses, (Figure 4.8) which are usually smaller, contain some swollen macrophages and are surrounded by gliosis and a few *Toxoplasma* cysts (Navia *et al.*, 1986b). Old toxoplasmic lesions often contain calcifications and cholesterol crystals (Figure 4.7). Immunocytochemistry is useful for detecting parasites when they are rare (Huang and Chou, 1988). In many patients who have been treated for cerebral toxoplasmosis months or years before death, toxoplasmic cysts are frequently found near microglial nodules or isolated. CNS toxoplasmosis was often associated with other opportunistic infections or with HIV encephalitis (Navia *et al.*, 1986b; Ibars *et al.*, 1987; Lucht *et al.*, 1987) before the systematic treatment of toxoplasmosis.

**Treatment**

There are two periods for therapy of toxoplasmic encephalitis: the first period, primary therapy, is administered during the acute phase; the second period, maintenance therapy, is administered after the clinical and neuroradiological responses are obtained. Maintenance therapy is maintained for life, since the rate of relapse is unacceptably high when treatment is stopped.

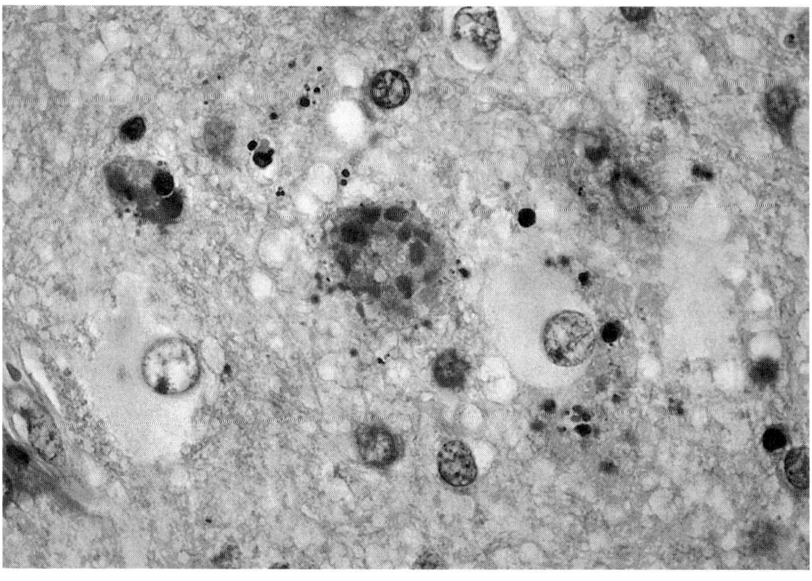

**Figure 4.8** Chronic toxoplasmic abscess showing a cyst associated with microglial cells and astrocytes. (Paraffin section; H&E; ×1500.)

*Primary therapy* (Table 4.8)

The diagnosis of toxoplasmic encephalitis is rarely based on detection of the parasite in pathological specimens, by culture of blood or a biopsy sample. As a consequence, treatment of toxoplasmic encephalitis is generally presumptive and based on a combination of clinical manifestations and abnormal CT or MRI findings. A favourable response to challenge therapy is the main diagnostic argument. Serological tests are of no value in the decision to treat (Eyles and Coleman, 1955; Leport *et al.*, 1988; Danneman *et al.*, 1992; Leport *et al.*, 1993a).

The standard first-line treatment for a patient with no known allergy to sulphonamides is based on the pyrimethamine–sulphadiazine combination. This combination blocks the folic acid metabolism of *T. gondii* and is synergistic *in vitro* and *in vivo* in experimental models of toxoplasmosis (Eyles and Coleman, 1953, 1955; Cook and Jacobs, 1958). The serum concentration of pyrimethamine is highly variable in patients receiving the same dose (Cavallito *et al.*, 1978; Weiss *et al.*, 1988a; Leport *et al.*, 1992); nevertheless serum concentrations increase with increasing dose of the drug (Leport *et al.*, 1992). The CSF concentration of the drug is 10–25% of the serum concentration and some data show that pyrimethamine may concentrate in the brain (Leport *et al.*, 1989a).

Pyrimethamine is administered orally, with a loading dose of 100–200 mg for the first 24 hours, then 50–75 mg daily in a single intake. Sulphadiazine is administered orally at a dose of 4–6 g/day in three or four fractions. Folinic acid (leucovorin calcium) is prescribed to prevent or correct the marrow toxicity of

**Table 4.8** Treatment of toxoplasmic encephalitis

| Therapy preference | Acute therapy | Maintenance therapy |
|---|---|---|
| First choice | Pyrimethamine 50 mg/day plus sulphadiazine 4 g/day | Pyrimethamine 25 mg/day plus sulphadiazine 2 g/day |
| Second choice | Pyrimethamine 50 mg/day plus clindamycin 2.4 g/day | Pyrimethamine 25 mg/day plus clindamycin 1.2 g/day |
| Alternatives | Pyrimethamine 50–75 mg/day plus dapsone 50–100 mg/day*<br>Pyrimethamine 75 mg/day plus clarithromycin 2 g/day*<br>Pyrimethamine 75 mg/day plus azithromycin 500 mg/day*<br>Atovaquone 750 mg four times daily*<br>Pyrimethamine 50 mg/day plus atovaquone 750 mg four times daily* | Pyrimethamine 50–100 mg/day*<br>Pyrimethamine 25 mg/day plus dapsone 25–50 mg/day*<br>Pyrimethamine plus azithromycin*†<br>Atovaquone 750 mg four times daily*<br>Minocycline plus clarithromycin*† |

* No validation in large-scale studies.

† No reported clinical data.

pyrimethamine (Kaufman and Geisler, 1960; Niyongabo *et al.*, 1991). The optimal initial dose of folinic acid remains to be established, but treatment usually starts with 20 or 25 mg/day and can be increased to 50 mg/day in case of cytopenia but there is no evidence showing that higher doses prevent or reverse haematotoxicity (Leport *et al.*, 1993a).

Corticosteroids are used for patients with clinical signs of intracranial hypertension or evidence of marked cerebral oedema on neuroimaging. Methylprednisolone can be given at a dose of 60–100 mg/day for 2–3 days and then tapered; mannitol can also be used or added. When corticosteroids are used, the course should be as brief as possible.

Anticonvulsants are prescribed to patients with seizures at presentation. Phenobarbitone is not recommended because of its multiple interactions with other drugs and neither is phenytoin given its potential haematotoxicity. Sodium valproate is the most widely used anticonvulsant, but it should be noted that full activity is only reached after 48 hours of treatment. Benzodiazepines are recommended for emergency use. The benefit of the prophylactic use of anticonvulsant agents in the absence of seizures has not been established and is thus not recommended (Leport *et al.*, 1993b).

Adequate hydration and alkalization of urine is recommended to avoid sulphonamide crystalluria, which could induce nephrotoxicity (Oster *et al.*, 1990; Simon *et al.*, 1990; Molina *et al.*, 1991).

The optimum duration of treatment has not been established in controlled trials but, empirically, a minimum of 3 weeks is necessary. If a full clinical recovery has not been achieved or if abnormalities persist on CT or MRI, it is recommended to continue treatment for a total of 4–6 weeks, until the optimal clinical and radiological response is obtained.

Of patients with toxoplasmic encephalitis 70–90% have an initial favourable course with the pyrimethamine–sulphadiazine combination (Eyles and Coleman, 1955; Navia *et al.*, 1986a; Leport *et al.*, 1988), but untoward reactions limit the duration of this type of regimen in as many as 35% of patients (Haverkos, 1987; Leport *et al.*, 1988; Guichard *et al.*, 1991) necessitating its discontinuation and administration of another drug, usually clindamycin. In case of previous allergy to sulphonamides, clindamycin is an alternative to sulphadiazine, which is only used in combination with pyrimethamine. The efficacy of clindamycin has been demonstrated in two prospective studies (Eyles and Coleman, 1955; Katlama, 1991). The recommended dose ranges from 2.4 to 4.8 g/day orally in four fractions or, if necessary, intravenously.

In the absence of reliable data, it does not seem necessary to modify the strategy defined above when patients have previously received prophylaxis. It is theoretically possible that chronic administration of chemoprophylaxis for toxoplasmosis may lead to the emergence of strains with diminished susceptibility or may modify clinical and neuroradiological findings, but this has never been reported in practice. Close monitoring should reveal any atypical features that arise during treatment and which may call for brain biopsy (see above).

*Clinical and neuroradiological end-points for the efficacy of primary therapy*
The disappearance or improvement of clinical manifestations is the first sign that treatment is effective. Fever usually abates during the first few days of treatment and neurological manifestations begin to improve after 7–10 days. In a recent study, a quantifiable neurological assessment was used prospectively to evaluate the clinical outcome of 49 patients with toxoplasmic encephalitis who were receiving a clindamycin–pyrimethamine regimen. The data showed that 71% of the patients responded to therapy; among these patients, 86% had improvement at day 7 and 91% at day 14. In the 29% of non-responders, neurological manifestations progressed or new manifestations developed during the first 12 days of therapy (Luft *et al.*, 1993). Neuroradiological study should be performed 2–4 weeks after the beginning of therapy or earlier in case of poor response to therapy.

*Approach to side-effects*

*In a patient on pyrimethamine–sulphadiazine.* Side-effects occur on pyrimethamine–sulphadiazine in 60–70% of patients, leading to withdrawal of one or both drugs in 20–30% of cases. The main side-effects are:

(1) dermatological (20–40%), with rash of variable severity and fever in some cases;
(2) haematological: leuconeutropenia (10–30%), thrombocytopenia (10–15%) and occasionally anaemia;
(3) crystalluria, colic or even renal impairment due to sulphadiazine precipitation;
(4) gastrointestinal disorders;
(5) hepatic cytolysis.

The management of skin eruptions depends on their severity. If the rash is only moderate it can be treated symptomatically and it may be possible to continue the treatment. If the skin reaction is severe and febrile, sulphadiazine must be stopped. If sulphadiazine withdrawal leads to the disappearance of the rash, this drug is most likely responsible and treatment can be continued with the pyrimethamine–clindamycin combination. If, on the contrary, sulphadiazine withdrawal does not lead to an improvement, then pyrimethamine is probably responsible and must be withdrawn. A similar approach is adopted in the case of haematotoxicity, with the aim of identifying the culprit drug. Crystalluria calls for sulphadiazine withdrawal. Gastrointestinal disorders should first be treated symptomatically, but may require interruption of one or other drug if they persist.

*In a patient on pyrimethamine–clindamycin.* Side-effects of pyrimethamine–clindamycin are also observed in about 60% of cases. The most frequent are skin rashes (30%), in which case the same approach as for pyrimethamine–sulphadiazine should be adopted. Diarrhoea (20%) may point to pseudomembranous colitis due to *Clostridium difficile*, which should be tested for in the stools along with its toxin. If the diarrhoea is severe and/or persistent, it is best to withdraw clindamycin and prescribe oral vancomycin (Jacobson *et al.*, 1991). Antiparasitic treatment should be continued with experimental combinations, as in patients who do not tolerate either of the two combinations, but it is advisable to confirm the allergy to sulphadiazine first.

*Treatment of patients tolerating neither standard combination.* Available alternatives have not been thoroughly tested in the clinical setting. This is the case with the new macrolides such as clarithromycin and azithromycin (Araujo *et al.*, 1988, 1992; Chang and Pechere, 1988). The same applies to atovaquone, which is now available for use in combination (Masur *et al.*, 1991). Other alternatives have not been tested in controlled clinical trials, and include doxycycline, dapsone and 5-fluorouracil. Combinations of these drugs have not yet been tested.

### *Maintenance treatment*

*First-line maintenance treatment.* Maintenance treatment is essential after an acute episode of toxoplasmosis, as more than 50% of patients otherwise relapse due to reactivation of cysts, which are not eradicated by existing curative treatments. There is no regimen that is completely effective and safe. The pyrimethamine–sulphadiazine combination is the first choice for maintenance treatment (Leport *et al.*, 1989b; Madlener *et al.*, 1992; Renold *et al.*, 1992) and patients on this regimen do not need further prophylaxis for *Pneumocystis carinii*; the combination is sufficient to prevent both opportunistic infections (Heald *et al.*, 1991). The recommended doses are pyrimethamine 25–50 mg/day and sulphadiazine 2–3 g/day. Folinic acid is generally used to reduce the frequency of haematotoxicity. Although no optimal dose has been established, a cumulative weekly dose of 50–75 mg of folinic acid appears to be adequate. Maintenance treatment must be started at the end of primary therapy and be continued for life.

The European trial ENTA 04 demonstrated the efficacy of pyrimethamine (25 mg/day) plus sulphadiazine (2 g/day) in 83 patients monitored for a median of 14 months; the relapse rate was only 7% (Katlama, 1991; Katlama *et al.*, 1991).

Other forms of prophylaxis have been proposed, notably intermittent pyrimethamine (25 mg/day) and sulphadiazine (2 g/day) administered twice weekly. This maintenance regimen seems to have a trend towards a higher rate of relapses (Pendrol *et al.*, 1990; Daniel, 1992; Renold *et al.*, 1992).

The safety of pyrimethamine–sulphadiazine appears to be better at maintenance doses than during the curative phase. This may also be related to the generally early occurrence of side-effects with pyrimethamine–sulphadiazine, which leads to the selection of patients tolerating the combination.

In the ENTA 04 trial, about 20% of patients receiving pyrimethamine–

sulphadiazine developed side-effects during maintenance treatment. As during the curative phase, the most frequent adverse reaction was cutaneous hypersensitivity (12% of cases). Pyrimethamine–sulphadiazine was rarely haematotoxic in this study (< 5% of cases) (Katlama *et al.*, 1991).

In general, all clinical or biological adverse effects potentially related to pyrimethamine–sulphadiazine must be investigated to determine attribution; the superior efficacy of this treatment over its alternatives justifies attempts to keep patients on the combination. For example, it is recommended that the incriminated drug is suspended for a few days before withdrawing it permanently, in order to determine its responsibility if side-effects develop.

In the case of haematological disorders, pyrimethamine–sulphadiazine treatment should only be modified if the apparent side-effect persists after increasing the dose of folinic acid and after adjusting the doses of other potentially haematotoxic drugs (e.g. replacing ganciclovir by foscarnet, zidovudine by didanosine, etc.).

As regards skin rash, treatment can be maintained for 2–4 days in the absence of gravity signs, hypersensitivity manifestations being treated symptomatically (bearing in mind that they can resolve spontaneously). The persistence of a skin rash or its extension to the mucous membrane calls for withdrawal of sulphadiazine.

Desensitization methods based on a very gradual increase in the (initially low) sulphadiazine dose may enable 'intolerant' patients to overcome hypersensitivity (Tenant-Flowers *et al.*, 1991). In addition to preventing the recurrence of cerebral toxoplasmosis, the pyrimethamine–sulphadiazine combination effectively prevents *Pneumocystis carinii* pneumonia (PCP) (Heald *et al.*, 1991).

*Second-line treatment.* In the case of severe or persistent side-effects with pyrimethamine–sulphadiazine, the pyrimethamine–clindamycin combination can be used. It is less effective in secondary prevention than pyrimethamine–sulphadiazine (Katlama *et al.*, 1991; Leport *et al.*, 1991); in the ENTA 04 trial the frequency of documented relapse of cerebral toxoplasmosis was 28% with pyrimethamine–clindamycin but only 5% with pyrimethamine–sulphadiazine (Katlama *et al.*, 1991).

Clindamycin is administered orally, usually at a minimal dose of 1200 mg/day, in combination with 25–50 mg/day of pyrimethamine. The side-effects of pyrimethamine–clindamycin are gastrointestinal in about 15% of cases (diarrhoea, nausea and vomiting), rash in 2% of cases and neutropenia in 3% of cases (Leport *et al.*, 1989a; Katlama *et al.*, 1991).

Pseudomembranous colitis is the most severe side-effect of the pyrimethamine–clindamycin combination. It should be sought for whenever diarrhoea develops or worsens, even if there is another identified cause (e.g. cryptosporidiosis, microsporidiosis, etc.). Rectoscopy and tests for *C. difficile* or its toxin are the mainstays of diagnosis. Given the lesser efficacy of pyrimethamine–clindamycin and the similar frequency of side-effects compared with pyrimethamine–sulphadiazine, the contraindications of sulphadiazine should be reassessed during treatment. In particular, intolerance during the curative phase may not recur during maintenance with lower doses.

The pyrimethamine–clindamycin combination does not prevent PCP (Girard *et al.*, 1989; Leport *et al.*, 1989a). Patients intolerant of sulphonamides are usually given pentamidine aerosols.

*Other alternatives.* The regimens for alternative maintenance therapy have not been completely or systematically evaluated and a number of agents alone or in association have been used. Patients intolerant of sulphadiazine can theoretically receive the dapsone–pyrimethamine combination. Dapsone is highly active on *Toxoplasma in vitro*, and is synergistic with pyrimethamine in mice. In addition, the efficacy of dapsone–pyrimethamine has been demonstrated in combined prophylaxis of PCP and toxoplasmosis (Girard *et al.*, 1993). However, the efficacy and tolerability of this combination has not been tested prospectively in clinical trials as maintenance treatment for toxoplasmosis. Pyrimethamine monotherapy at a dose of 50–100 mg/day prevented recurrences of toxoplasmosis in an open retrospective study (Maslo *et al.*, 1992), but must only be given to patients who fail to tolerate any of the available combinations.

Atovaquone, which has been approved recently for treatment of mild to moderate *P. carinii* infection in patients intolerant to co-trimoxazole, is active against the tachyzoite and cyst forms of *T. gondii* both *in vitro* and *in vivo* (Araujo *et al.*, 1991) but has not been tested as maintenance therapy for a sufficient period of time. There is some experimental and clinical evidence that this compound should not be used alone for toxoplasmosis (Araujo *et al.*, 1993); the combination of atovaquone and folinic inhibitors is effective *in vitro* (Comley and Sterling, 1995). Synergy between atovaquone and sulphadiazine has been demonstrated *in vitro* but the combination has not been tested in the clinical setting. Azithromycin and clarithromycin, alone or in combination with pyrimethamine, have not been assessed as maintenance therapy.

## PROPHYLAXIS

### *Primary prophylaxis*

In most Western countries, one-third or more of patients who are seropositive for *T. gondii* will develop toxoplasmic encephalitis (Beaman *et al.*, 1992), with a short-term mortality rate exceeding 10%; 40–50% of survivors have sequelae (Pedrol *et al.*, 1990). Since 1989, primary prophylaxis against PCP has become widely used and the need for combined prophylaxis against PCP and toxoplasmosis has led to a number of trials. It is now possible to establish guidelines for the primary prophylaxis of toxoplasmosis.

Two parameters are predictive of the development of visceral (usually cerebral) toxoplasmosis during HIV infection: a previous *Toxoplasma* infection (indicated by serology) and the severity of the immune deficiency (indicated by the $CD4^+$ T-cell count).

*Previous infection (serology).* Virtually all episodes of visceral toxoplasmosis occur in patients who are seropositive for *T. gondii* (Girard *et al.*, 1993; Israelski *et al.*, 1993). Exceptions may be related to loss of pre-existing antibody in extreme immunosuppression and primary infection, but the risk of primary infection is low (annual seroconversion rate 0.7–1.4%) (Wallace *et al.*, 1993). The use of *Toxoplasma* serology to define patients requiring primary prophylaxis calls for two standardized techniques and strict interpretation of results. When both of the most frequently used tests are positive (e.g. > 8 IU for indirect immunofluorescence, exceeding thresholds for enzyme-linked immunosorbent assay (ELISA)), the serology is positive indicating a previous infection. If both tests are negative, the serology is negative indicating the absence of previous infection. Finally, when only one test is positive, or when the titre of both tests is borderline, the serology should be re-evaluated. A previous, stored serum sample may be useful, since some patients may lose their antibodies when immunosuppression becomes severe (Renold *et al.*, 1992). If doubt persists, the patients are considered at risk of toxoplasmosis reactivation.

*Severity of the immune deficiency ($CD4^+$ T-cell count).* The risk of reactivation is proportional to the severity of the immune deficiency: 75–80% of cases of cerebral toxoplasmosis occur in patients with $CD4^+$ T-cell counts $< 100\ ml^{-1}$; however, 10% of cases of cerebral toxoplasmosis occur in patients whose $CD4^+$ T-cell counts exceed $200\ ml^{-1}$ (Renold *et al.*, 1992). Patients with $CD4^+$ T-cell counts $< 100\ ml^{-1}$ and positive toxoplasmic serology have an estimated risk of cerebral toxoplasmosis of 18–40% after 12–18 months (Ginard *et al.*, 1993) whatever the titre of anti-*Toxoplasma* antibodies (Table 4.9).

*Guidelines*

These guidelines were established during an Expert Conference on Toxoplasmosis and HIV infection held in Paris in 1993 (Hirschel *et al.*, 1993). With the goal of combined prophylaxis in mind, patients at risk for visceral toxoplasmosis are those with positive *Toxoplasma* serology and $CD4^+$ T-cell counts $< 200\ ml^{-1}$, analogous to the guidelines for PCP.

*Patients with $CD4^+$ T-cell count $\geq 200\ ml^{-1}$.* No anti-*Toxoplasma* prophylaxis is given whatever the anti-*Toxoplasma* serology, but monitor the $CD4^+$ T-cell count every 3–4 months when it approaches $200\ ml^{-1}$. For patients in whom serology is negative for toxoplasmosis, advise on hygiene and diet and repeat serology every 6 months.

*Patients with $CD4^+$ T-cell count $< 200\ ml^{-1}$.* When there is positive anti-*Toxoplasma* serology, administer toxoplasmosis prophylaxis. When there is

**Table 4.9** Twelve-month incidence (%) of toxoplasmosis (AGS)

| Patient selection (reference) | CD4⁺ T-cell count < 200 ml⁻¹ | CD4⁺ T-cell count < 200 ml⁻¹ plus positive serology | CD4⁺ T-cell count < 100 ml⁻¹ | CD4⁺ T-cell count < 100 ml⁻¹ plus positive serology |
|---|---|---|---|---|
| ARC/AIDS (Dournon *et al.*, 1988) | 16 | | 19 | |
| CD4⁺ T-cell count <200 mm³ (Hischel *et al.*, 1991) | | 16 | | |
| CD4⁺ T-cell count <200 mm³ (Girard *et al.*, 1993) | 8 | 12 | | 22 |
| AIDS (Chiriani *et al.*, 1992) | 15 | | | 28 |

negative anti-*Toxoplasma* serology, do not administer toxoplasmosis prophylaxis, advise on hygiene and diet and repeat *Toxoplasma* serology every 6 months.

*Regimens for prophylaxis*

The aim of prophylaxis in HIV-infected patients is to ensure effective, stable and well-tolerated protection, at least against the two major opportunistic infections: PCP and toxoplasmosis (Table 4.10). At present, the choice is principally limited to two drug combinations: trimethoprim–sulphamethoxazole (co-trimoxazole) and dapsone–pyrimethamine. The known efficacy of these two combinations is based on results from various sources. In the case of co-trimoxazole, non-randomized retrospective or prospective studies failed to show efficacy in an intention-to-treat analysis (Carr *et al.*, 1992; Hardy *et al.*, 1992; May *et al.*, 1992; Reynes *et al.*, 1992; Schneider *et al.*, 1992; Oksenhendler *et al.*, 1994; Bozzette *et al.*, 1995). The efficacy of dapsone–pyrimethamine has been investigated in two randomized prospective trials (Girard *et al.*, 1993; Opravil *et al.*, 1995).

*Trimethoprim–sulphamethoxazole (co-trimoxazole).* Since 1991, studies have suggested that co-trimoxazole administered as prophylaxis for PCP also prevents toxoplasmosis (Carr *et al.*, 1992; Oksenhendler *et al.*, 1994). In the absence of randomization, it remains difficult to rule out an inclusion bias that might reduce the risk of toxoplasmosis in patients given co-trimoxazole. Moreover, because of the low seroprevalence of *T. gondii* in the majority of controlled trials of co-trimoxazole (namely those conducted in the USA), the protective effect was difficult to demonstrate, but a trend existed (Hardy *et al.*, 1992; Schneider *et al.*, 1992). No recommendations can be made as to the minimal effective dose since those used vary widely, from 480 to 1920 mg/day; however a dose of 960 mg/day (one double-strength tablet per day) is the most usual since it has been proposed for the prophylaxis of PCP, the setting in which most trials were conducted. Tolerance of co-trimoxazole varies from one study to another and depends partly on the dose and, in some studies, on selection bias (patients intolerant to co-trimoxazole were excluded).

Most side-effects (digestive and cutaneous) appear between days 10 and 30 of treatment (Gordin *et al.*, 1984; Coopman *et al.*, 1993) and seem to develop earlier with higher doses (May *et al.*, 1992). Although the mechanisms of these side-effects is not fully understood (Carr *et al.*, 1994; Koopmans *et al.*, 1995), it is important to note that a high number of patients can be treated with this drug because the untoward reactions are often mild and transitory (Putterman *et al.*, 1990). The addition of folinic acid is not beneficial at the doses used for prophylaxis. Analysis on an intention-to-treat basis revealed no significant difference in the incidence of toxoplasmosis when co-trimoxazole was compared with other forms of prophylaxis (Hardy *et al.*, 1992; May *et al.*, 1992; Podzamczer *et al.*, 1993). This may be explained by the high incidence of side-effects in the co-trimoxazole group leading to changes in the original treatment, the small number of patients included, and a low incidence of *Toxoplasma*

**Table 4.10** Potential regimens for primary prophylaxis of toxoplasmosis and *Pneumocystis carinii* pneumonia (PCP): advantages and disadvantages

| Regimens | Advantages | Disadvantages |
|---|---|---|
| Co-trimoxazole | Largely prescribed (PCP)<br>Efficacy in retrospective studies<br>First-line prophylaxis for PCP | High incidence of side-effects<br>Optimal dosage unknown |
| Dapsone–pyrimethamine (+ folinic acid) | Effective for prevention of PCP<br>Efficacy assessed by intention-to-treat analysis | High incidence of side-effects<br>Drug interaction with rifampin and didanosine |
| Pyrimethamine–Sulfadoxine | Weekly administration | High incidence of side-effects |
| Pyrimethamine–Sulphadiazine | Efficacy for acute treatment of toxoplasmosis<br>Efficacy for prevention of PCP | High intolerance rate means no evaluation |
| Macrolides | Well tolerated | Poorly effective in experiments<br>Uneffective against PCP<br>Poorly evaluated |
| Atovaquone | *In vitro* and experimental efficacy against *T. gondii* and *P. carinii*<br>Better tolerated? | Unevaluated |

infection. However, if one examines the treatment the patients effectively received, it is rare to find toxoplasmosis developing in a patient on co-trimoxazole (Oksenhendler *et al.*, 1994).

*Dapsone–pyrimethamine.* One trial has demonstrated the efficacy of the combination of dapsone (50 mg/day) and pyrimethamine (50 mg/week) with supplementary folinic acid (25 mg/week) (Girard *et al.*, 1993). Intention-to-treat analysis was significant only for this trial. In another study, similar results were obtained with a different dose (dapsone 200 mg/week plus pyrimethamine 75 mg/week); the reported difference appeared only in the undertreatment analysis (Opravil *et al.*, 1995). Studies using a lower dose of dapsone–pyrimethamine (dapsone 100 mg/week plus pyrimethamine 25 mg/week) found no efficacy against toxoplasmosis (Mallolas *et al.*, 1993). The rate of discontinuation of treatment for intolerance is 24–30% with effective doses (Girard *et al.*, 1993; Opravil *et al.*, 1995). Most treatment discontinuations for intolerance (cutaneous, digestive or haematological) occur during the first 3 months of therapy.

The two combinations (co-trimoxazole and dapsone-pyrimethamine) have not been compared. Co-trimoxazole, however, is used more often than dqpsone-pyrimethamine as first-line primary prevention of PCP. This is because it has several advantages including: simple prescription; the fact that practitioners are familiar with it; probable efficacy against bacterial pathogens; as well as the absence of interaction with didanosine. Unfortunately, after one year, about 25% of patients will have stopped taking co-trimoxazole (May *et al.*, 1992), mainly because of rashes and cytopenias. The dapsone-pyrimethamine combination is as effective as aerosolized pentamidine in preventing PCP and also prevents toxoplasmosis, but side-effects are similar to those of co-trimoxazole (Reynes *et al.*, 1992; Girard *et al.*, 1993). Although dapsone-pyrimethamine and co-trimoxazole have not been compared directly, one might argue that: (a) dapsone-pyrimethamine is as effective as pentamidine aerosols in prevention of PCP (Girard *et al.*, 1993); (b) co-trimoxazole is more effective than pentamidine aerosols (Hardy *et al.*, 1992; Schneider *et al.*, 1992); and therefore (c) co-trimoxazole should also be more effective than dapsone-pyrimethamine. Co-trimoxazole is now the recommended first-line choice for the primary prophylaxis of toxoplasmosis.

A major problem remains the search for an alternative for patients who tolerate neither co-trimoxazole nor dapsone–pyrimethamine, this group representing 15–20% of all patients eligible for prophylaxis (Blum *et al.*, 1992). Dapsone used alone appears to be ineffective (Slavin *et al.*, 1992) and the combination of dapsone and trimethoprim has yet to be evaluated. Pyrimethamine was studied in one placebo-controlled double-blind study of 544 patients seropositive for *T. gondii*. Intention-to-treat analysis suggested that pyrimethamine 50 mg/day with 15 mg of folinic acid thrice weekly did not influence the rate of occurrence of toxoplasmosis, but when the analysis was restricted to the period when patients were receiving their assigned drug it was shown that the rate of toxoplasmic encephalitis was significantly lower among those who tolerated pyrimethamine compared with those receiving placebo. However, patients who stopped taking the drug because of rash were at higher risk for subsequent toxoplasmic encephalitis, an unexplained phenomenon (Leport *et al.*, 1993).

The combination of pyrimethamine and sulphadiazine and of pyrimethamine and sulfadoxine (Köppen *et al.*, 1992) are effective against both infections but fears of toxicity hinder their use of primary prophylaxis. Among the macrolides, clarithromycin alone appears to lack efficacy and roxithromycin has been only tentatively evaluated. Clindamycin has been abandoned (Jacobson *et al.*, 1992) and atovaquone has not yet been assessed.

Further studies are needed to find new drugs and/or regimens that are both effective and well tolerated.

## OTHER PARASITIC INFECTIONS

These are extremely rare in Europe, but the increasing number of people who travel to endemic countries should be borne in mind when HIV-infected patients do not respond to antitoxoplasmic therapy.

*Trypanosoma cruzi* infection (Chagas' disease) is frequent in South America and has been observed in association with HIV infection. Most cases have been recorded in Brazil (Chimelli *et al.*, 1992; Oddó *et al.*, 1992; Rosemberg *et al.*, 1992; Metze and Maciel, 1993) and Chile (Oddó *et al.*, 1992). Fatal meningoencephalitis caused by reactivation of Chagas' disease was seen in some patients (Rosemberg *et al.*, 1992; Metze and Maciel, 1993). Acute Chagas' disease was observed in some cases (Ferreira *et al.*, 1991; Metze and Maciel, 1993).

*Acanthamoeba* may induce granulomatous brain lesions. On CT, multiple hypodense (Anzil *et al.*, 1991) or enhancing (Gardner *et al.*, 1991) lesions have been observed. The outcome is usually rapidly fatal. Gross examination showed multiple haemorrhagic abscesses (Gardner *et al.*, 1991). Immunofluorescence may be useful to identify the trophozoites as *Acanthamoeba*.

## VIRAL INFECTIONS

### Progressive multifocal leucoencephalopathy

Improvement in the survival of individuals with HIV infection is mainly due to control of opportunistic infections, many of which affect the CNS and cause mental deterioration and severe neurological deficits. One such agent of opportunistic infection is JC virus, which is aetiologically linked with PML, a severe subacute demyelinating disease of the CNS. Originally reported as a rare complication of immunodepression, PML is far more prevalent among AIDS patients, with estimates of incidence ranging from 4 to 7%. The incidence is expected to increase since it remains one of the few opportunistic infections with no known therapy.

PML (which should actually be termed progressive multifocal leucoencephalitis) is a common viral opportunistic infection of the CNS caused by the JC strain of polyoma virus (Aksamit *et al.*, 1985), resulting in devastating demyelinating lesions that predominate in the cerebral hemispheres. PML is characterized by the occurrence of major neurological deficits, eventually leading to death usually in a matter of months. First identified in 1958 by Aström *et al.* in three patients with chronic leukaemia or Hodgkin's disease as a complication of conditions inducing immunodeficiency, PML was extremely rare before the outbreak of the epidemic of HIV infection, but has since become one of the major neurological complications in patients with immunodeficiency induced by this agent (Berger *et al.*, 1991; Lang *et al.*, 1989). This subacute encephalopathy occurs in patients with severe immunodepression (Krupp *et al.*, 1985; Quinlivan *et al.*, 1992). In patients with AIDS (Scaravilli *et al.*, 1989; von Einsiedel *et al.*, 1993), PML is the second most common viral opportunistic infection of the CNS after CMV infection. PML is found in 4% of autopsy cases in the USA (Kure *et al.*, 1991), 6% in Switzerland (Lang *et al.*, 1989), 5% and 0.5% in France (Gray *et al.*, 1988; Matthiessen *et al.*, 1992), 0.8% in Brazil (Chimelli *et al.*, 1992) and 5% in Austria (Budka *et al.*, 1987).

*Clinical presentation*

Clinical manifestations of PML are related to lesions of the white matter of the brain (Price *et al.*, 1983). In a recent personal series, 11 patients, nine men and two women, aged 28–62 years (mean age 36 years) were affected. In six patients PML was the first opportunistic infection; three of these patients were first seen by neurologists because PML revealed HIV infection as well. In the other five patients, the first manifestations of PML occurred after a mean interval of 1 year (5–24 months) after another manifestation of AIDS. The mean $CD4^+$ T-cell count was 57 $ml^{-1}$ (range 3–194). The main neurological manifestations at onset include hemiparesis with facial or limb weakness, aphasia, dysarthria, hemianopsia and ataxia (Holmann *et al.*, 1991). Occasionally patients may present with blindness due to lesions of the optic nerve or the chiasma, with pontocerebellar syndrome with deafness, or with involuntary movements. The course of PML is subacute, without symptoms of intracranial hypertension. Mental deterioration, flaccid hemiplegia, major ataxia, difficulty in swallowing and loss of vision gradually make these patients bedridden. There is no fever related to PML. These patients usually die from their neurological problems within a few weeks or months (Miller *et al.*, 1984; Holmann *et al.*, 1991). Data from recent studies have shown that the mean survival time after diagnosis of HIV-associated PML is around 3.5 months. However, subacute forms may cause death in a few weeks; conversely, prolonged survival up to 30 months has been reported (Berger and Mucke, 1988; Laforêt *et al.*, 1994). In our series, patients with the highest $CD4^+$ T-cell count had the longest survival time. An unusual relapsing course, mimicking multiple sclerosis, has been reported (Dupuis *et al.*,

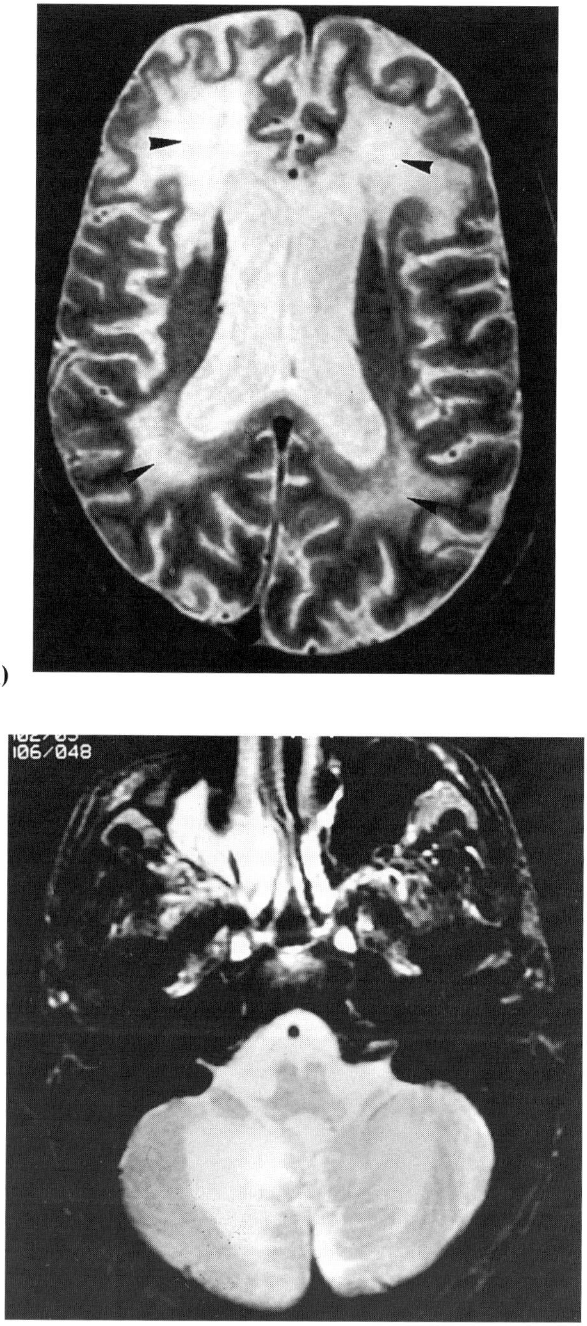


(a)

(b)

**Figure 4.9** (a) $T_2$-weighted MRI showing high-intensity signal in the frontal and occipital white matter of a patient with PML (arrowheads). (b) $T_2$-weighted MRI showing high-intensity signal in the white matter of the cerebellum in a patient with PML.

1986). Two cases of PML were reported in children with AIDS (Van der Steenhoven *et al.*, 1990; Berger *et al.*, 1991).

*Diagnosis*

Brain MRI shows characteristic lesions in the majority of cases. The typical aspect includes the presence of asymmetric, non-enhancing, hypointense white-matter lesions on $T_1$-weighted images without mass effect (Lipton *et al.*, 1988). The lesions may be unique or multiple focal areas of abnormal high-intensity signal on $T_2$-weighted images (Figure 4.9) (Levy JD *et al.*, 1986; Trotot *et al.*, 1990). In some patients the subcortical lesions also affect part of the adjacent cortex, with a necrotic appearance. Brain CT images, although less spectacular, show hypodense, non-contrast-enhancing lesions of the white matter without mass effect (Figure 4.10).

The use of brain biopsy to confirm the diagnosis of PML has been advocated by several authors, since brain sampling allows morphological examination of the lesions and detection of JC virus in glial cells by immunochemistry or *in situ* DNA hybridization. Brain sampling also permits the exclusion of other diagnoses, such as lymphoma, cerebral toxoplasmosis or other, less common opportunistic infections. However, patients are usually in poor condition with a life expectancy of a few weeks or months, with severe neurological handicap and, frequently, blood dyscrasia. Considering the risk of cerebral haemorrhages

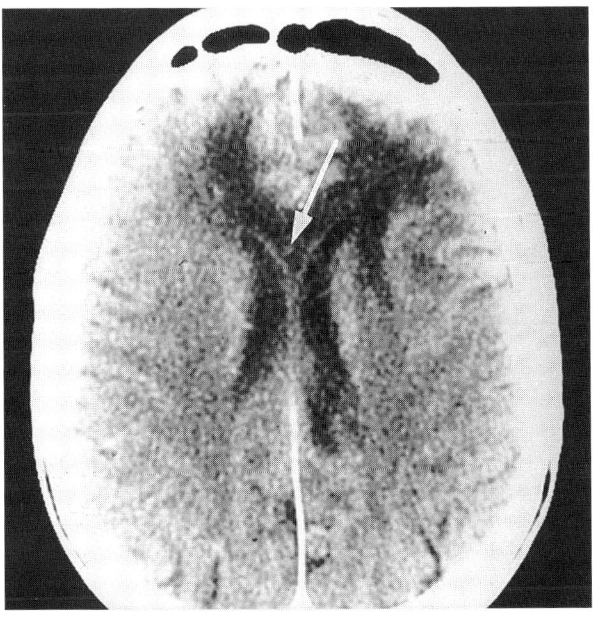

**Figure 4.10** CT image with contrast showing a non-enhancing hypodense lesion of the frontal white matter and corpus callosum (arrow) in an HIV-infected patient with PML.

induced by brain biopsy, even with stereotactic techniques, and the lack of efficient treatment, we do not advise performance of brain biopsy to confirm PML. Occasionally, cerebral toxoplasmosis may present with mental impairment and widespread hyperintensity of the white matter on $T_2$-weighted images without mass effects. In such patients, in whom the diagnosis of PML has been considered, spectacular improvement of the clinical condition can be achieved by a few weeks of specific antitoxoplasmic treatment. In countries where toxoplasmosis is common, we recommend systematic treatment with antitoxoplasmic drugs for 4 weeks, with clinical testing and neuroimaging at the end of the treatment, before the diagnosis of PML is made.

Detection of JC viral DNA by PCR in blood and CSF has been available for a few years. Initial reports of PCR analysis in PML have shown the high specificity of this method (Telenti *et al.*, 1990). Negative results do not exclude the diagnosis of PML, on account of the low sensitivity of PCR (Telenti *et al.*, 1990; Tornatore *et al.*, 1992). It seems that only CSF analysis has diagnostic value, with PCR being positive in 16–37% of histologically proven cases of PML (Aksamit *et al.*, 1987; Telenti *et al.*, 1992). Using PCR technology, JC viral DNA was found in peripheral lymphocytes of 89% of HIV-infected patients with brain-biopsy-proven PML, 38% of HIV-seropositive patients without PML and in no control patients (Tornatore *et al.*, 1992). In the CSF, JC viral DNA was detected in only 27% of the patients (Tornatore *et al.*, 1992). Whether or not PCR detection of JC virus will be reliable enough to allow evaluation of treatments for PML remains to be demonstrated.

*Therapeutic trials*

Some beneficial effect of treatment of PML with cytosine arabinoside has been claimed (Portegies *et al.*, 1991), but has not been confirmed by controlled studies. Treatment of PML with interferon $\alpha$ seemed to induce clinical stabilization or improvement (Tashiro *et al.*, 1986), but the heterogeneity of inclusion criteria and of the therapeutic modalities does not allow firm conclusions to be drawn. In a recent study of 10 patients treated with interferon $\alpha$ (Laforêt *et al.*, 1994), we could only conclude that the patients with the longest survival time were those with the highest number of $CD4^+$ T cells and those in whom PML was the first manifestation of AIDS. No conclusion could be drawn as to the effect of interferon $\alpha$, which would be minor at best. One study has mentioned the relative efficacy of azidodeoxythymidine (Conway *et al.*, 1990).

*Pathology*

The JC virus has been identified in oligodendrocytes and a few astrocytes, but not in neurones, macrophages or endothelial cells (Aksamit *et al.*, 1985; Anders *et al.*, 1986; Ironside *et al.*, 1989). The JC virus is latent in the kidney, bone marrow and spleen (Houff *et al.*, 1988; Tornatore *et al.*, 1992) and in the brain of some elderly patients (Lipton, 1991; Mori *et al.*, 1991).

Macroscopic examination of the brain of patients with PML shows areas of demyelination in the subcortical white matter, sometimes associated with

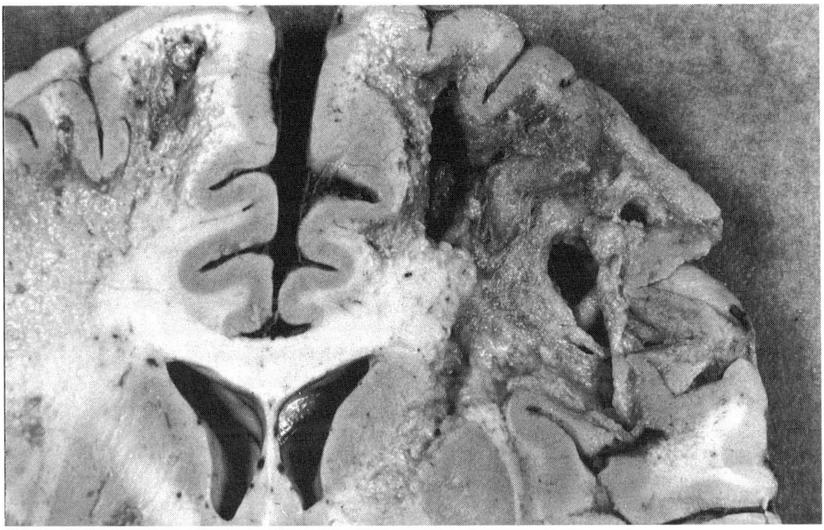

**Figure 4.11** Vertical section of the frontal lobes of a patient with asymmetric necrotizing PML.

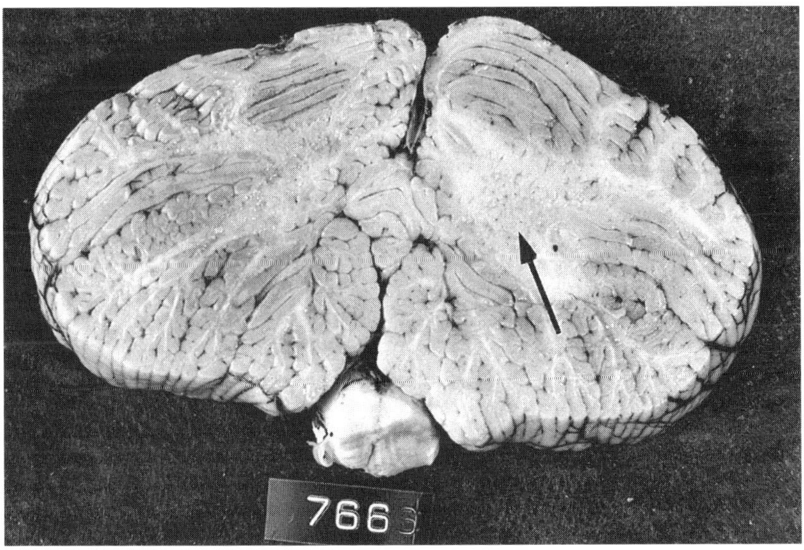

**Figure 4.12** Necrosis of the white matter (arrow) and preservation of the cortex in the cerebellum and medulla of the same patient as in Figure 4.2.

necrosis (Figure 4.11). The grey matter looks preserved. The lesions of the white matter may be found in the frontal, temporal or occipital lobes (Kure *et al.*, 1991; von Einsiedel *et al.*, 1993), occasionally in the cerebellum and pons (Figure 4.12) (Knobler *et al.*, 1986; Vinters *et al.*, 1987; Lipton *et al.*, 1988; Anders *et al.*, 1990; Kuchelmeister *et al.*, 1993a). Myelin staining shows irregular, large or small unstained areas (Figure 4.13). Demyelination is the most prominent abnormality on light microscopic examination (Figure 4.14); axons seem to be more preserved than the myelin sheath. Foamy macrophages are present, associated with large 'bizarre' reactive astrocytes in the subcortical white matter or the deep cortex (Figure 4.15). Oligodendrocytes with dense nuclear amphophil inclusions are found usually in the vicinity of necrotic or demyelinated areas (Figure 4.16). The cortex and deep grey matter may be involved in some cases (Kuchelmeister *et al.*, 1993a). Proliferation of Rosenthal fibres may be observed (Vuia, 1976). Perivascular inflammatory cells are uncommon (Schmidbauer *et al.*, 1990). Such lymphocytes are T cells (Hair *et al.*, 1992). Myelin-associated glycoprotein (MAG) and myelin basic protein (MBP) are severely altered in demyelinated regions associated with little staining for JC virus; however, in surrounding areas infected oligodendrocytes are numerous, MAG staining is decreased and MBP staining is normal (Itoyama *et al.*, 1982). Changes in MAG distribution could be an indicator of early oligodendroglial abnormalities (Itoyama *et al.*, 1982). In some cases, MGCs containing HIV antigen are associated with PML lesions (Koyanagi *et al.*, 1987; Vazeux *et al.*, 1990). The papovavirus can be detected by immunocytochemistry (Figure 4.17) and by *in situ* hybridization in oligodendrocytes and the nucleus of some 'bizarre' astrocytes (Aksamit *et al.*, 1990; Schmidbauer *et al.*, 1990; von Einsiedel *et al.*, 1993). Coinfection with HIV may occur (Vazeux *et al.*, 1990; Kuchelmeister *et al.*, 1993a) (Figure 4.18). In these coinfected brains, necrotic

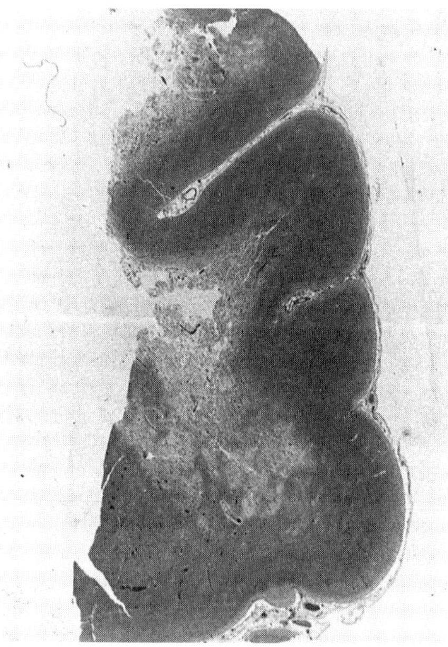

**Figure 4.13** Necrosis of the white matter and preservation of the cortex in the left frontal lobe of the same patient as in Figure 4.1. (Paraffin section; H&E.)

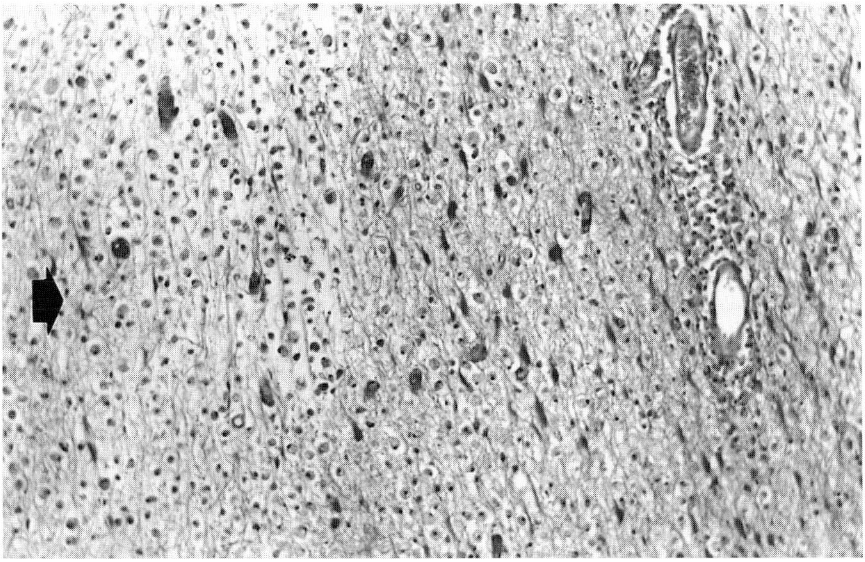

**Figure 4.14** Massive demyelination (arrowhead) and relative preservation of the axons in the white matter of a patient with PML. (Paraffin section; H&E; ×260.)

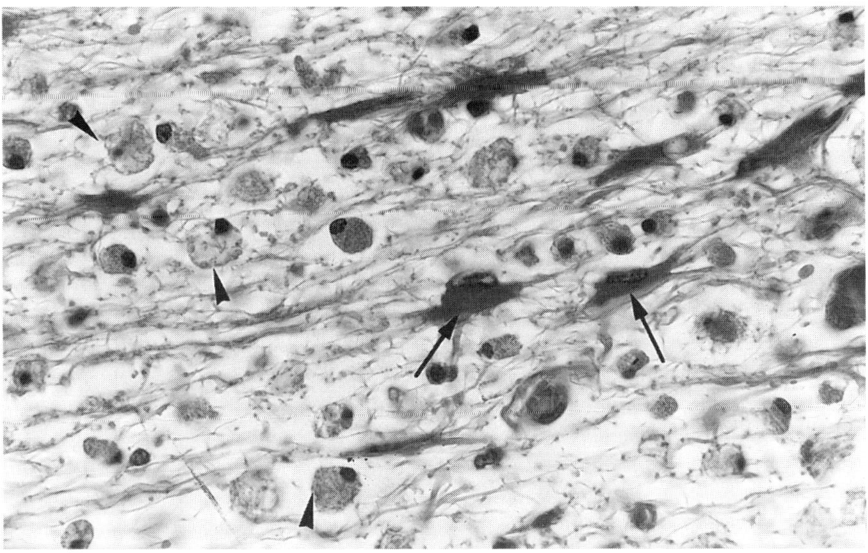

**Figure 4.15** 'Bizarre' astrocytes (arrows) and macrophages (arrowheads) in the white matter of a patient with PML. (Paraffin section; H&E; ×1060.)

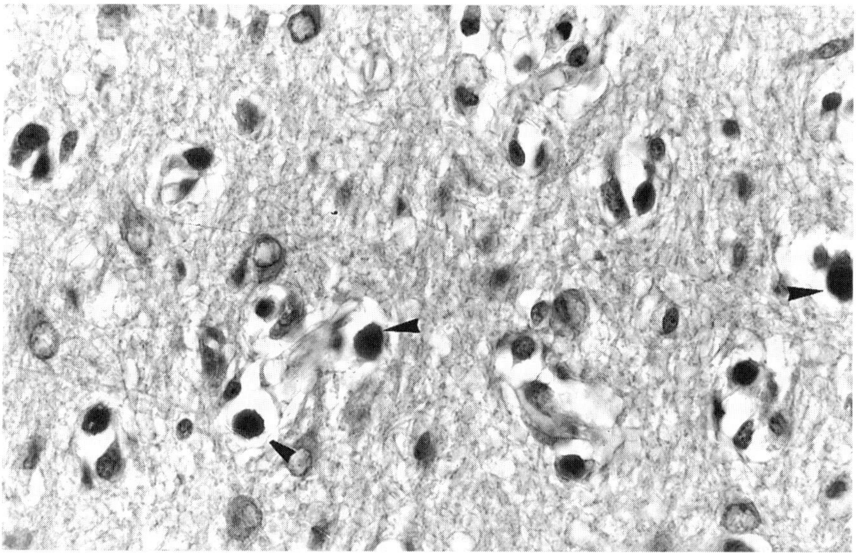

**Figure 4.16** Dense intranuclear inclusions in oligodendrocytes (arrowheads) in the white matter of the same patient as in Figure 4.15. (Paraffin section; H&E; ×1060.)

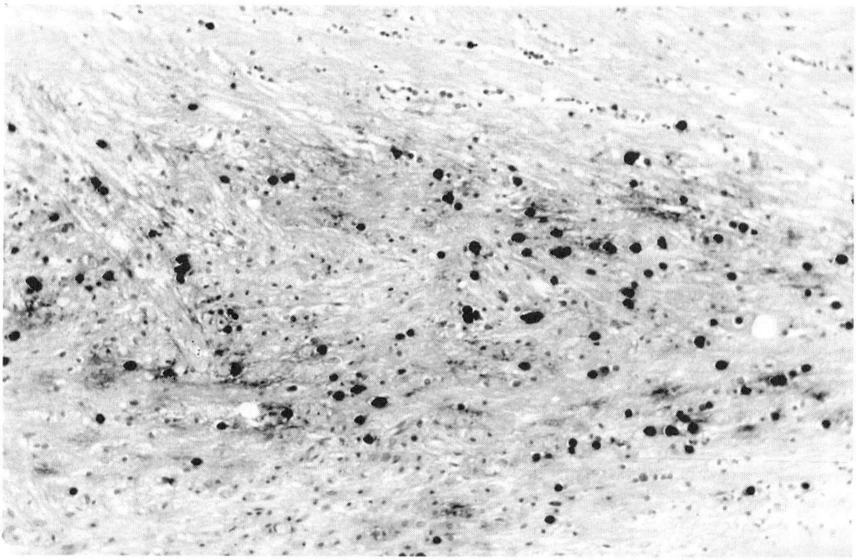

**Figure 4.17** Immunocytochemistry with a polyclonal SV40 antibody staining papovavirus inclusions in oligodendrocytes in the white matter of a patient with PML. (Paraffin section; DAB; ×260.)

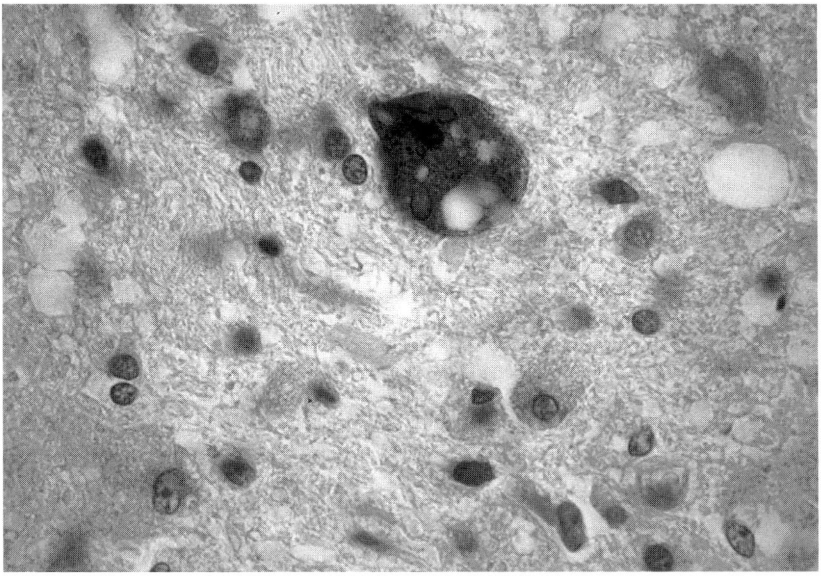

**(a)**

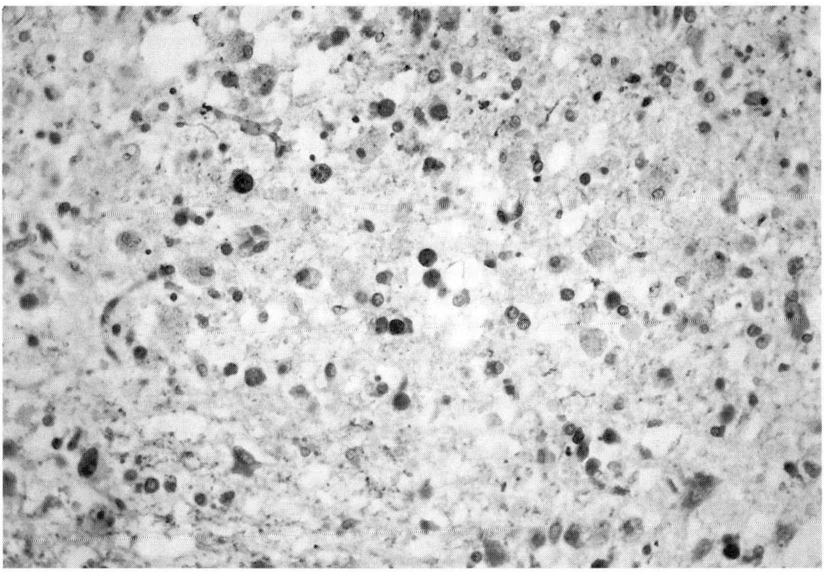

**(b)**

**Figure 4.18** (a) Multinucleated giant cell stained by an HIV gp41 antibody in the frontal white matter of a patient with HIV and PML encephalitis. (Paraffin section; DAB; ×1000.) (b) Papovavirus inclusions in oligodendrocytes stained by an SV40 antibody in the same patient as in (a). (Paraffin section; DAB; ×300.)

lesions seem more prominent than usual in PML (Vazeux *et al.*, 1990; see Table 4.7). Electron microscopy can demonstrate intranuclear spherical and filamentous viral particles in oligodendrocytes (Orenstein and Janotta, 1988), but JC virus can also replicate in astrocytes in culture (Major and Vacante, 1989). In addition to HIV encephalitis, PML can be associated with other opportunistic infections, such as *T. gondii* (Chimelli *et al.*, 1992) or *Histoplasma capsulatum* (Weidenheim *et al.*, 1992).

The immunopathogenesis of PML is still unclear. In patients with profound immunodepression, the latent JC virus in the kidney follows a haematogenous route to enter the brain (Aksamit *et al.*, 1990). Demyelinated areas are usually located in the vicinity of blood vessels (de la Monte *et al.*, 1987). The JC virus could penetrate the blood–brain barrier via infected macrophages (Wiley *et al.*, 1988). High levels of class I and II MHC antigens are expressed in macrophage/microglia in demyelinating lesions of PML, suggesting a delayed-type immune response to JC virus within the CNS (Achim and Wiley, 1992). The HIV tat protein can activate the JC virus late promoter in glial cells (Tada *et al.*, 1990). The presence of both viruses may increase the effects of each other (Koyanagi *et al.*, 1987; Vazeux *et al.*, 1990).

*Summary*

PML represents one of the major neurological problems in immunosuppressed patients. Thanks to modern neuroimaging methods and molecular biology the diagnosis of PML can be achieved by non-invasive methods. Exclusion of other treatable opportunistic infections is the main objective in such patients, since PML remains the last opportunistic infection of the nervous system for which there is no known treatment.

**Cytomegalovirus infection**

CMV infection of the CNS has been observed in the normal host, in newborn infants and in transplant recipients (Bale, 1984; Cohen and Corey, 1985).

*Clinical presentation*

CMV encephalitis occurs as a late and terminal complication in patients who have had AIDS for more than 1 year (Jacobson *et al.*, 1988; Kalayjian *et al.*, 1993; Holland *et al.*, 1994). A large proportion of patients with CMV encephalitis have had previous CMV retinitis or lung infection (Fiala *et al.*, 1993). In most cases, disorientation, confusion and lethargy develop within 2 weeks, together with involvement of cranial nerves and motor deficits. Death occurs in a median of 4 weeks after the initial manifestation, in spite of ganciclovir therapy (Kalayjian *et al.*, 1993; Holland *et al.*, 1994; McCutchan, 1995). CMV can also induce myeloradiculitis with a rapidly progressive flaccid paraplegia associated with sphincter incontinence (Jeantils *et al.*, 1986; Chimelli *et al.*, 1990). Multifocal lesions of the CNS progressing rapidly to flaccid paraplegia, and coma due to multiple brain and spinal cord lesions, often characterize the clinical manifestations.

*Investigations*

Non-specific changes are observed on CT and MRI. Usually CT shows cortical atrophy and enlargement of the ventricles but fails to detect specific changes (Post *et al.*, 1986). MRI seems to be more sensitive and may reveal multifocal lesions despite normal CT (Masdeu *et al.*, 1988), with periventricular (Figure 4.19) and meningeal enhancement with gadolinium (Kalayjian *et al.*, 1993; Holland *et al.*, 1994).

In some patients CSF analysis can reveal elevation of proteins, hypoglycorrhachia and pleocytosis with polymorphonuclear cells (Kalayjian *et al.*, 1993); however, CSF analysis may be normal (Fiala *et al.*, 1993). CMV is rarely detected by culture methods (Edwards *et al.*, 1985; Jeantils *et al.*, 1986; Kalayjian *et al.*, 1993). Several papers have demonstrated that PCR is useful for detecting CMV DNA in the CSF of patients with CMV infection of the CNS (Cinque *et al.*, 1992; Gozlan *et al.*, 1992; Wolf and Spector, 1992; Holland *et al.*, 1994), especially in patients with myeloradiculitis (Clifford *et al.*, 1993). PCR seems to have a higher diagnostic value than detection of intrathecal antibody synthesis (Weber *et al.*, 1994).

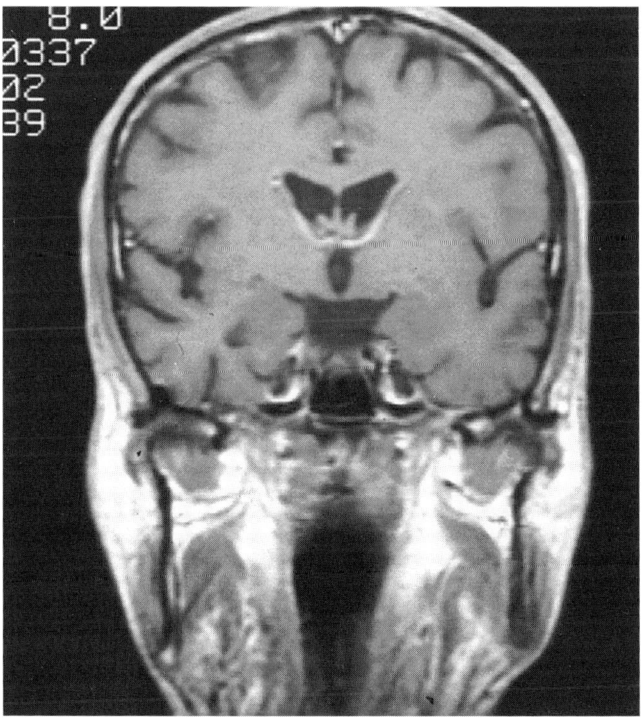

**Figure 4.19** Sagittal MRI with gadolinium showing enhancement of the periventricular area in a patient with CMW ventriculitis.

*Pathology*

The pathological examination is currently the only way to prove the diagnosis of CMV encephalopathy. Only a few stereotactic biopsies have been carried out in such encephalopathies and most cases were diagnosed at autopsy. CMV encephalitis is the most frequent opportunistic infection after toxoplasmosis, the incidence ranging from 7 to 26% in large autopsy series (see Table 4.7). CMV encephalitis with microglial nodules has been previously described in organ-transplant recipients (Bale, 1984). AIDS patients with CMV infection of the CNS have also been found to have ventriculitis, necrotizing encephalitis, myelitis, radiculomyelitis, focal demyelination of the brain and spinal cord, and vasculitis (Morgello *et al.*, 1987; Grafe and Wiley, 1989; Vinters *et al.*, 1989). The gross pathology is normal in many cases. Periventricular necrosis with haemorrhagic foci is observed (Figure 4.20) (Morgello *et al.*, 1987). Small focal softening and grey discolorations are usually present in the white matter (Figure 4.21) (Morgello *et al.*, 1987). Necrosis of the white matter is rare (Morgello *et al.*, 1987) (Figure 4.22). Microglial nodules are detected in a variable proportion of cases, usually in the subcortical grey matter (Morgello *et al.*, 1987). Microglial nodules contain macrophages, rod cells and sometimes CMV inclusion-bearing cells (Morgello *et al.*, 1987; Vinters *et al.*, 1989). A diffuse necrotizing ventriculitis was present in all our patients with CMV encephalopathy: the ependymal cells had disappeared or in some areas had Cowdry type A intranuclear inclusions (Figure 4.23). Lipid-laden macrophages, MGCs containing cytomegalic inclusions and rare lymphocytes were present in the subependymal region. Any part of the CNS can be affected. The presence of CMV-infected cells can be proved by characteristic morphological features (Figure 4.23), by immunolabelling (Figure 4.24), *in situ* hybridization (Schmidbauer *et al.*, 1989) and electron microscopy (Wiley and Nelson, 1988). Infected cells comprise glial cells, neurones (Figure 4.25), endothelial cells, smooth muscle cells, oligodendrocytes and macrophages (Booss *et al.*, 1989; Schmidbauer *et al.*, 1989; Vinters *et al.*, 1989; Walker *et al.*, 1989). In our patients, most cells with CMV inclusions were ependymal cells or neurones. *In vitro* studies have demonstrated that CMV can infect neural cells (McCarthy *et al.*, 1991). CMV infection of macrophage/microglial cells has been demonstrated in cultures and animals models (Booss *et al.*, 1989; Pulliam, 1991).

CMV encephalopathy is the only opportunistic infection in most patients, but in some cases is associated with other types of neuropathology including HIV encephalitis, HSV, VZV, *Toxoplasma*, *Cryptococcus*, candidosis, PML and primary cerebral lymphoma (see Table 4.9; Morgello *et al.*, 1987; Vinters *et al.*, 1989).

*Treatment*

Three drugs are used in patients with suspected CMV encephalitis, polyradiculoneuritis or retinitis: ganciclovir (Michon *et al.*, 1988; Novak *et al.*,

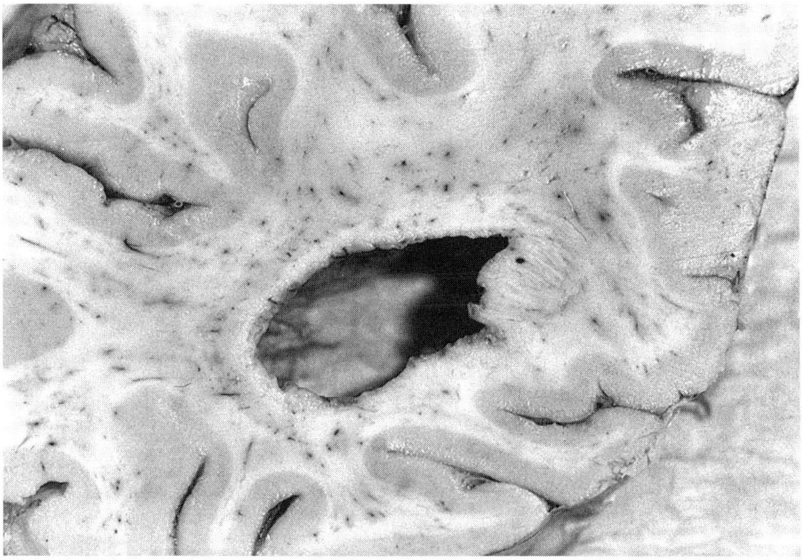

**Figure 4.20** Section of occipital horn showing irregular ependymal wall in a patient with CMV ventriculitis.

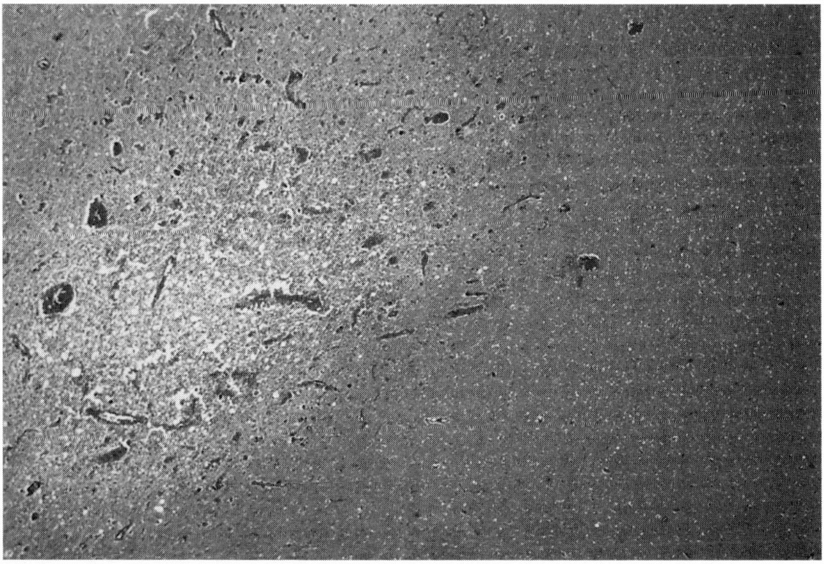

**Figure 4.21** Focal necrosis of the white matter in a patient with CMV encephalitis. (Paraffin section; H&E; ×60.)

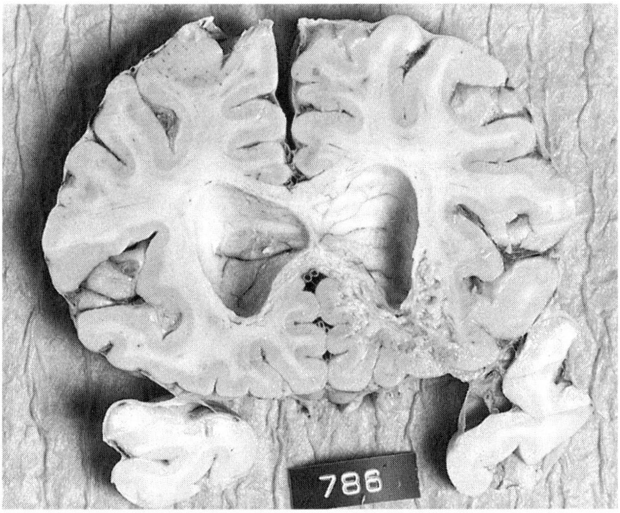


**(a)**

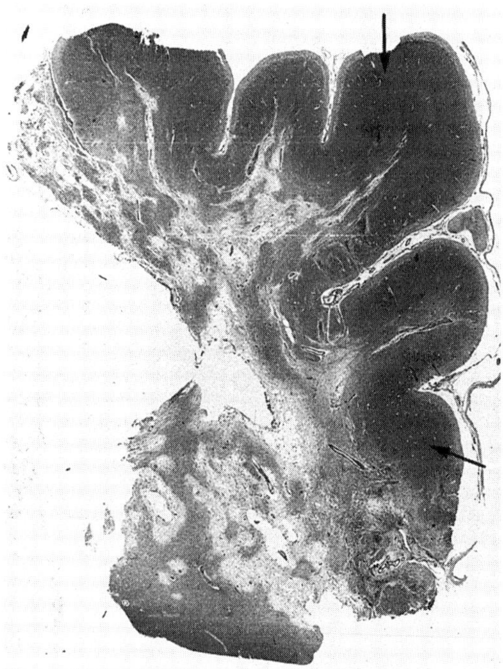

**(b)**

**Figure 4.22** (a) Necrosis of the white matter and enlargement of the ventricles in the frontal lobes of a patient with CMV encephalitis. (b) Necrosis of the white matter and relative preservation of the cortex (arrows) in the frontal lobe of a patient with CMV encephalitis. (Paraffin section; H&E.)

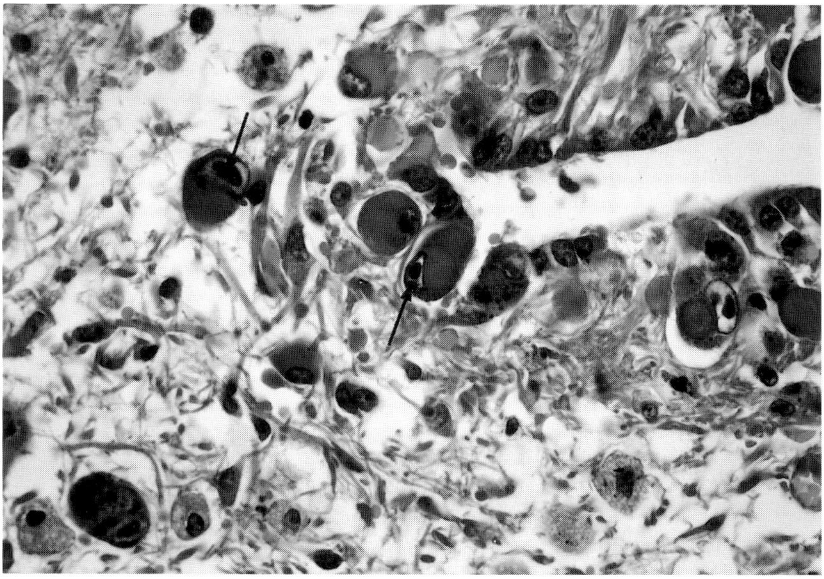

**Figure 4.23** Necrosis of the ependymal layer and cytomegalic inclusions of some ependymal cells (arrows) in the fourth ventricle of a patient with CMV ventriculitis. (Paraffin section; H&E; ×990.)

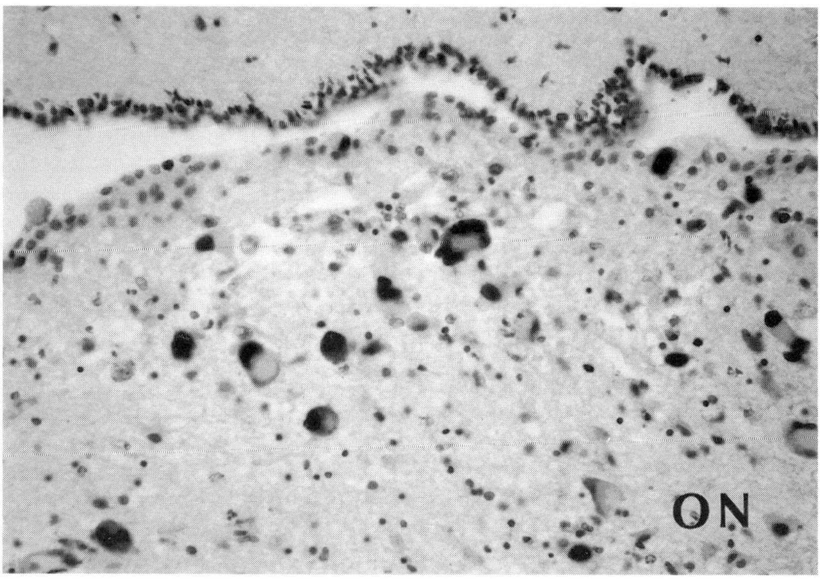


**Figure 4.24** Infiltration of the proximal part of the optic nerve (ON) by cytomegalic cells recognized by a CMV antibody in a patient with CMV encephalitis. (Paraffin section; DAB; × 490.)

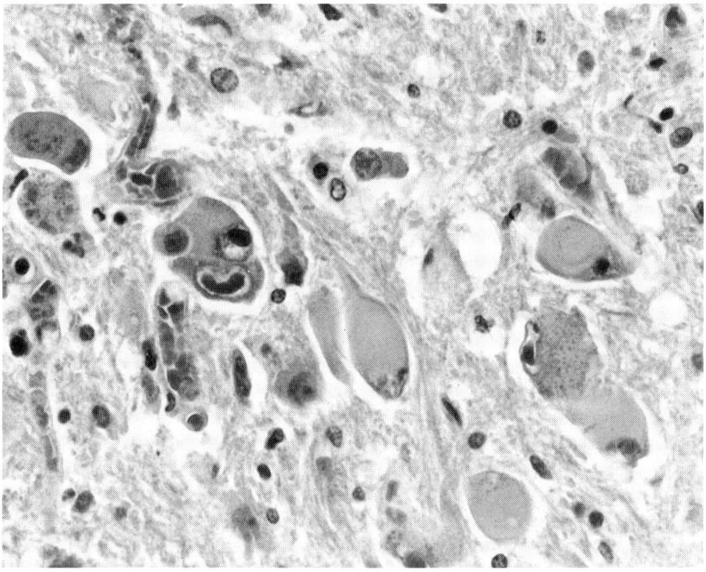

**Figure 4.25** Motor neurones containing owl-eye nuclear cytomegalic inclusions in the spinal cord of a patient with CMV encephalomyelitis. (Paraffin section; H&E; ×1020.)

1989), foscarnet (Michon *et al.*, 1988) and cidofovir. Ganciclovir and foscarnet are usually administered by daily intravenous infusions; oral capsules of ganciclovir are available (Oral Ganciclovir European and Australian Cooperative Study Group, 1995). A 2-week dosing regimen may be given with cidofovir. Ganciclovir can cross the blood–brain barrier better than foscarnet (Jacobson and Mills, 1988). Side-effects of ganciclovir are neutropenia, thrombocytopenia and neuropsychiatric disturbances (Michon *et al.*, 1988); the side-effect of foscarnet is nephrotoxicity (Michon *et al.*, 1988). In a series of patients with retinitis, survival was higher with foscarnet but tolerance was lower (Jabs *et al.*, 1992). The combination of the two drugs induced a transient improvement in a patient with CMV meningoencephalitis (Enting *et al.*, 1992). Ganciclovir resistance was suspected in patients who developed encephalitis during therapy for retinitis or in the absence of response to therapy (Drew *et al.*, 1991; Elbright and Crane, 1991; Berman *et al.*, 1992; Kim and Hollander, 1993). Both drugs may be relatively effective in polyradiculoneuritis (Kim and Hollander, 1993). Therapy always failed when necrotic lesions had occurred in the CNS, especially in myelitis (Jacobson *et al.*, 1988). One report mentioned an improvement of suspected encephalitis with foscarnet, but no pathological examination was carried out (Nicoli *et al.*, 1992). Nevertheless, once initiated, the treatment must be administered indefinitely, intravenously during the first weeks and with the oral form later. Only very early or preventive therapy could be useful in CMV infection of the CNS. Recent studies of oral ganciclovir for the prevention of CMV disease in AIDS indicate a significant reduction of CMV infection in the patients who received the drug (Drew *et al.*, 1995; Spector *et al.*, 1996).

**Varicella-zoster and herpes simplex infection**
In addition to CMV, other herpes viruses may infect the CNS including VZV (Ryder *et al.*, 1986; Gilden *et al.*, 1988; Chrétien *et al.*, 1993) and HSV types 1 and 2 (Dix *et al.*, 1985; Devinski *et al.*, 1991; Tan *et al.*, 1993).

*VZV*
Subacute or progressive VZV encephalitis can occur a few months after a cutaneous zoster in immunosuppressed patients (Gilden *et al.*, 1988). Neurological impairment is subacute, with progressive memory loss, confusion, sensorimotor deficits, general epileptic seizures and coma (Gray *et al.*, 1992). Pathological examinations found multifocal necrosis and ventriculitis associated with intranuclear Cowdry type A inclusions in glial cells, endothelial cells, macrophages, neurones and oligodendroglia (Ryder *et al.*, 1986; Rosenblum, 1989). The presence of VZV was confirmed by immunocytochemistry, electron microscopy and PCR (Gilden *et al.*, 1988; Gray *et al.*, 1992).

*HSV types 1 and 2*
HSV type 1 (Tan *et al.*, 1993) or type 2 (Dix *et al.*, 1985; Laskin *et al.*, 1987; Gateley *et al.*, 1990) encephalitis are rare in patients with AIDS. The clinical presentation and the pathological features of HSV encephalitis are similar to those in patients without immunosuppression. HSV myelitis may occur (Britton *et al.*, 1985). Some patients have improved with acyclovir (Dix *et al.*, 1985).

## FUNGAL INFECTIONS

A variety of fungal infections may occur in patients with AIDS. They include *Cryptococcus neoformans*, *Candida albicans* and *Aspergillus fumigatus*, which are ubiquitous (Anders *et al.*, 1986; Budka *et al.*, 1987; Rhodes, 1993) (see Table 4.7), or other fungi restricted to some geographic areas like histoplasmosis and coccidioidomycosis in the southern USA (Vinters and Anders, 1990) or South America (Chimelli *et al.*, 1992).

**Aspergillus fumigatus**
Anecdotal cases of CNS aspergillosis have been reported for adults (Lang *et al.*, 1989; Vinters and Anders, 1990; Kure *et al.*, 1991; Rodriguez-Arrondo *et al.*, 1991; Chimelli *et al.*, 1992) and children (Kozlowski *et al.*, 1990; Lacroix *et al*, 1993) with AIDS. In most cases, multiple abscesses were found at autopsy. Meningitis or meningoencephalitis may be present (Snider *et al.*, 1983).

**Candida albicans**
A few reports have mentioned meningoencephalitis or abscesses due to *C. albicans* (Budka *et al.*, 1987; Kure *et al.*, 1991). In all cases, autopsy showed necrotic areas containing yeasts and pseudohyphae (Levy *et al.*, 1988; Kure *et al.*, 1991) (Figure 4.26).

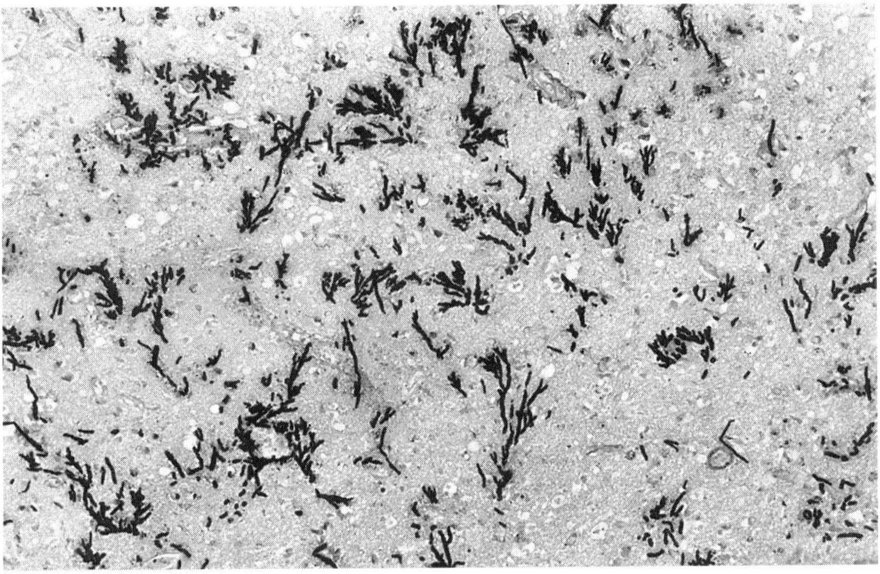

**Figure 4.26** *Candida albicans*: multiple pseudohyphae (stained by a silver technique) in a frontal abscess of a patient who also had HIV encephalitis. (Paraffin section; Grocott; ×260.)

***Cryptococcus neoformans***
Meningoencephalitis or abscesses associated with *Cryptococcus* infection occur frequently in the AIDS population (Levy *et al.*, 1988) and are found more often in the USA and Brazil than in Europe (Zuger *et al.*, 1986; Budka *et al.*, 1987; Chimelli *et al.*, 1992; Matthiessen *et al.*, 1992; Rhodes, 1993). Meningitis is the more frequent neurological localization (Kovacs *et al*, 1985; Zuger *et al.*, 1986) and may be the initial presentation of AIDS, as in one of our patients (Giberson and Kalyan-Raman, 1987). CSF examination shows an elevated white cell count, low glucose levels and elevated protein levels; india ink preparation demonstrates the cryptococcomas (Zuger *et al.*, 1986). Detection of the cryptococcal antigen in the CSF may determine the diagnosis; treatment is with amphotericin B combined with flucytosine (Zuger *et al.*, 1986). Occasional brain abscesses have been observed in patients with focal neurological abnormalities (Kovacs *et al.*, 1985; Zuger *et al.*, 1986; Graefin von Einsiedel *et al.*, 1992) (Figure 4.27). Cryptococcal meningitis may be associated with other opportunistic

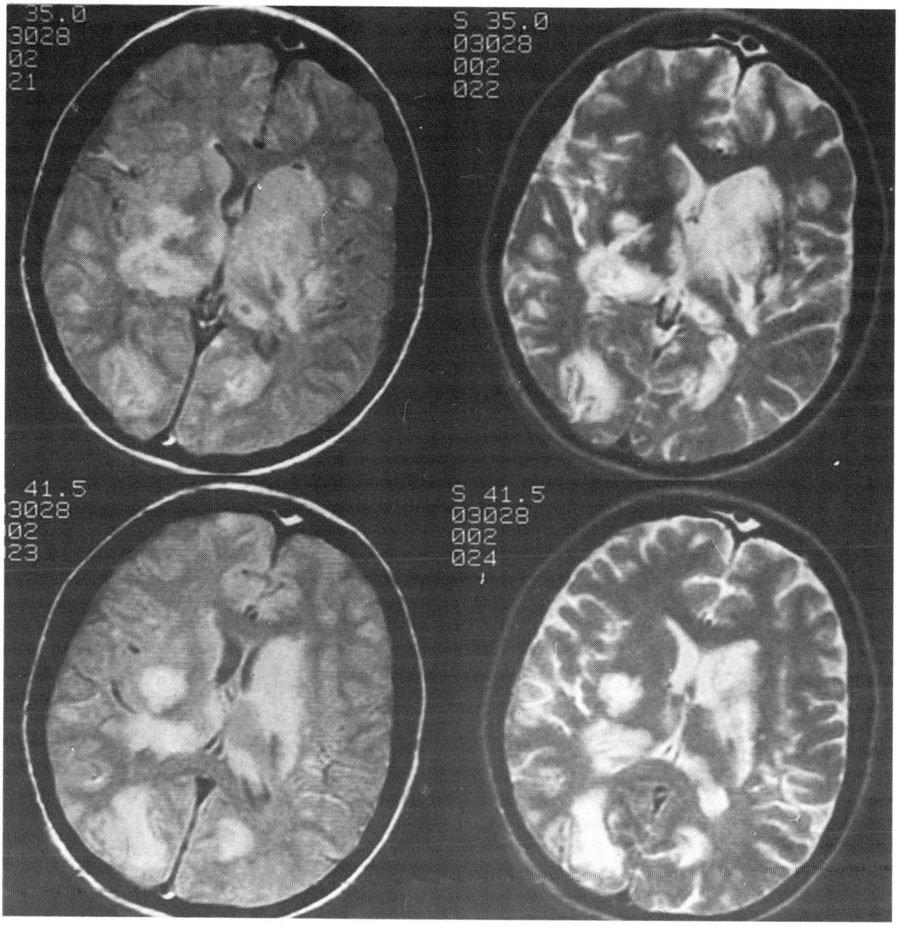


**Figure 4.27** $T_1$-(left) and $T_2$-(right) weighted MRI of a patient with *Cryptococcus* meningoencephalitis.

infections, such as toxoplasmosis (Lucht *et al.*, 1987) or PML (see Table 4.7). The granulomatous lesions infiltrate the Virchow–Robin spaces and the parenchyma. The microorganisms are associated with macrophages and giant cells (Figures 4.28 and 4.29).

### *Coccidioides immitis*

In California, meningitis and brain abscesses due to coccidioidomycosis have been reported in patients with AIDS (Bronnimann *et al.*, 1987; Jarvik *et al.*, 1988b; Levy *et al.*, 1988).

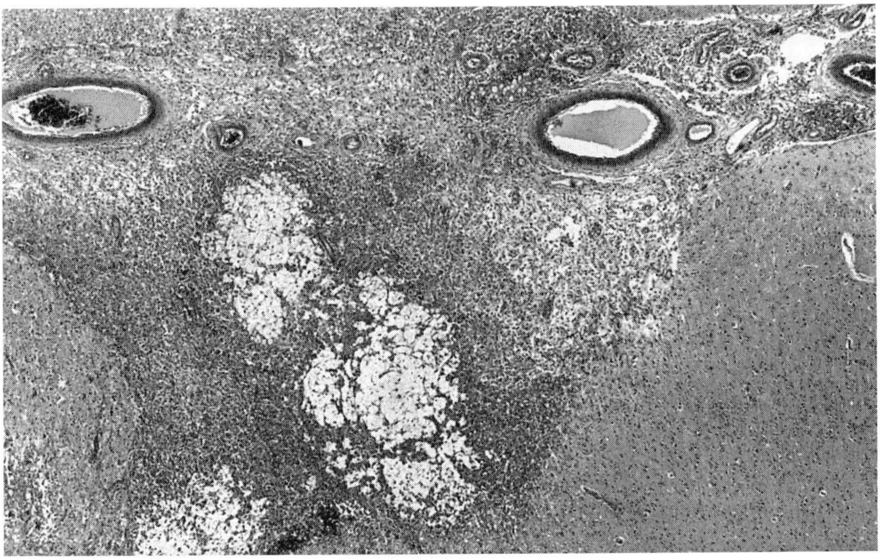

**Figure 4.28** Granulomatous meningoencephalitis associated with cryptococci in the temporal lobe. (Paraffin section; H&E; ×70.)

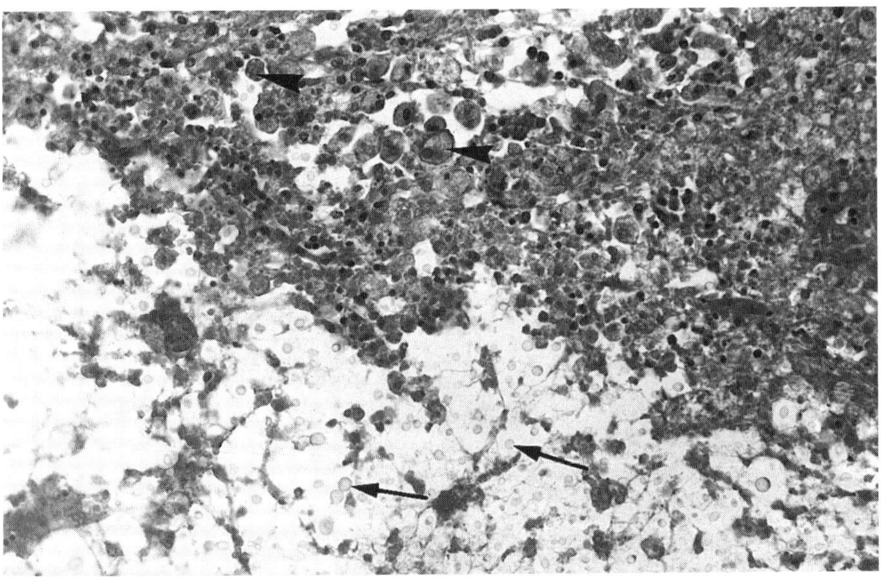

**Figure 4.29** Higher magnification of the same abscess as in Figure 4.28 showing cryptococci with a dense core (arrows) surrounded by a clear capsule and macrophages (arrowheads). (Paraffin section; H&E; ×530.)

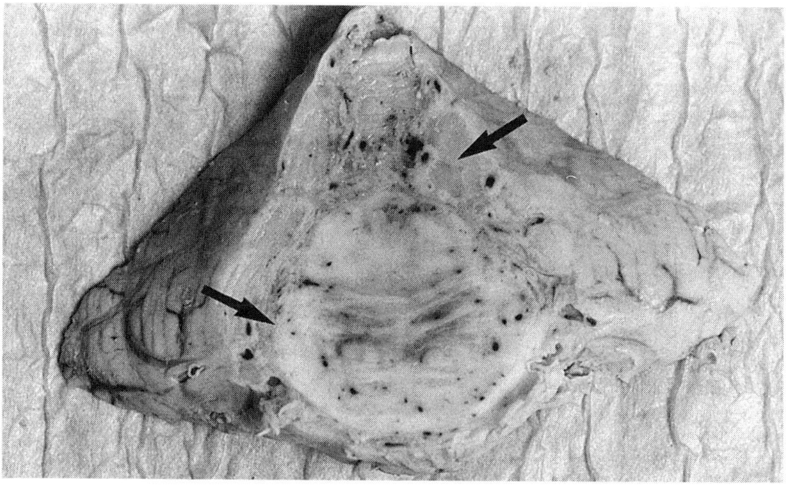

**Figure 4.30** Transverse section of the pons and cerebellum of a patient with *Mycobacterium tuberculosis* meningitis. The meninges around the pons are thickened (arrows); those of the cerebellum are spared.

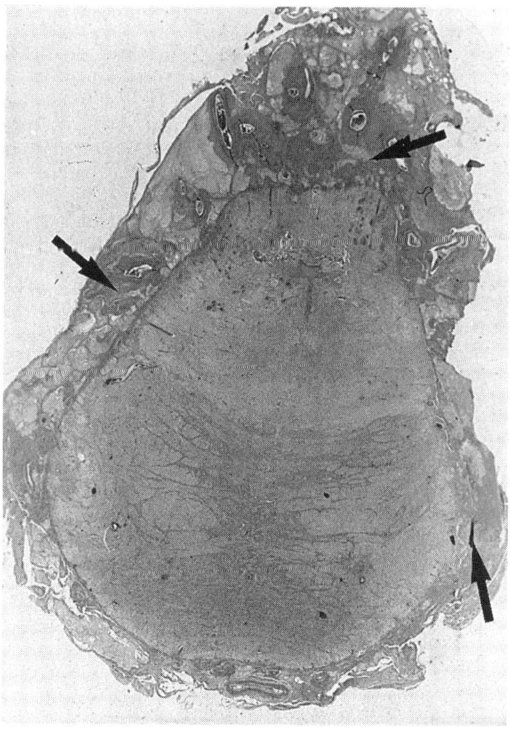

**Figure 4.31** Spectacular thickening of the meninges (arrows) in the pons of the same patient as in Figure 4.30. (Paraffin section; H&E.)

### *Histoplasma caspulatum*

Several cases of meningitis or granulomatous encephalitis related to *H. caspulatum* have been observed (Bonner *et al.*, 1984; Wheat *et al.*, 1985; Anders *et al.*, 1986; Chimelli *et al.*, 1992).

## BACTERIAL INFECTIONS

Although less common than opportunistic viral and parasitic infections, different types of bacteria may infect the CNS or meninges during the course of HIV infection (Johns *et al.*, 1987). Most of them are treatable if the diagnosis is made early enough.

### Syphilis

Some cases of syphilitic meningoradiculitis have emerged in association with HIV infection (Kato *et al.*, 1987; Whiteside *et al.*, 1987; Lanska and Lanska, 1989) and prospective studies suggest an increased prevalence of neurosyphilis in patients with HIV infection (Holtom *et al.*, 1992; Katz *et al.*, 1993), most patients having asymptomatic neurosyphilis (Berger, 1991). HIV infection can alter the natural history of neurosyphilis by concurrent infection (Berry *et al.*, 1987a). Positivity of VDRL (Venereal Disease Reference Laboratory) test in the CSF may be delayed (Feraru *et al.*, 1990). Neurological relapse may occur after benzathine penicillin treatment for early syphilis (Berry *et al.*, 1987b; Johns *et al.*, 1987) or for neurosyphilis. High doses of penicillin are suggested by some authors (Whiteside *et al.*, 1987). Recent studies on the response of symptomatic neurosyphilis to high-dose intravenous penicillin G in patients with HIV infection showed that therapy may fail and neurosyphilis may occur in patients with early syphilis and HIV infection. However, failure of treatment could not be predicted since patients with clear failure of treatment did not have the highest RPR (rapid plasma reagin) or VDRL titres at diagnosis and their $CD4^+$ T-cell counts were not the lowest (Musher *et al.*, 1990; Gordon *et al.*, 1994).

### *Mycobacterium tuberculosis*

Tuberculous meningitis is the most frequent neurological complication of *M. tuberculosis* in patients with HIV infection (Kure *et al.*, 1991; Berenguer *et al.*, 1992; Matthiessen *et al.*, 1992). Most patients are drug abusers (Bishburg *et al.*, 1986; Berenguer *et al.*, 1992) or Haitians (Levy *et al.*, 1988). The meningitis may occur as the first manifestation of AIDS (Berenguer *et al.*, 1992). Clinical symptoms and response to therapy are similar to tuberculous meningitis (Kure *et al.*, 1991; Berenguer *et al.*, 1992). In some cases, the CSF remains acellular (Laguna *et al.*, 1992), which may occasionally occur in non-HIV-infected patients. One of our patients, who was not known to be HIV positive at the time of admission, was admitted comatose and died within 24 hours. CT showed ventricular enlargement and contrast enhancement of the posterior fossa. Post-mortem examination showed spectacular thickening of the meninges around

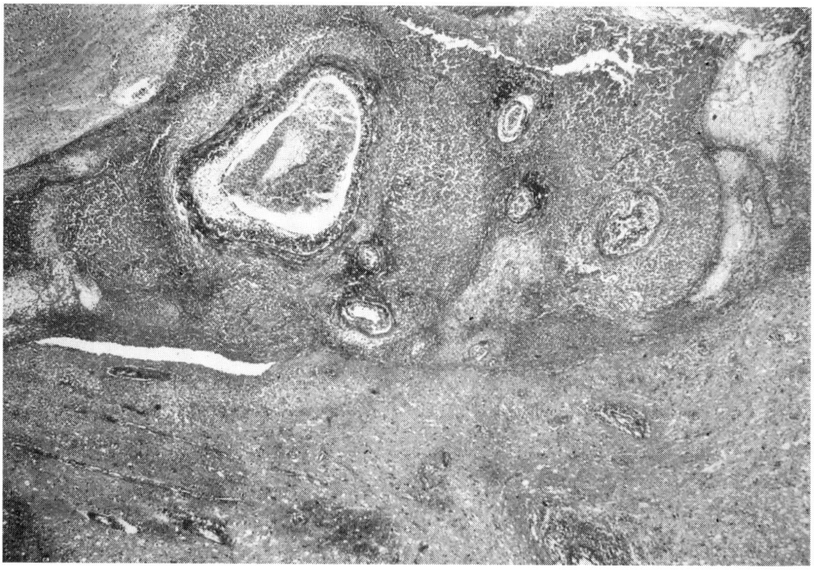

**(a)**

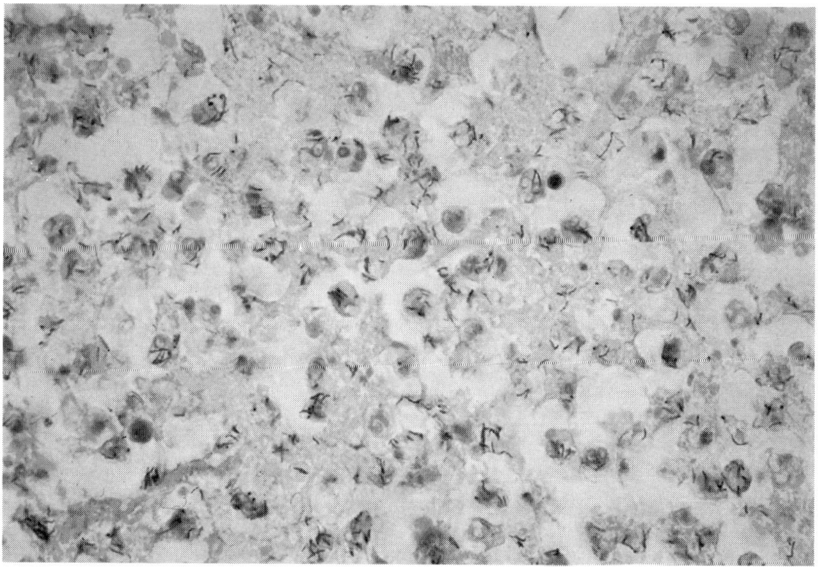

**(b)**

**Figure 4.32** (a) Thickening of the leptomeninges associated with proliferation of vessels in a patient with *Mycobacterium tuberculosis* meningitis around the brainstem. (Paraffin section; H&E; ×60.) (b) Higher magnification of the leptomeninges showing numerous acid-fast bacilli isolated or in macrophages. (Paraffin section; Ziehl stain; ×1530.)

the brainstem (Figures 4.30 and 4.31) with numerous acid-fast bacilli in the meninges and the Virchow spaces (Figure 4.32). Cerebral abscesses and tuberculomas may develop in the brain and spinal cord (Bishburg *et al.*, 1986; Kure *et al.*, 1991; Melhem and Wang, 1992). Diagnosis is usually made after death.

*Mycobacterium avium-intracellulare* and *Mycobacterium kansasii* have occasionally been encountered (Levy *et al.*, 1988; Matthiessen *et al.*, 1992).

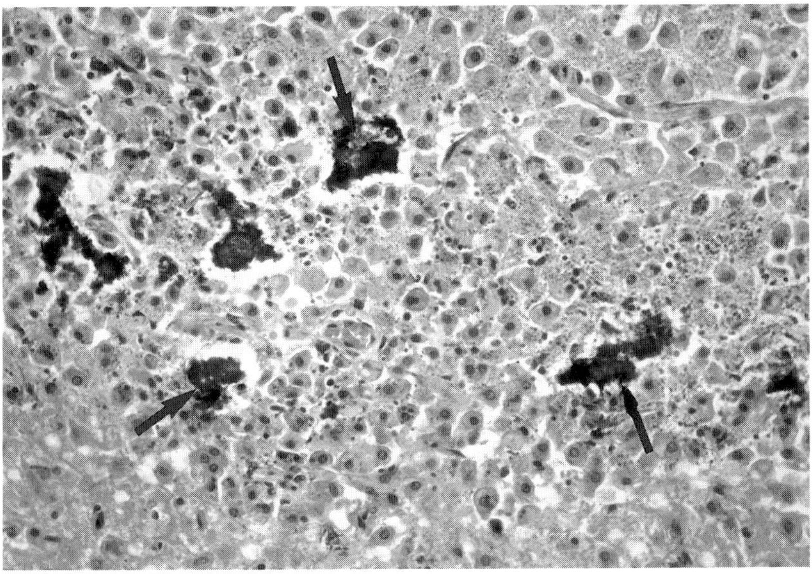

**Figure 4.33** Old brain abscess with macrophages and calcifications (arrows). No organism was detected. (Paraffin section; H&E; ×480.)

### Other bacterial infections

Cerebral abscesses due to *Nocardia* may be observed in patients with HIV infection (Sharer and Kapila, 1985; Adair *et al.*, 1987). *Listeria monocytogenes* may be responsible for meningitis (Decker *et al.*, 1991) and brain abscesses (Harris *et al.*, 1989). As reported by others (Kure *et al.*, 1991; Chimelli *et al.*, 1992), in our experience multiple brain abscesses or microabscesses are present at autopsy without identifiable organisms (Figure 4.33).

## REFERENCES


Achim CL and Wiley CA (1992) Expression of major histocompatibility complex antigens in the brains of patients with progressive multifocal leukoencephalopathy. *Journal of Neuropathology and Experimental Neurology* **51**: 257–263.

Adair JC, Beck AC, Apfelbaum RI and Baringer JR (1987) Nocardial cerebral abscesses in the acquired immunodeficiency syndrome. *Archives of Neurology* **44**: 548–550.

Aksamit AJ, Mourrain P, Sever JL and Major EO (1985) Progressive multifocal leukoencephalopathy: investigation of three cases using *in situ* hybridization with JC virus biotinylated DNA probe. *Annals of Neurology* **18**: 490–496.

Aksamit AJ, Major EO, Ghatak NR *et al.* (1987) Diagnosis of progressive multifocal leukoencephalopathy by brain biopsy with biotin labelled DNA: DNA *in situ* hybridization. *Journal of Neuropathology and Experimental Neurology* **46**: 556–566.

Aksamit AJ, Gendelman HE, Orenstein JM and Pezeshkpour GH (1990) AIDS-associated progressive multifocal leukoencephalopathy (PML): comparison to non-AIDS PML with *in situ* hybridization and immunocytochemistry. *Neurology* **40**: 1073–1078.

Alonso R, Heiman-Patterson T and Mancall EL (1984) Cerebral toxoplasmosis in acquired immune deficiency syndrome. *Archives of Neurology* **41**: 321–323.

Anders KH, Guerra WF, Tomiyasu U *et al.* (1986) The neuropathology of AIDS: UCLA experience and review. *American Journal of Pathology* **124**: 537–558.

Anders KH, Holden JL, Becker PS and Vinters HV (1990) Focal pontine leukoencephalopathy. A review of ten cases. *Journal of Neuropathology and Experimental Neurology* **49**: 315.

Anger S, Maero E, Blanco JC *et al.* (1992) Early diagnosis of toxoplasmic encephalitis in AIDS patients by dot blot hybridization analysis. *Journal of Clinical Microbiology* **30**: 3286–3287.

Anzil AP, Rao C, Wrzolek MA, Visvesvara GS, Sher JH and Kozlowski PB (1991) Amoebic meningoencephalitis in a patient with AIDS caused by a newly recognised opportunistic pathogen, *Leptomyxid amoeba. Archives of Pathology and Laboratory Medicine* **115**: 21–25.

Araujo FG, Guptil DR and Remington JS (1988) Azithromycin, a macrolide antibiotic with potent activity against *Toxoplasma gondii. Antimicrobial Agents and Chemotherapy* **32**: 755–757.

Araujo FG, Huskinson J and Remington JS (1991) Remarkable *in vitro* and *in vivo* activities of the hydroxynaphthoquinone 566C80 against tachyzoites and tissue cysts of *Toxoplasma gondii. Antimicrobial Agents and Chemotherapy* **35**: 293–299.

Araujo FG, Lin T and Remington JS (1992) Synergistic combination of azithromycin and sulfadiazine for treatment of toxoplasmosis in mice. *European Journal of Clinical Microbiology and Infectious Diseases* **11**: 71–72.

Araujo FG, Lin T and Remington JS (1993) The activity of atovaquone (566C80) in murine toxoplasmosis is markedly augmented when used in combination with pyrimethamine or sulfadiazine. *Journal of Infectious Diseases* **167**: 494–497.

Aspock H and Hassl A (1990) Parasitic infections in HIV patients in Austria: first results of a long-term study. *Zentralblatt fur Bakteriologie* **272**: 540–546.

Aström KE, Mancall EL and Richardson EP (1958) Progressive multifocal leukoencephalopathy. *Brain* **81**: 93–111.

Bale JF (1984) Human cytomegalovirus infection and disorders of the nervous system. *Archives of Neurology* **41**: 310–320.

Beaman MH, Luft BJ, Remington JS (1992) Prophylaxis for toxoplasmosis in AIDS. *Annals of Internal Medicine* **117**: 163 64.

Beaman MH, McCabe RE, Wong SY and Remington JS (1994) *Toxoplasma gondii.* In: *Principles and Practice of Infectious Diseases* (eds GL Mandell, RG Douglas and JE Bennett), 4th edn, pp. 2455–2474. New York: Churchill Livingstone.

Berenguer J, Moreno S, Laguna F *et al.* (1992) Tuberculosa meningitis in patients infected with the human immunodeficiency virus. *New England Journal of Medicine* **326**: 668–672.

Berger JR (1991) Neurosyphilis in human immunodeficiency virus type 1-seropositive individuals: a prospective study. *Archives of Neurology* **48**: 700–702.

Berger JR and Mucke L (1988) Prolonged survival and partial recovery in AIDS-associated progressive multifocal leukoencephalopathy. *Neurology* **38**: 1060–1064.

Berger JR, Albrecht J, Tornatore C *et al.* (1991). Progressive multifocal leukoencephalopathy in an HIV-1 infected child (abstract). Presented at HIV Infection Basic and Clinical Frontiers, a satellite conference prior to the VII International Conference on AIDS, Padova, Italy.

Berman S, Kim R, Hook E *et al.* (1992) Cytomegalovirus encephalitis in patients receiving glanciclovir for cytomegalovirus retinitis. 7th Conference on AIDS. Florence, Italy.

Berry CD, Hooton TM, Collier AV *et al.* (1987a) Neurosyphilis and HIV infection. *New England Journal of Medicine* **317**: 1475.

Berry CD, Hooton TM, Collier AV *et al.* (1987b) Neurologic relapse after benzathine penicillin therapy for secondary syphilis in a patient with HIV infection. *New England Journal of Medicine* **316**: 1587–1589.

Bishburg E, Sunderam G, Reichman LB *et al.* (1986) Central nervous system tuberculosis with the acquired immunodeficiency syndrome and its related complex. *Annals of Internal Medicine* **105**: 210–213.

Blas C and Meary E (1991) La neuro-imagerie dans les infections par le VIH et les infections opportunistes. In *Manifestations Neurologiques et Infections Rétrovirales: SIDA et Autres Rétroviroses* (eds G Said and AG Saimot), pp. 77–97. Paris: Pradel.

Blum RN, Miller LA, Gaggini, Cohn DL (1992) Comparative trial of dapsone versus trimethoprim/sulfamethoxazole for primary prophylaxis of *Pneumocystis carnii* pneumonia. *Journal of Acquired Immune Deficiency Syndrome* **5**: 341–47.

Bonner JR, Alexander J, Dismukes WE *et al.* (1984) Disseminated histoplasmosis in patients with the acquired immunodeficiency syndrome. *Achives of Internal Medicine* **144**: 2178.

Booss J, Dann PR, Griffith BP and Kim JH (1989) Host defense response to cytomegalovirus in the central nervous system. *American Journal of Pathology* **134**: 71–78.

Bougnoux ME, Nicaise P, Heyerc F *et al.* (1990) Diagnostic de la toxoplasmose cérébrale chez les sidéens. Valeur de la recherche d'anticorps dans le liquide céphalorachidien. *Presse Medicale* **19**: 1751–1753.

Bozzette SA, Finkelstein DM, Spector SA *et al.* (1995) A randomized trial of three antipneumocystis agents in patients with advanced human immunodeficiency virus infection. *New England Journal of Medicine* **332**: 693–699.

Britton CB, Mesa-Tejada R, Fenoglio CM *et al.* (1985) A new complication of AIDS: thoracic myelitis caused by herpes simplex virus. *Neurology* **35**: 1071–1074.

Bronnimann DA, Adam RD, Galgani JN *et al.* (1987) Disseminated coccidioidomycosis in the acquired immunodeficiency syndrome. *Annals of Internal Medicine* **106**: 372.

Budka H, Costanzi G, Cristina S *et al.* (1987) Brain pathology induced by infection with the human immunodeficiency virus (HIV): 100 autopsy cases. *Acta Neuropathologica* **75**: 185–198.

Burns DK, Risser RC and White CL (1991) The neuropathology of HIV infection: the Dallas experience. *Journal of Neuropathology and Experimental Neurology* **50**: 323.

Carr A, Tindall B, Brew BJ *et al.* (1992) Low-dose trimethoprmsulfamethoxazole prophylaxis for toxoplasmic encephalitis in patients with AIDS. *Annals of Internal Medicine* **117**: 106–11.

Carr A, Gross AS, Hoskins JM *et al.* (1994) Acetylation phenotype and cutaneous hypersensitivity to trimethoprim-sulphamethoxazole in HIV-infected patients. *AIDS* **8**: 333–337.

Cavallito JC, Nichol CA, Brenckman Jr WD *et al.* (1978) Lipid-soluble inhibitors of dihydrofolate reductase. I. Kinetics, tissue distribution and extent of metabolism of pyrimethamine, metroprime, and etoprine in the rat, dog, and man. *Drug Metabolism and Disposition* **6**: 329–337.

Chang HR and Pechere JC (1988) *In vitro* effects of four macrolides (roxithromycin, spiramycin, azithromycin, CP-62,93 and A-56,268) on *Toxoplasma gondii*. *Antimicrobial Agents and Chemotherapy* **32**: 524–529.

Chappell ET, Guthrie BL and Orenstein J (1992) The role of stereotactic biopsy in the management of HIV-related focal brain lesions. *Neurosurgery* **30**: 825–829.

Chatterton JMW (1992) Pregnancy. In: *Human Toxoplasmosis* (eds Do Ho–Yen and AWL Joss), pp. 144–183. Oxford: Oxford University Press.

Chimelli L, de Freitas MRG, Bazin AR *et al.* (1990) Encéphalo-myélo-radiculite à cytomégalovirus au cours du syndrome d'immuno-déficience acquise. *Revue Neurologique* **146**: 354–360.

Chimelli L, Rosemberg S, Hahn MD *et al.* (1992) Pathology of the central nervous system in patients infected with the human immunodeficiency virus (HIV): a report of 252 autopsy cases from Brazil. *Neuropathology and Applied Neurobiology* **18**: 478–488.

Chiriani A, Tullio CP, Orefice G *et al.* (1992) Probability of developing cerebral toxoplasmosis in patients with AIDS in relation to serology for anti-*Toxoplasma gondii*. VIIIth International Conference on AIDs, Amsterdam 1992.

Chrétien F, Gray F, Lescs MC *et al.* (1993) Acute varicella-zoster virus ventriculitis and meningo-myelo-radiculitis in acquired immunodeficiency syndrome. *Acta Neuropathologica* **86**: 659–665.

Cimino C, Lipton RB, Williams A *et al.* (1991) The evaluation of patients with human immunodeficiency virus-related disorders and brain mass lesions. *Archives of Internal Medicine* **151**: 1381–1384.

Cinque P, Vago L, Brytting M *et al.* (1992) Cytomegalovirus infection of the central nervous system in patients with AIDS: diagnosis by DNA amplification from cerebrospinal fluid. *Journal of Infectious Diseases* **166**: 1408–1411.

Cinque P, Brytting M, Vago L *et al.* (1993) Epstein–Barr virus DNA in cerebral fluid from patients with AIDS-related primary lymphoma of the central nervous system. *Lancet* **342**: 398–401.

Ciricillo SF and Rosenblum ML (1990) Use of CT and MR imaging to distinguish intracranial lesions and to define the need for biopsy in AIDS patients. *Journal of Neurosurgery* **73**: 720–724.

Clifford DB, Buller RS, Mohammed S *et al.* (1993) Use of polymerase chain reaction to demonstrate cytomegalovirus DNA in CSF of patients with human immunodeficiency virus infection. *Neurology* **43**: 75–79.

Clumeck N (1991) Some aspects of the epidemiology of toxoplasmosis and pneumocystosis in AIDS in Europe. *European Journal of Clinical Microbiology and Infectious Diseases* **10**: 177–178.

Clumeck N, Sonnet J, Taelman H *et al.* (1984) Acquired immunodeficiency syndrome in African patients. *New England Journal of Medicine* **310**: 492–497.

Cochereau-Massin I, LeHoang P and Lautier-Frau M (1992) Ocular toxoplasmosis in human immunodeficiency virus-infected patients. *American Journal of Ophthalmology* **114**: 130–135.

Cohen JI and Corey GR (1985) Cytomegalovirus infection in the normal host. *Medicine* **64**: 100–114.

Cohn J, McMeeking A, Cohen W, Jacobs J and Holzman RS (1989) Evaluation of the policy of empirical treatment of suspected *Toxoplasma* encephalitis in patients with the acquired immunodeficiency syndrome. *American Journal of Medicine* **86**: 521–527.

Comley JCW and Sterling AM (1995) Effect of atovaquone and atovaquone drug combinations on prophylaxis of *Pneumocystis carinii* pneumonia in SCID mice. *Antimicrobial Agents and Chemotherapy*, **39**: 806–811.

Conway B, Halliday WC and Brunham RC (1990) Human immunodeficiency virus-associated progressive multifocal leukoencephalopathy: apparent response to 3′-azido-3′deoxythymidine. *Review of Infectious Diseases* **12**: 479–482.

Cook MK and Jacobs L (1958) *In vitro* investigations on the action of pyrimethamine against *Toxoplasma gondii*. *Journal of Parasitology* **44**: 280–288.

Coopman SA, Johnson RA, Platt R, Stern RS (1993) Cutaneous disease and drug reactions in HIV infection. *New England Journal of Medicine* **328**: 1670–1674.

Crowe SM, Carlin JB, Stewart KI *et al.* (1991) Predictive value of CD4 lymphocyte numbers for the development of opportunistic infections and malignancies in HIV-infected persons. *Journal of Acquired Immune Deficiency Syndromes* **4**: 770–776.

Daniel P (1992) Randomised daily vs twice weekly maintenance therapy with sulfadiazine pyrimethamine for cerebral toxoplasmosis in AIDS patients. Preliminary results. *VIII International Conference on AIDS, Amsterdam, The Netherlands, 19–24 July*, Abstract B126.

Dannemann B, McCutchan JA, Israelski D *et al.* (1992) Treatment of toxoplasmic encephalitis in patients with AIDS: a randomised trial comparing pyrimethamine plus clindamycin to pyrimethamine plus sulfadiazine. *Annals of Internal Medicine* **116**: 33–43.

Decker CF, Simon GL, DiGiola RA and Tuazon CU (1991) *Listeria monocytogenes* infections in patients with AIDS: report for five cases and review. *Review of Infectious Diseases* **13**: 413–417.

de la Monte SM, Ho DD, Schooley RT *et al.* (1987) Subacute encephalomyelitis of AIDS and its relation to HTLV-III infection. *Neurology* **37**: 562–569.

De La Paz R and Enzmann D (1988) Neuroradiology of acquired immunodeficiency syndrome. In: *AIDS and the Nervous System* (ed. ML Rosenblum), pp. 21–154. New York: Raven Press.

Dement SH, Cox MC and Gupta PK (1987) Diagnosis of central nervous system. *Toxoplasma gondii* from the cerebrospinal fluid in a patient with acquired immunodeficiency syndrome. *Diagnostic Cytopathology* **3**: 148–151.

Derouin F, Thulliez Ph and Garin YJF (1991) Intérêt et limites de la sérologie de toxoplasmose chez les sujets VIH+. *Pathologie Biologie* **39**: 255–259.

Devinski O, Cho E-S, Petito CK and Price RW (1991) Herpes zoster myelitis. *Brain* **114**: 1811–1196.

Dina TS (1991) Primary central nervous system lymphoma versus toxoplasmosis in AIDS. *Radiology* **179**: 823–828.

Dix RD, Waitzmann DM, Follansbee S *et al.* (1985) Herpes simplex virus type 2 encephalitis in two homosexual men with persistent lymphadenopathy. *Annals of Neurology* **17**: 203–206.

Dournon E, Matheron S, Rozenbaum W *et al.* (1988) Effects of zidovudine in 365 consecutive patients with AIDS or AIDS-related complex. Lancet **1988(ii)**: 1297–1300.

Drew WL, Miner RC, Busch DF *et al.* (1991) Prevalence of resistance in patients receiving ganciclovir for serious cytomegalovirus infection. *Journal of Infectious Diseases* **163**: 716–719.

Drew WL, Ives D, Lalezari JP *et al.* (1995) Oral ganciclovir as maintenance treatment for cytomegalovirus retinitis in patients with AIDS. *New England Journal of Medicine* **333**: 615–620.

Dubey JP (1986) A review of toxoplasmosis in pigs. *Veterinary Parasitology* **19**: 181–223.

Dubey JP and Beattie CP (1988) *Toxoplasmosis of Animals and Man*. Boca Raton, Florida: CRC Press.

Dumas N, Cazaux M and Seguela JP (1991) Épidémiologie de la toxoplasmose chez la mère et l'enfant en Afrique tropicale. *Bulletin de la Societe de Pathologie Exotique et de ses Filiales* **84**: 645–658.

Dupouy-Camet J, Lavareda de Souza S, Maslo C *et al.* (1993) Detection of *Toxoplasma gondii* in venous blood from AIDS patients by polymerase chain reaction. *Journal of Clinical Microbiology* **31**: 1866–1869.

Dupuis M, Fernandez Xavier FG, Gonsette RE and Brucher JM (1986) Progressive multifocal leukoencephalopathy mimicking multiple sclerosis as the sole clinical manifestation of acquired immunodeficiency syndrome. *Acta Neurologica Belgica* **86**: 285–296.

Edwards KR and Pendlebury WW (1987) Central nervous system lymphomas versus toxoplasmosis in a patient with AIDS. *New England Journal of Medicine* **317**: 1540.

Edwards RH, Messing R and McKendall RR (1985) Cytomegalovirus meningoencephalitis in a homosexual man with Kaposi's sarcoma: isolation of CMV from CSF cells. *Neurology* **35**: 560–562.

Elbright JR and Crane LR (1991) Ganciclovir-resistant cytomegalovirus. *AIDS* **5**: 604.

Eliaszewicz M, Lecomte I and De Sa M (1990) Relation between decreasing serial CD4 lymphocyte count and outcome of toxoplasmosis in AIDS patients: a basis for primary prophylaxis. *VI International Conference on AIDS, San Francisco, California, 20–24 June*, Abstract ThB 481.

Enting R, de Gans J, Reiss P *et al.* (1992). Ganciclovir/foscarnet for cytomegalovirus meningoencephalitis in AIDS (letter). *Lancet* **340**: 559–560.

European Centre for the Epidemiological Monitoring of AIDS (WHO-EC Collaborating Centre on AIDS) (1994) *AIDS Surveillance in Europe*. Quarterly report no. 44.

European Centre for the Epidemiological Monitoring of AIDS (WHO-EC Collaborating Centre on AIDS) (1995) *AIDS Surveillance in Europe*. Quarterly report no. 45.

Eyles DE and Coleman N (1953) Synergistic effect of sulfadiazine and daraprim against experimental toxoplasmosis in the mouse. *Antibiotics and Chemotherapy* **3**: 483–490.

Eyles DE and Coleman N (1955) An evaluation of the curative effects of pyrimethamine and sulfadiazine, alone and in combination in experimental mouse toxoplasmosis. *Antibiotics and Chemotherapy* **5**: 529–539.

Farkash AE, MacCabee PJ, Sher JH, Landesman SH and Hotson G (1986) CNS toxoplasmosis in acquired immune deficiency syndrome: a clinical–pathological–radiological review of 12 cases. *Journal of Neurology, Neurosurgery and Psychiatry* **49**: 744–748.

Feldman HA (1965) A nation-wide serum survey of United States military recruits, 1962. VI: *Toxoplasma* antibodies. *American Journal of Epidemiology* **81**: 385–391.

Feldman HA (1982) Epidemiology of *Toxoplasma* infection. *Epidemiologic Reviews* **4**: 204–213.

Feraru ER, Aronow HA and Lipton RB (1990) Neurosyphilis in AIDS patients: initial CSF VDRL may be negative. *Neurology* **40**: 541–543.

Ferreira S, Nishioka S, de Rocha A *et al.* (1991) Acute fatal *Tryanosoma cruzi* meningoencephalitis in a human immunodeficiency virus-positive haemophiliac patient. *American Journal of Tropical Medicine and Hygiene* **45**: 723–727.

Fiala M, Singer EJ, Graves MC *et al.* (1993) AIDS dementia complex complicated by cytomegalovirus encephalopathy. *Journal of Neurology* **240**: 223–231.

Friedman D (1991) Neuro-ophthalmic manifestations of human immunodeficiency virus infection. *Neurologic Clinics* **9**: 55–72.

Gardner HA, Martinez AJ, Visvesvara GS and Sotrel A (1991) Granulomatous amoebic encephalitis in an AIDS patient. *Neurology* **41**: 993–995.

Gastaut JL, Nicoli F, Somma-Mauvais H *et al.* (1992) Hémichorée-hémiballisme et toxoplasmose au cours du SIDA. *Revue Neurologique* **148**: 785–788.

Giberson TP and Kalyan-Raman K (1987) Cryptococcal meningitis: initial presentation of acquired immunodeficiency syndrome. *Annals of Emergency Medicine* **16**: 802–804.

Gilden DH, Murray RS, Wellish BS *et al.* (1988) Chronic progressive varicella-zoster virus encephalitis in an AIDS patient. *Neurology* **38**: 1150–1153.

Gill PS, Graham RA, Boswell W, Meyer P, Krailo M and Levine AM (1986) A comparison of imaging, clinical and pathologic aspects of space-occupying lesions within the brain in patients with acquired immune deficiency syndrome. *American Journal of Physiologic Imaging* **1**: 134–141.

Girard PM, Lepretre A, Detruchig P, Matheson S, Conlard JP (1989) Failure of pyrimethamine-dindamycin combination for prophylaxis of *Pneumocystis carinii* pneumonia. *Lancet* **1989,ii**: 1459.

Girard PM, Landman R, Gaudebout CL *et al.* (1993) Dapsone–pyrimethamine compared with aerosolized pentamidine as primary prophylaxis against *Pneumocystis carinii* pneumonia and toxoplasmosis. *New England Journal of Medicine* **328**: 1514–1520.

Glaser CA, Angulo FJ and Rooney JA (1994) Animal-associated opportunistic infections among persons infected with the human immunodeficiency virus. *Clinical Infectious Diseases* **18**: 14–24.

Gordin FM, Simon GL, Wotsy CB, Mills J (1984) Adverse reactions to trimethoprim-sulphamethoxazle in patients with the acquired immunodeficiency syndrome. *Annals of Internal Medicine* **100**: 495–499.

Gordon SM, Eaton ME, George R *et al.* (1994) The response of symptomatic neurosyphilis to high-dose intravenous penicillin G in patients with human immunodeficiency virus infection. *New England Journal of Medicine* **331**: 1469–1473.

Gozlan J, Salord JM, Roullet E *et al.* (1992) Rapid detection of cytomegalovirus DNA in cerebrospinal fluid of AIDS patients with neurologic disorders. *Journal of Infectious Diseases* **166**: 1416–1421.

Graefin von Einsiedel R, Fiala M and Vinters HV (1992) Severe granulomatous meningoencephalitis with CNS cryptococcosis (abstract). *Journal of Neuropathology and Experimental Neurology* **51**: 375.

Grafe MR and Wiley CA (1989) Spinal cord and peripheral nerve pathology in AIDS: the roles of cytomegalovirus and human immunodeficiency virus. *Annals of Neurology* **25**: 561–566.

Grant IH, Gold JMW, Rosenblum M *et al.* (1990) *Toxoplasma gondii* serology in HIV-infected patients: the development of central nervous system toxoplasmosis in AIDS. *AIDS* **4**: 519–521.

Gray F, Gherardi R, Keohane C *et al.* (1988) Pathology of the central nervous system in 40 cases of acquired immune deficiency syndrome (AIDS). *Neuropathology and Applied Neurobiology* **14**: 365–380.

Gray F, Gherardi R, Wingate E *et al.* (1989) Diffuse 'encephalitic' cerebral toxoplasmosis in AIDS. Report of four cases. *Journal of Neurology* **236**: 273–277.

Gray F, Mohr M, Rozenberg F *et al.* (1992) Varicella-zoster virus encephalitis in acquired immunodeficiency syndrome: report of four cases. *Neuropathology and Applied Neurobiology* **18**: 502–514.

Grob U, Roggenkamp A, Janitschke K and Heesemann J (1992) Improved sensitivity of the polymerase chain reaction for detection of *Toxoplasma grondii* in biological and human clinical specimens. *European Journal of Clinical Microbiology and Infectious Diseases* **11**: 33–39.

Guichard A, Zamora L, Caumes E *et al.* (1991) Cutaneous side-effects: a major problem in the treatment of toxoplasmosis encephalitis. *VII International Conference on AIDS, Florence,* Abstract MB2188.

Hair LS, Nuovo G, Powers JM *et al.* (1992) Progressive multifocal leukoencephalopathy in patients with human immunodeficiency virus. *Human Pathology* **23**: 663–667.

Handler M, Ho V, Whelan M and Budzilovitch G (1983) Intracerebral toxoplasmosis in patients with acquired immune deficiency syndrome. *Journal of Neurosurgery* **59**: 994–1001.

Hardy WD, Veinberg J, Finkelstein D. *et al.* (1992) A controlled trial of trimethoprim-sulfamethoxazole or aerosolized pentamidine for secondary prophylaxis of *Pneumocystis carinii* penumonia in patients with the acquired immunodeficiency syndrome. AIDS Clinical Trials Group Protocol 021. *New England Journal of Medicine* **327**: 1842–1848.

Harris JO, Marquez J, Serdloff MA and Magana IA (1989) *Listeria* brain abscess in the acquired immunodeficiency syndrome. *Archives of Neurology* **46**: 250.

Harris TM, Smith RR, Bognanno JR and Edwards MK (1990) Toxoplasmic myelitis in AIDS: gadolinium-enhanced MR. *Journal of Computer Assisted Tomography* **14**. 809–811.

Hauser WE, Luft BJ, Conley BK *et al.* (1982) Central nervous system toxoplasmosis in homosexual and heterosexual adults. *New England Journal of Medicine* **307**: 498–499.

Haverkos HW (1987) Assessment of therapy for *Toxoplasma* encephalitis. The toxoplasmic encephalitis study group. *American Journal of Medicine* **82**: 907–914.

Heald A, Flepp M, Chave J-P *et al.* (1991) Treatment of cerebral toxoplasmosis protects against *Pneumocystis carinii* pneumonia in patients with AIDS. *Annals of Internal Medicine* **115**: 760–763.

Herskovitz S, Siegel SE, Schneider AT, Nelson SJ, Goodrich JT and Lantos G (1989) Spinal cord toxoplasmosis in AIDS. *Neurology* **39**: 1552–1553.

Hirschel B, Lazzarin A, Chopard P *et al.*, (1991) A controlled study of inhaled pentamidine for primary prevention of *Pneumocystis carinii* pneumonia. *New England Journal of Medicine* **324**: 1079–1083.

Hirschel B, Landman R and Oksenhendler E (1993) Prophylaxie primaire de la toxoplasmose au cours de l'infection par le VIH. Eléments de recommandation. *Médecine et Maladies Infectieuses (Spécial)* **23**: 731–760.

Holland GN, Engstrom RE Jr, Glasgow BJ *et al.* (1988) Ocular toxoplasmosis in patients with the acquired immunodeficiency syndrome. *American Journal of Ophthalmology* **106**: 653–667.

Holland NR, Power C, Mathews VP *et al.* (1994) Cytomegalovirus encephalitis in acquired immunodeficiency syndrome (AIDS). *Neurology* **44**: 507–514.

Holliman RE, Johnson JD and Sawa D (1990) Diagnosis of cerebral toxoplasmosis in association with AIDS using the polymerase chain reaction. *Scandinavian Journal of Infectious Diseases* **22**: 243–244.

Holmann RC, Janssen RS, Buehler JW *et al.* (1991) Epidemiology of progressive multifocal leukoencephalopathy in the United States: analysis of national mortality and AIDS surveillance data. *Neurology* **41**: 1733–1736.

Holtom PD, Larsen RA, Leal ME and Leedom JM (1992) Prevalence of neurosyphilis in human immunodeficiency virus-infected patients with latent syphilis. *American Journal of Medicine* **93**: 9–12.

Horowitz S, Bentson JR, Bentson DF *et al.* (1983) CNS toxoplasmosis in acquired immunodeficiency syndrome. *Archives of Neurology* **40**: 649–652.

Houff SA, Major EO, Katz DA *et al.* (1988) Involvement of JC virus-infected mononuclear cells from the bone marrow and spleen in the pathogenesis of progressive multifocal leukoencephalopathy. *New England Journal of Medicine* **318**: 301–305.

Hu DJ, Fleming PL, Jones JL and Ward JW (1995) Epidemiology of protozoal opportunistic infections (POI) among persons with AIDS in the United States. *34th Interscience Conference on Antimicrobial Agents and Therapy Orlando*, Abstract I 161.

Huang TE and Chou SM (1988) Occlusive hypertrophic arteritis as the cause of discrete necrosis in CNS toxoplasmosis in the acquired immunodeficiency syndrome. *Human Pathology* **19**: 1210–1214.

Ibars IB, Matias-Guiu J, Cervera C and Puiggros AC (1987) Cryptococcal meningitis and cerebral toxoplasmosis in AIDS: another case report. *Journal of Neurology, Neurosurgery and Psychiatry* **50**: 116–118.

Ironside JW, Lewis FA, Blythe D and Wakefield EA (1989) The identification of cells containing JC papova virus DNA in progressive multifocal leukoencephalopathy by combined *in situ* hybridization and immunocytochemistry. *Journal of Pathology* **157**: 291–297.

Israelski D and Remington JS (1988) Toxoplasmic encephalitis in patients with AIDS. *Infectious Disease Clinics of North America* **2**: 429–444.

Israelski DM and Remington JS (1993) Toxoplasmosis in patients with cancer. *Clinical Infectious Diseases* **17** (Suppl. 2): S423-S435.

Israelski DM, Chmiel JS, Poggensee L, Phair JP and Remington JS (1993) Prevalence of *Toxoplasma* infection in a cohort of homosexual men at risk of AIDS and toxoplasmic encephalitis. *Journal of Acquired Immune Deficiency Syndromes* **6**: 414–418.

Itoyama Y, Webster HD, Sternberger NH *et al.* (1982) Distribution of papovavirus, myelin-associated glycoprotein, and myelin basic protein in progressive multifocal leuko-encephalopathy lesions. *Annals of Neurology* **11**: 396–407.

Jabs DA, Davis MD, Meinert CL *et al.* (1992) Mortality in patients with AIDS treated with either foscarnet or ganciclovir for cytomegalovirus retinitis. *New England Journal of Medicine* **326**: 213–220.

Jackson MH and Hutchison WM (1989) The prevalence and source of *Toxoplasma* infection in the environment. *Advances in Parasitology* **28**: 55–105.

Jacobson MA and Mills J (1988) Serious cytomegalovirus disease in the acquired immunodeficiency syndrome (AIDS). *Annals of Internal Medicine* **108**: 585–594.

Jacobson MA, Mills J, O'Donnel J *et al.* (1988) Failure of antiviral therapy for acquired immunodeficiency syndrome-related cytomegalovirus myelitis. *Archives of Neurology* **45**: 1090–1092.

Jacobson MA, Besch CL, Child B *et al.* (1991) Randomized study of clindamycin (C) or pyrimethamine (P) prophylaxis for toxoplasmic encephalitis (toxoplasmic encephalitis) in patients with advanced HIV disease. *31st Interscience Conference on Antimicrobial Agents and Chemotherapy*, Abstract 298.

Jacobson MA, Besch CL, Child C *et al.* (1992) Toxicity of clindamycin as prophylaxis for AIDS-associated toxoplasmic encephalitis. Programs for Clinical Research on AIDS. *Lancet* **339**: 333–4.

Jarvik JG, Hesselink JR, Kennedy C *et al.* (1988a) Acquired immunodeficiency syndrome. Magnetic resonance patterns of brain involvement with pathologic correlation. *Archives of Neurology* **45**: 731–736.

Jarvik JG, Hesselink JR, Wiley C *et al.* (1988b) Coccidioidomycotic brain ABCs in an HIV-infected man. *Western Journal of Medicine* **149**: 83.

Jeannel D, Niel G, Costagliola D, Danis B, Traore BM and Gentilini M (1988) Epidemiology of toxoplasmosis among pregnant women in the Paris area. *International Journal of Epidemiology* **17**: 595–602.

Jeantils V, Lemaitre MO, Robert J *et al.* (1986) Subacute polyneuropathy with encephalopathy in AIDS with human cytomegalovirus pathogenicity? *Lancet* **ii**: 1039.

Johns DR, Tierney M and Felsenstein D (1987) Alteration in the natural history of neurosyphilis by concurrent infection with the human immunodeficiency virus. *New England Journal of Medicine* **316**: 1569–1572.

Kalayjian RC, Cohen ML, Bonomo RA and Flanigan TP (1993) Cytomegalovirus ventriculoencephalitis in AIDS. A syndrome with distinct clinical and pathologic features. *Medicine* **72**: 67–77.

Katlama C (1991) Evaluation of the efficacy and safety of clindamycin plus pyrimethamine for induction and maintenance therapy of toxoplasmic encephalitis in AIDS. *European Journal of Clinical Microbiology and Infectious Diseases* **10**: 189–191.

Katlama C, De Witt S, Guichard A *et al.* (1991) Pyrimethamine–clindamycin (P/C) versus pyrimethamine–sulfadiazine (P/S) in *Toxoplasma* encephalitis (toxoplasmic encephalitis) in AIDS. A randomised prospective multicentric European study. *VII International Conference on AIDS, Florence*, Abstract WB 30.

Kato T, Hirano A, Llena JF, Dembitzer HM (1987) Neuropathology of the acquired immune deficiency syndrome (AIDS) in 53 autopsy cases with particular emphasis on microglial nodules and multinucleated giant cells. *Acta Neuropathology* **73**: 287–294.

Katz D and Berger JR (1989) Neurosyphilis in AIDS. *Archives of Neurology* **46**: 895–901.

Katz D, Berger JR, Duncan KC (1993) Neurosyphilis. A comparative study of the effects of infection with human immunodeficiency virus. *Archives of Neurology* **50**: 243–249.

Kaufman HE and Geisler PH (1960) The hematologic toxicity of pyrimethamine (Daraprim) in man. *Archives of Ophthalmology* **64**: 140–146.

Kayser C, Campbell R, Sartoriuous C and Bartlett M (1990) Toxoplasmosis of the conus medullaris in a patient with haemophilia A-associated AIDS. *Journal of Neurosurgery* **73**: 951–953.

Khuong MA, Matheron S, Marche C, De Truchis P, Coulaud JP and Saimot AG (1990) Diffuse toxoplasmic encephalitis (toxoplasmic encephalitis) without abscess in AIDS patients. *30th Interscience Conference on Antimicrobial Agents and Chemotherapy, Atlanta, Georgia, 21–24 October*, Abstract 1157.

Kim YS and Hollander H (1993) Polyradiculopathy due to cytomegalovirus: report of two cases in which improvement occurred after prolonged therapy and review of the literature. *Clinical Infectious Diseases* **17**: 32–37.

Knobler RL, Lublin FD, Northrup BE *et al.* (1986) Progressive leukoencephalopathy in the posterior fossa of patients with AIDS. *Neurology* **36** (Suppl. 1): 206.

Koopmans PP, Van der Ven AJ, Vree TB, Van der Meer JWM (1995) Pathogenesis of hypersensitivity reactions to drugs in patients with HIV infection: allergic or toxic? *AIDS* **9**: 217–222.

Köppen S, Grunewald T, Jautzke G, Gottschalle, J, Pohle HD, Ruf B (1992) Prevention of *Pneumocystis carinii* penumonia and toxoplasmic encephalitis in human immunodeficiency virus infected patients: a clinical approach comparing aerosolized pentamidine and pyrimethamine-sulfadoxine. *Clinical Investigations* **70**: 508–512.

Kovacs JA, Kovacs AA, Polis M *et al.* (1985) Cryptococcosis in the acquired immunodeficiency syndrome. *Annals of Internal Medicine* **103**: 533–538.

Koyanagi Y, Miles S, Mitsuyasu RT *et al.* (1987) Dual infection of the central nervous system by AIDS viruses with distinct cellular tropisms. *Science* **236**: 819–822.

Kozlowski PB, Sher JH, Dickson DW *et al.* (1990) Central nervous system in pediatric HIV infection: a multicenter study. In: *Brain in Pediatric AIDS* (eds PB Kozlowski, DA Snider, PM Vietze and HM Wisniewski), Basel: Karger. 132–146.

Krupp LB, Lipton RB, Swerdlow ML *et al.* (1985) Progressive multifocal leukoencephalopathy: clinical and radiographic features. *Annals of Neurology* **17**: 344–349.

Kuchelmeister K, Bergmann M, Angeli G and Masini T (1993a) Progressive multifocal leukoencephalopathy (PML) in the acquired immunodeficiency syndrome (AIDS). A neuropathological autopsy study of 21 cases. *Pathology, Research and Practice* **189**: 163–173.

Kuchelmeister K, Bergmann M and Gullotta F (1993b) Cellular changes in the cerebellar granular layer in AIDS-associated PML. *Neuropathology and Applied Neurobiology* **19**: 398–401.

Kupfer MC, Zee CS, Colletti PM, Boswell WD and Rhodes R (1990) MRI evaluation of AIDS-related encephalopathy: toxoplasmosis vs lymphoma. *Magnetic Resonance Imaging* **8**: 51–57.

Kure K, Llena JF, Lyman WD *et al.* (1991) Human immunodeficiency virus-1 infection of the nervous system: an autopsy study of 268 adult, pediatric, and fetal brains. *Human Pathology* **22**: 700–710.

Lacroix C, Vazeux R, Brousse N *et al.* (1993) Etude neuropathologique de 10 enfants infectés par le VIH. *Revue Neurologique* **149**: 37–45.

Laforêt P, Matheron S, Adams D *et al.* (1994) Progressive multifocal leucoencephalopathy in AIDS. Treatment with alpha-interferon. *Journal of Neurology* **241**: S4.

Laguna F, Adrados M, Ortaga A and Gonzales-Lahoz JM (1992) Tuberculous meningitis with acellular cerebrospinal fluid in AIDS patients. *AIDS* **6**: 1165–1167.

Lang W, Miklossy J, Deruaz JP *et al.* (1989) Neuropathology of the acquired immune deficiency syndrome (AIDS): a report of 135 consecutive autopsy cases from Switzerland. *Acta Neuropathologica* **77**: 379–390.

Lanska MJ and Lanska DJ (1989) Treatable causes of meningomyeloradiculitis in individuals infected with human immunodeficiency virus. *Archives of Neurology* **46**: 722–723.

Lantos PL, McLaughlin JE, Scholz GL *et al.* (1989) Neuropathology of the brain in HIV infection. *Lancet* **ii**: 309–311.

Lavrard I, Roux P, Poirot JF, Olivier JL, Lemarchand B and Marteau M (1992) Pulmonary toxoplasmosis: detection of *Toxoplasma gondii* DNA by polymerase chain reaction in bronchoalveolar lavage and induced sputum. *VIII International Conference on AIDS, Amsterdam, The Netherlands, 19–24 July*, Abstract B121.

Lebech M, Lebech AM, Nelsing S, Vuust J, Mathiesen L and Petersen E (1992) Detection of *Toxoplasma gondii* DNA by polymerase chain reaction in cerebrospinal fluid from AIDS patients with cerebral toxoplasmosis. *Journal of Infectious Diseases* **165**: 982–983.

Leport C, Raffi F, Matheron S *et al.* (1988) Treatment of central nervous system toxoplasmosis with pyrimethamine/sulfadiazine combination in 35 patients with acquired immunodeficiency syndrome. *American Journal of Medicine* **84**: 94–100.

Leport C, Bastuji-Garin S, Perrone C, Salmon D, Marche C and Bricaire F (1989a) An open study of the pyrimethamine–clindamycin combination in AIDS patients with brain toxoplasmosis. *Journal of Infectious Diseases* **160**: 557–558.

Leport C, Tournerie C, Raguin G *et al.* (1989b) Long-term follow-up of patients with AIDS on maintenance therapy for toxoplasmosis. *European Journal of Clinical Microbiology* **160**: 312–320.

Leport C, Meulemans A, Robine D *et al.* (1989c) Penetration of pyrimethamine into human brain tissue after a single dose administration. *29th Interscience Conference on Antimicrobial Agents and Chemotherapy, Houston, September*, Abstract 248.

Leport C, Tournerie C, Raguin G, Fernandez-Martin J, Niyongabo T and Vildé JL (1991) Long term follow-up of patients with AIDS on maintenance therapy for toxoplasmosis. *European Journal of Microbiology and Infectious Diseases* **10**: 192–193.

Leport C, Meulemans A, Robine D *et al.* (1992) Levels of pyrimethamine in serum and penetration into brain tissue in humans. *AIDS* **6**: 1040–1041.

Leport C, Ambroise-Thomas P, Chene G *et al.* (1993a) Traitement d'attaque, in: *Toxoplasmose et infection HIV. Etat des Connaissances et recommondations en Mai 1993. Médecine et Maladies Infectieuses (Spécial)* **23**: 719–723.

Leport C, Ambroise-Thomas P, Chene G, Katlama C, Raffi F and Vilde JL (1993b) Propositions consensuelles pour le traitement de la toxoplasmose chez les patients infectés par le virus de l'immunodéfience humaine (VIH). *Annales de Medecine Interne* **144**: 53–56.

Leport C, Morlat P, Chene G *et al.* (1993c) Pyrimethamine for primary prophylaxis of toxoplasmosis in HIV patients. A double-blind randomized trial. The First National Conference on Human Retroviruses and Related Infections. Washington, Abstract 36.

Levy JD, Cottingham KL, Campbell RJ *et al.* (1986) Progressive multifocal leukoencephalopathy and magnetic resonance imaging. *Annals of Neurology* **19**: 399–401.

Levy RM and Bredesen DE (1992) Central nervous system dysfunction in acquired immunodeficiency syndrome. *Medicine* **71**: 224–239.

Levy RM, Bredesen DE and Rosenblum ML (1985) Neurological manifestations of the acquired immunodeficiency syndrome (AIDS): experience at UCSF and review of the literature. *Journal of Neurosurgery* **62**: 475–495.

Levy RM, Rosenblum S and Perrett LV (1986) Neuroradiological findings in the acquired immunodeficiency syndrome (AIDS): a review of 200 cases. *American Journal of Neuroradiology* **7**: 833–839.

Levy RM, Janssen RS, Bush TJ and Rosenblum ML (1988) Neuroepidemiology of acquired immunodeficiency syndrome. In: *AIDS and the Nervous System* (ed ML Rosenblum), pp. 13–27. New York: Raven Press.

Levy RM, Mills CM, Posin JP, Moore SG, Rosenblum ML and Bredesen DE (1990) The efficacy and clinical impact of brain imaging in neurologically symptomatic AIDS patients: a prospective CT/MRI study. *Journal of Acquired Immune Deficiency Syndromes* **3**: 469–471.

Lipton HL (1991) Is JC virus latent in brain? *Annals of Neurology* **29**: 433–434.

Lipton RB, Krupp L, Horoupian D *et al.* (1988) Progressive multifocal leukoencephalopathy of the posterior fossa in an AIDS patient: clinical, radiographic and evoked potential findings. *European Neurology* **28**: 258–261.

Lucht F, Jaubert J, Huppert J *et al.* (1987) Cryptococcal meningitis and cerebral toxoplasmosis in a patient with acquired immunodeficiency syndrome. *Journal of Neurology, Neurosurgery and Psychiatry* **50**: 116.

Luft BJ (1989) *Toxoplasma gondii*. In: *Parasitic Infections in the Compromised Host* (eds PD Walzer and RM Genta), pp. 179–279. New York: Marcel Dekker.

Luft BJ and Remington JS (1985) Toxoplasmosis of the central nervous system. In: *Current Topics in Infectious Diseases*, Vol. 6 (eds JS Remington and MN Swartz), pp. 315–358. New York: McGraw-Hill.

Luft BJ and Remington JS (1988) Toxoplasmic encephalitis. *Journal of Infectious Diseases* **157**: 1–6.

Luft BJ and Remington JS (1992) Toxoplasmic encephalitis in AIDS. *Clinical Infectious Diseases* **15**: 211–222.

Luft BJ, Conley FK and Remington JS (1983) Outbreak of central nervous system toxoplasmosis in Western Europe and North America. *Lancet* **i**: 781–784.

Luft BJ, Brooks RG, Conley FK *et al.* (1984) Toxoplasmic encephalitis in patients with AIDS. *Journal of the American Medical Association* **252**: 913–917.

Luft BJ, Hafner R, Korzun AH *et al.* (1993) Toxoplasmic encephalitis in patients with the acquired immunodeficiency syndrome. *New England Journal of Medicine* **329**: 995–1000.

McCabe RE and Remington JS (1990) *Toxoplasma gondii*. In: *Principles and Practice of Infectious Diseases* (eds GL Mandell, RG Douglas and JE Bennett), 3rd edn, pp. 2090–2103. New York: Churchill Livingstone.

McCarthy M, Resnick L, Taub F *et al.* (1991) Infection of human neural cell aggregate cultures with a clinical isolate of cytomegalovirus. *Journal of Neuropathology and Experimental Neurology* **50**: 441–450.

McCutchan JA (1995) Clinical impact of cytomegalovirus infections of the nervous system in patients with AIDS. *Clinical Infectious Diseases* **21** (Suppl. 2): S196–S201.

Madlener L, Enzensberger W, Herdt P *et al.* (1992) Neurological outcome and follow-up after successful treatment of CNS toxoplasmosis. *VIII International Conference on AIDS, Amsterdam, The Netherlands, 19–24 July*, Abstract B122.

Major E, Vacante DA (1989) Human fetal astrocytes in cultures support the growth of the neurotropic polyomavirus JCV. *Journal of Neuropathology and Experimental Neurology* **48**: 425–436.

Mallolas J, Zamora L, Gatell JM *et al.* (1993) Primary prophylaxis for *Pneumocystis carinii* pneumonia: a randomized trial comparing cotrimoxazole, aerosolized pentamidine and dapsone plus pyrimethamine. *AIDS* **7**: 59–64.

Manji H, Sweeney B, Connolly S *et al.* (1995) Movement disorders in AIDS: infective, neoplastic and iatrogenic causes. *Parkinsonism and Related Disorders* **1**: 13–19.

Masdeu JC, Small CB, Weiss L *et al.* (1988) Multifocal cytomegalovirus encephalitis in AIDS. *Annals of Neurology* **23**: 97–99.

Maslo C, Matheron S, Saimot AG *et al.* (1992) Cerebral toxoplasmosis: assessment of maintenance therapy. *VIII International Conference on AIDS, Amsterdam, The Netherlands, 19–24 July*, Abstract POB 3218.

Masur H, O'Neil D, Feuersteinb I *et al.* (1991) 566C80 is effective as salvage treatment for *Toxoplasma* encephalitis. *VII International Conference on AIDS, Florence*, Abstract WB 31.

Matheron S, Dournon E, Garakhanian S, Leport C, Detruchis P and Gaudebout C (1990) Prevalence of toxoplasmosis in 365 AIDS and ARC patients before and during zidovudine treatment. *VI International Conference on AIDS, San Francisco, California, 20–24 June*, Abstract B476.

Matthiessen L, Marche C, Labrousse F, Trophilme D, Fontaine C and Vedrenne C (1992) Etude neuropathologique de l'encéphale de 174 patients morts du SIDA dans un hôpital parisien, de 1982 à 1988. *Annales de Medecine Interne* **143**: 43–49.

Mattos JP, Ross ALZ, Correa RB and Novis S (1993) Involuntary movements and AIDS. Reports of seven cases and review of the literature. *Archivos de Neuro-Psiquiatrica* **51**: 491–497.

May TL, Benscart C, Leclercq P *et al.* (1992) Trimethoprim-sulfamethoxazole versus aerosolized pentamidine for primary prophylaxis of *Pneumocystis carinii* pneumonia: a prospective randomized, controlled clinical trial. Program and Abstracts of the 32nd Interscience Conference on Antimicrobial Agents and Chemotherapy, Anaheim 1992, Abstract 1471.

Mehren M, Burns PJ, Mamani F, Levy CS and Laureno R (1988) Toxoplasmic myelitis mimicking intramedullary spinal cord tumor. *Neurology* **38**: 1648–1650.

Melhem ER and Wang H (1992) Intramedullary spinal cord tuberculoma in a patient with AIDS. *AJNR* **13**: 986–988.

Metze K and Maciel JA (1993) AIDS and Chagas' disease. *Neurology* **43**: 447.

Michon C, Girard PM, Ngovan J *et al.* (1988) Traitement des infections à cytomégalovirus de l'immunodéprimé. *Annales de Medecine Interne* **139**: 511–515.

Miller JR, Barrett RE, Britton CB *et al.* (1984) Progressive multifocal leukoencephalopathy in a male with T-cell immune deficiency. *New England Journal of Medicine* **307**: 1436–1438.
Milligan SA, Katz MS, Craven PC, Strandberg DA, Russell IJ and Becker RA (1984) Toxoplasmosis presenting as panhypopituitarism in a patient with the acquired immune deficiency syndrome. *American Journal of Medicine* **77**: 760–764.
Molina JM, Belenfant X, Doco-Lecompte T *et al.* (1991) Sulfadiazine-induced crystalluria in AIDS patients with *Toxoplasma* encephalitis. *AIDS* **5**: 587–589.
Moret H, Guichard M, Matheron S *et al.* (1993) Virological diagnosis of progressive multifocal leukoencephalopathy: detection of JC virus DNA in cerebrospinal fluid and brain tissue of AIDS patients. *Journal of Clinical Microbiology* **31**: 3310–3313.
Morgello S, Cho E-S, Nielsen S *et al.* (1987) Cytomegalovirus encephalitis in patients with acquired immunodeficiency syndrome an autopsy study of 30 cases and a review of the literature. *Human Pathology* **18**: 289–197.
Mori M, Kurata H, Tafima M and Shimada H (1991) JC virus detection by *in situ* hybridization in brain tissue from elderly patients. *Annals of Neurology* **29**: 428–432.
Morlat Ph, Ragnaud JM, Gin H, Lacoste, Beylot and Aubertin J (1993) La toxoplasmose cérébrale au cours du SIDA. *Medecine Maladies Infectieuses* **23**: 183–189.
Moskowitz LB, Hensley GT, Chan JC, Gregorios J and Conley FK (1984) The neuropathology of acquired immune deficiency syndrome. *Archives of Pathology and Laboratory Medicine* **108**: 867–872.
Moulignier A, Pialoux G, Mikol J *et al.* (1993) CT-guided stereotactic brain biopsy in 68 neuroradiologically symptomatic AIDS patients. *VIII International Conference on AIDS, Amsterdam*, Abstract PO-B16–1724.
Musher DM, Hamill RJ and Baughn RE (1990) Syphilis, the response to penicillin therapy, neurosyphilis and the effect of human immunodeficiency virus infection. *Annals of Internal Medicine* **113**: 872–881.
Navia BA, Petito CK, Gold JWM *et al.* (1986a) Cerebral toxoplasmosis complicating AIDS: clinical and neuropathological findings in 27 patients. *Annals of Neurology* **19**: 224–238.
Navia BA, Cho E-S, Petito CK *et al.* (1986b) The AIDS dementia complex: II. Neuropathology. *Annals of Neurology* **19**: 525–535.
Ndumbe P, Andela A, Nkemnkeng-Asong J *et al.* (1992) Prevalence of infections affecting the child among pregnant women in Yaounde, Cameroon. *Medical Microbiology and Immunology* **181**: 127–130.
Nicoli F, Dhiver C, Chave B *et al.* (1992) Leuco-encéphalite diffuse régressive sous foscarnet au cours d'un SIDA. *Presse Medicale* **21**: 436.
Niyongabo T, Leport C and Vilde JL (1991) Utilité de l'acide folinique dans les cytopénies induites par les médicaments antiparasitaires au cours du SIDA. *Presse Medicale* **34**: 1677–1681.
Novak IS, Trujillo JR, Rivera VM *et al.* (1989) Ganciclovir in the treatment of CMV infection in AIDS patients with neurologic complications. *Neurology* **39** (Suppl. 1): 379–380.
Oddó D, Casanova M, Acuña G *et al.* (1992) Acute Chagas' disease (trypanosomiasis americana) in acquired immunodeficiency syndrome. Report of two cases. *Human Pathology* **23**: 41–44.
Oksenhendler E, Cadranel J, Sarfati C *et al.* (1990) *Toxoplasma gondii* pneumonia in patients with the acquired immunodeficiency syndrome. *American Journal of Medicine* **88**: 18N–21N.
Oksenhendler E, Charreau I, Tournerie C *et al.* (1994) *Toxoplasma gondii* infection in advanced HIV infection. *AIDS* **8**: 483–487.
Opravil M, Hirschel B, Lazzarin A *et al.* (1995) Once-weekly administration of dapson/pyrimethamine vs aerosolized pentamidine as combined prophylaxis for *Pneumocystis carinii* pneumonia and toxoplasmic encephalitis in human immunodeficiency virus-infected patients. *Clinical Infectious Diseases* **20**: 531–541.
Oral Ganciclovir European and Australian Cooperative Study Group (1995) Intravenous versus oral ganciclovir. European/Australian comparative study of efficacy and safety in the prevention of cytomegalovirus retinitis recurrence in patients with AIDS. *AIDS* **9**: 471–477.
Orenstein JM, Janotta F (1988) Human immunodeficiency virus and papovavirus infections in acquired immunodeficiency syndrome: an ultrastructural study of three cases. *Human Pathology* **19**: 350–361.
Oster S, Hutchison F and McCabe R (1990) Resolution of acute renal failure in toxoplasmic encephalitis despite continuance of sulfadiazine. *Reviews of Infectious Diseases* **12**: 618–620.
Ostertun B, Dewes W, Suss H, Steudel A, Brassel H and Harder T (1988) MR tomography of non-tumor diseases of the brain and cervical cord. *ROFO* 148: 408–414.
Overhage JM, Greist A and Brown DR (1990) Conus medullaris syndrome resulting from

*Toxoplasma gondii* infection in a patient with the acquired immunodeficiency syndrome. *American Journal of Medicine* **89**: 814–815.

Parke DW and Font RL (1986) Diffuse toxoplasmic retinochoroiditis in a patient with AIDS. *Archives of Ophthalmology* **104**: 571–575.

Parmley S, Goebel F and Remington J (1992) Detection of *Toxoplasma gondii* in cerebrospinal fluid from AIDS patients by polymerase chain reaction. *Journal of Clinical Microbiology* **30**: 3000–3002.

Pedrol E, Gonzalez-Clemente J, Gatell JM *et al.* (1990) Central nervous system toxoplasmosis in AIDS patients: efficacy of an intermittent maintenance therapy. *AIDS* **4**: 511–517.

Petito CK, Cho E-S, Lemann W *et al.* (1986) Neuropathology of acquired immunodeficiency syndrome (AIDS): an autopsy review. *Journal of Neuropathology and Experimental Neurology* **45**: 635–646.

Pfefferkorn ER (1990) Cell biology of *Toxoplasma gondii.* In: *Modern Parasite Biology: Cellular, Immunological, and Molecular Aspects* (ed. DJ Wyler), pp. 26–50. New York: WH Freeman.

Podzamczer D, Santin M, Jimenez J, Casanova A, Bolao F, Gudiol GRF (1993) Thrice-weekly co-trimoxazole is better than weekly dapsone-pyrimethamine for the primary prevention of *Pneumocystis carinii* pneumonia in HIV-infected patients. *AIDS* **7**: 501–506.

Portegies P, Algra PR, Hollak CEM *et al.* (1991) Response to cytarabine in progressive multifocal leukoencephalopathy in AIDS. *Lancet* **337**: 680–681.

Porter SB and Sande M (1992) Toxoplasmosis of the central nervous system in the acquired immunodeficiency syndrome. *New England Journal of Medicine* **327**: 1643–1648.

Post MJD, Hensley GT, Moskowitz LB *et al.* (1986) Cytomegalic inclusion virus encephalitis in patients with AIDS: CT, clinical, and pathological correlation. *American Journal of Roentgenology* **146**: 1229–1234.

Potasman I, Resnick L, Luft BJ and Remington JS (1988) Intrathecal production of antibodies against *Toxoplasma gondii* in patients with toxoplasmic encephalitis and the acquired immunodeficiency syndrome (AIDS). *Annals of Internal Medicine* **108**: 49–51.

Price RW, Nielsen S, Horten B *et al.* (1983) Progressive multifocal leukoencephalopathy: a burn-out case. *Annals of Neurology* **13**: 485–490.

Pulliam L (1991) Cytomegalovirus preferentially infects a monocyte derived macrophage/ microglial cell in human brain cultures: neuropathology differs between strains. *Journal of Neuropathology and Experimental Neurology* **50**: 432–440.

Putterman C, Rahav G, Shalit M, Rubinow A (1990) Treating through hypersensitivity to co-trimoxazole in AIDS patients. *Lancet* **2**: 52.

Quinlivan EB, Norris M, Bouldin TW *et al.* (1992) Subclinical central nervous system infection with JC virus in patients with AIDS. *Journal of Infectious Diseases* **166**: 80–85.

Raffi F (1993) Quelles sont les indications de la biopsie cérébrale? *Medicine Maladies Infectieuses* **23**: 700–703.

Redfield RR, Wright DC and Tramont EC (1986) The Walter Reed staging classification for HTLV II/LAV infection. *New England Journal of Medicine* **314**: 131–132.

Remington JS and Cavanaugh EN (1965) Isolation of the encysted form of *Toxoplasma gondii* from human skeletal muscle and brain. *New England Journal of Medicine* **293**: 1308–1310.

Remington JS and Desmonts G (1990) Toxoplasmosis. In *Infectious Diseases of the Fetus and New-born Infant* (eds JS Remington and Jo Klein), pp. 89–195. Philadelphia: WB Saunders.

Remington JS, Efron B, Cavanaugh E *et al.* (1970) Studies on toxoplasmosis in El Salvador. Prevalence and incidence of toxoplasmosis as measured by the Sabin–Feldman dye test. *Transactions of the Royal Society of Tropical Medicine and Hygiene* **64**: 252–267.

Renold C, Sugar A, Chave JP *et al.* (1992) *Toxoplasma* encephalitis in patients with the acquired immunodeficiency syndrome. *Medicine* **71**: 224–239.

Reynes J, Atoni N, Lassonnery M *et al.* (1992) Cotrimoxazole (TMPISMX) in primary prophylaxis of cerebral toxoplasmosis in HIV-infected patients. 3rd European Conference on Clinical Aspects and Treatment of HIV Infection. Paris 1992, Abstract P242.

Rhodes RH (1987) Histopathology of the central nervous system in the acquired immunodeficiency syndrome. *Human Pathology* **18**: 636–643.

Rhodes RH (1993) Histopathologic features in the central nervous system of 400 acquired immunodeficiency syndrome cases: implications of rates of occurrence. *Human Pathology* **24**: 1189–1198.

Rosemberg S, Chaves CJ, Higuchi ML, Lopes MB, Castro LH and Machado LR (1992) Fatal meningoencephalitis caused by reactivation of *Trypanosoma cruzi* infection in a patient with AIDS. *Neurology* **42**: 640–642.

Rosenblum MK (1989) Bulbar encephalitis complicating trigeminal zoster in the acquired immune deficiency syndrome. *Human Pathology* **20**: 292–295.

Ryder JW, Croen D, Kleinschmidt-DeMasters BK *et al.* (1986) Progressive encephalitis 3 months after resolution of cutaneous zoster in a patient with AIDS. *Annals of Neurology* **19**: 182–188.
Said G (1993) Indications de la biopsie cérébrale en présence de lésions intracraniennes au cours du SIDA. *Médecine et Maladies Infectieuses (Spécial)* **23**: 717.
Said G, Masnou P, Chemouilli P *et al.* (1996) Involuntary movements in patients with HIV infection. *Journal of Neurology* **243** (Suppl. 2): S22.
Sanchez-Ramos JR, Factor SA, Weiner WJ and Marquez J (1989) Hemichorea–hemiballismus associated with acquired immune deficiency syndrome and cerebral toxoplasmosis. *Movement Disorders* **4**: 266–273.
Scaravilli F, Ellis DS, Tovey G *et al.* (1989) Unusual development of polyoma virus in the brains of two patients with the acquired immune deficiency syndrome (AIDS). *Neuropathology and Applied Neurobiology* **15**: 407–418.
Schmidbauer M, Budka H, Ulrich W and Ambros P (1989) Cytomegalovirus (CMV) disease of the brain in AIDS and connatal infection: a comparative study by histology, immunocytochemistry and *in situ* DNA hybridization. *Acta Neuropathologica* **79**: 286–293.
Schmidbauer M, Budka H and Shah KV (1990) Progressive multifocal leukoencephalopathy (PML) in AIDS and in the pre-AIDS era: a neuropathological comparison using immunocytochemistry and *in situ* DNA hybridization for virus detection. *Acta Neuropathologica* **80**: 375–380.
Schneider MME, Hoepelman AIM, Eefintck Schattenkerle JKM *et al.* (1992) A controlled trial of aerosolized pentamidine or trimethoprimsulfamethoxazole as primary prophylaxis against *Pneumocystis carinii* pneumonia in patients with human immunodeficiency virus infections. *New England Journal of Medicine* **327**: 1836–1841.
Schoondemark R, Van de Ven ES, Galama J, Kaaijeveld C, Van Druten J, Menwissen J, Melchers W (1993) Value of the polymerase chain reaction for the detection of *Toxoplasma gondii* in cerebrospinal fluid from patients with AIDS. *Clinical Infectious Diseases* **16**: 661–666.
Selik RM, Starcher ET and Curran JW (1990) Opportunistic disease reported in AIDS patients: frequencies, associations, and trends. *Journal of Acquired Immune Deficiency Syndromes* **1**: 175–182.
Sharer LR and Kapila R (1985) Neuropathologic observations in the acquired immunodeficiency syndrome. *Acta Neuropathologica* **66**: 188–198.
Simon DI, Brosius FC and Rothstein DM (1990) Sulfadiazine crystalluria revisited. *Archives of Internal Medicine* **150**: 2379–2384.
Sinibaldi J and De Ramirez I (1992) Incidence of congenital toxoplasmosis in live Guatemalan newborns. *European Journal of Epidemiology* **8**: 516–520.
Slavin MA, Hoy JF, Stewart K *et al.* (1992) Oral dapsone versus nebulized pentamidine for *Pneumocystis carinii* pneumonia prophylaxis: an open randomized prospective trial to assess efficacy and hematological toxicity. *AIDS* **6**: 1169–1174.
Snider WD, Simpson DM, Nielsen S *et al.* (1983) Neurological complications of AIDS: analysis of 50 patients. *Annals of Neurology* **14**: 403–418.
Spector SA, McKinley GF, Lalezari JP *et al.* (1996) Oral ganciclovir for the prevention of cytomegalovirus disease in persons with AIDS. *New England Journal of Medicine* **334**: 1491–1497.
Stavrou D, Mehraein P, Mellert W *et al.* (1989) Evaluation of intracerebral lesions in patients with acquired immunodeficiency syndrome: neuropathological findings and experimental data. *Neuropathology and Applied Neurobiology* **15**: 207–222.
Strittmatter C, Lang W, Wiestler OD and Kleihues P (1992) The changing pattern of human immunodeficiency virus associated cerebral toxoplasmosis: a study of 46 postmortem cases. *Acta Neuropathologica* **83**: 475–481.
Suzuki Y, Israelski DM, Dannemann BR *et al.* (1988) Diagnosis of toxoplasmic encephalitis in patients with AIDS by using a new serologic method. *Journal of Clinical Microbiology* **26**: 2541–2543.
Tada H, Rappaport J, Lashgari M *et al.* (1990) Trans-activation of the JC virus late promoter by the tat protein of type 1 human immunodeficiency virus in glial cells. *Proceedings of the National Academy of Sciences USA* **87**: 3479–3483.
Tan SV, Guiloff RJ, Scaravilli F *et al.* (1993) Herpes simplex type I encephalitis in acquired immunodeficiency syndrome. *Annals of Neurology* **34**: 619–622.
Tashiro K, Doi S, Moriwaka F *et al.* (1986) Progressive multifocal leukoencephalopathy with magnetic resonance imaging verification and therapeutic trials with interferon. *Journal of Neurology* **234**: 427–429.
Telenti A, Aksamit AJ, Proper J and Smith TF (1990) Detection of JC virus DNA by polymerase chain reaction in patients with progressive multifocal leucoencephalopathy. *Journal of Infectious Diseases* **162**: 858–861.

Telenti A, Marshall WF, Aksamit AJ *et al.* (1992) Detection of JC virus by polymerase chain reaction in CSF from two patients with progressive multifocal leukoencephalopathy. *European Journal of Clinical Microbiology* **11**: 253–254.

Tenant-Flowers M, Boyle MJ, Carey J *et al.* (1991) Sulfadiazine desensibilisation in patients with AIDS and cerebral toxoplasmosis. *AIDS* **5**: 311–315.

Tolge CF and Factor SA (1991) Focal dystonia secondary to cerebral toxoplasmosis in a patient with acquired immune deficiency syndrome. *Movement Disorders* **6**: 69–72.

Tornatore C, Berger JR, Houff SA *et al.* (1992) Detection of JC virus DNA in peripheral lymphocytes from patients with and without progressive multifocal leukoencephalopathy. *Annals of Neurology* **31**: 454–462.

Toxoplasmose et Infection HIV (1993) Etat des connaissances et recommandations en Mai 1993. Sixième conférence en thérapeutique anti-infectieuse de la Société de Pathologie infectieuse de Langue Française. Conférence d'experts, Paris, 14 Mai 1993. *Médecine et Maladies Infectieuses (Spécial)* **23**.

Trotot PM, Vazeux R, Yamashita HK *et al.* (1990) MRI pattern of progressive multifocal leukoencephalopathy (PML) in AIDS. Pathological correlations. *Journal of Neuroradiology* **17**: 233–254.

Van der Steenhoven JJ, Dbaibo G, Boyko OB *et al.* (1990) Progressive multifocal leukoencephalopathy in paediatric acquired immunodeficiency syndrome (abstract). *Journal of Neuropathology and Experimental Neurology* **50**: 326.

Vazeux R, Cumont M, Girard PM *et al.* (1990) Severe encephalitis resulting from coinfection with HIV and JC virus. *Neurology* **40**: 944–948.

Vietzke WM, Gelderman AH, Grimley PM and Valsamis MP (1968) Toxoplasmosis complicating malignancy. *Cancer* **21**: 816–827.

Vinters HV and Anders KH (1990) *Neuropathology of AIDS*, pp. 79–84. Boca Raton, Florida: CRC Press.

Vinters HV, Anders KH and Barach P (1987) Focal pontine leukoencephalopathy in immunosuppressed patients. *Archives of Pathology and Laboratory Medicine* **111**: 192–196.

Vinters H, Kwok MK, Ho HW *et al.* (1989) Cytomegalovirus in the nervous system of patients with the acquired immune deficiency syndrome. *Brain* **112**: 245–268.

von Einsiedel RW, Fife TD, Askamit AJ *et al.* (1993) Progressive multifocal leukoencephalopathy in AIDS: a clinicopathologic study and review of the literature. *Journal of Neurology* **240**: 391–406.

Vuia O (1976) Progressive multifocal leukoencephalopathy and Rosenthal fibres. *European Neurology* **14**: 198–208.

Walker DG, Itagaki S, Berry K and McGeer PM (1989) Examination of brain of AIDS cases for human immunodeficiency virus and human cytomegalovirus nucleic acids. *Journal of Neurology, Neurosurgery and Psychiatry* **52**: 583–590.

Wallace MR, Rossetti RJ and Olson PE (1993) Cats and toxoplasmosis risk in HIV-infected adults. *Journal of the American Medical Association* **260**: 76–77.

Weber T, Beck R, Stark E *et al.* (1994) Comparative analysis of intrathecal antibody synthesis and DNA amplification for the diagnosis of cytomegalovirus infection of the central nervous system in AIDS patients. *Journal of Neurology* **241**: 407–414.

Weidenheim KN, Nelson SJ, Kure K *et al.* (1992) Unusual patterns of histoplasma capsulatum meningitis and progressive multifocal leukocephalopathy in a patient with the acquired human immunodeficiency virus. *Human Pathology* **23**: 581–586.

Weisberg LA, Greenberg J and Stazio A (1988) Computed tomographic findings in cerebral toxoplasmosis in adults. *Computerized Medical Imaging and Graphics* **12**: 379–383.

Weiss A, Margo CE, Ledford DK *et al.* (1986) Toxoplasmic retinochoroiditis as an initial manifestation of AIDS. *American Journal of Ophthalmology* **101**: 248–249.

Weiss LM, Harris C, Berger M *et al.* (1988a) Pyrimethamine concentrations in serum and cerebrospinal fluid during treatment of acute *Toxoplasma* encephalitis in patients with AIDS. *Journal of Infectious Diseases* **157**: 580–583.

Weiss LM, Udem SA, Tanowitz H and Wittner M (1988b) Western blot analysis of the antibody responses of patients with AIDS and *Toxoplasma* encephalitis: antigenic diversity among *Toxoplasma* strains. *Journal of Infectious Diseases* **157**: 7–13.

Wheat LJ, Slama TG and Zeckel ML (1985) Histoplasmosis in the acquired immunodeficiency syndrome. *American Journal of Medicine* **78**: 203.

Whelan MA, Kricheff I, Handler M *et al* (1983) Acquired immunodeficiency syndrome: cerebral computed tomographic manifestations. *Radiology* **149**: 477–484.

Whiteside C, Flynn N and Fitzgerald FT (1987) Neurosyphilis and HIV infection. *New England Journal of Medicine* **317**: 1473.

Wijdicks EFM, Borletfs JCC, Hoepelman AIM and Jansen GH (1991) Fatal disseminated hemorrhagic toxoplasmic encephalitis as the initial manifestation of AIDS. *Annals of Neurology* **29**: 683–686.

Wiley CA and Nelson JA (1988) Role of human immunodeficiency virus and cytomegalovirus in AIDS encephalitis. *American Journal of Pathology* **133**: 73–81.

Wiley CA, Grafe M, Kennedy C and Nelson JA (1988) Human immunodeficiency virus (HIV) and JC virus in acquired immunodeficiency syndrome (AIDS) patients with progressive multifocal leukoencephalopathy. *Acta Neuropathologica* **76**: 338–346.

Wolf DG and Spector SA (1992) Diagnosis of human cytomegalovirus central nervous system disease in AIDS patients by DNA amplification from cerebrospinal fluid. *Journal of Infectious Diseases* **166**: 1412–1415.

Wong B, Gold JWM, Brown AE *et al* (1984) Central-nervous-system toxoplasmosis in homosexual men and parenteral drug abusers. *Annals of Internal Medicine* **100**: 36–42.

Wong SY and Remington JS (1993) Biology of *Toxoplasma gondii*. *AIDS* **7**: 299–316.

Wong SY and Remington JS (1994) Toxoplasmosis in the setting of AIDS. In: *Textbook of AIDS Medicine* (eds S Broder, TC Merigan Jr and D Bolognesi), pp. 223–257. Baltimore: Williams and Wilkins.

Wong SY, Israelski DM and Remington JS (1995) AIDS-associated toxoplasmosis. In: *The Medical Management of AIDS* (eds MA Sande and PA Volberding), 4th edn, pp. 460–493. Philadelphia: WB Saunders.

Zangerle R, Allenberger F, Pohl P, Fritsch and Dierich MP (1991) High risk of developing toxoplasmic encephalitis in AIDS patients seropositive for *Toxoplasma gondii*. *Medical Microbiology and Immunology* **180**: 59–66.

Zimmer C, Daeschlein G, Patt S and Weigel K (1991) Strategy for diagnosis of *Toxoplasma gondii* in stereotactic brain biopsies. *Stereotactic and Functional Neurosurgery* **56**: 66–75.

Zimmer C, Marzheuser S, Patt S *et al.* (1992) Stereotactic brain biopsy in AIDS. *Journal of Neurology* **239**: 394–400.

Zuger A, Louie E, Holzman RS *et al* (1986) Cryptococcal disease in patients with the acquired immunodeficiency syndrome. *Annals of Internal Medicine* **104**: 234–240.

# 5

# *Spinal Cord Disorders in AIDS*

In addition to HIV-ADC, HIV infection can induce myelopathy often in association with brain lesions in both adults and children. Opportunistic infections or lymphomas, and less commonly vasculitis, can also induce spinal cord lesions in HIV-infected patients at the stage of immunodepression.

## MYELOPATHIES RELATED TO HIV

### Acute myelopathy

Transient paraplegia of a few days' or weeks' duration can be observed at the time of seroconversion with spontaneous, although partial, recovery (Denning *et al.*, 1987; Berger *et al.*, 1989; Chemouilli *et al.*, 1994).

### HIV-1 associated myelopathy

HIV-1 associated myelopathy was described in patients with ARC or AIDS, usually in association with vacuolar lesions in the posterior and lateral columns (Anders *et al.*, 1986; Budka *et al.*, 1991). In the first descriptions of HIV-associated myelopathy, this vacuolar myelopathy was compared with subacute combined degeneration (Goldstick *et al.*, 1985; Petito *et al.*, 1985; Singh *et al.*, 1986; Gray and Gherardi, 1990). HIV-1 associated myelopathy is characterized in most cases by lower limb weakness, sensory ataxia with increased deep tendon reflexes and, in the terminal stage, sphincter disturbances. It is currently impossible to ascertain the onset of spinal cord myelopathy. However, by the late stage of HIV infection, many of these patients also have higher function disorders and abnormal sensorimotor functions with sphincter disturbances, leading to suspected associated spinal cord lesions. Spinal cord lesions are often found at autopsy. MRI of the spinal cord gives normal results in this setting.

#### *Pathology*

The most frequent lesion observed in the spinal cord is a vacuolar myelopathy with demyelination and spongy changes of the pyramidal tracts and posterior

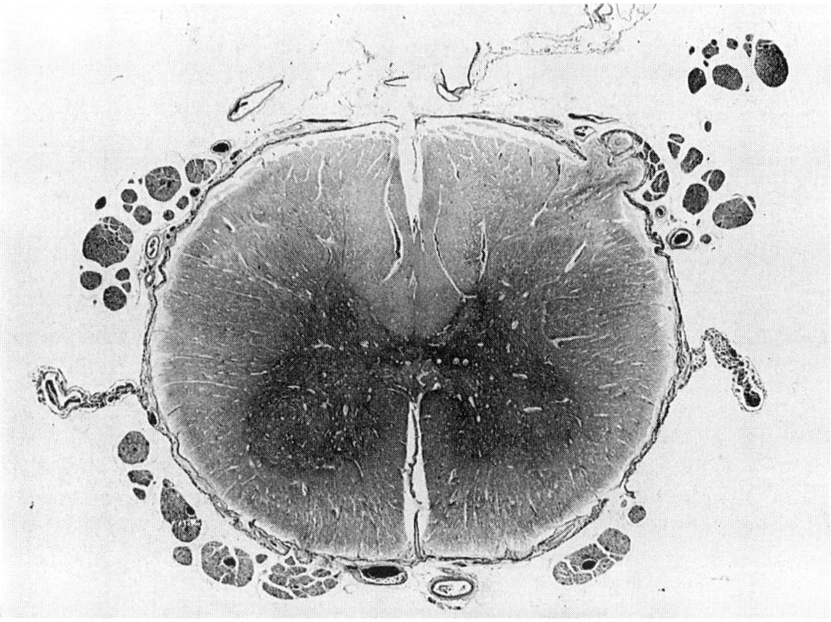

**Figure 5.1** Transverse section of the lumbar spinal cord of a patient with vacuolar myelopathy. (H&E; ×1100.)

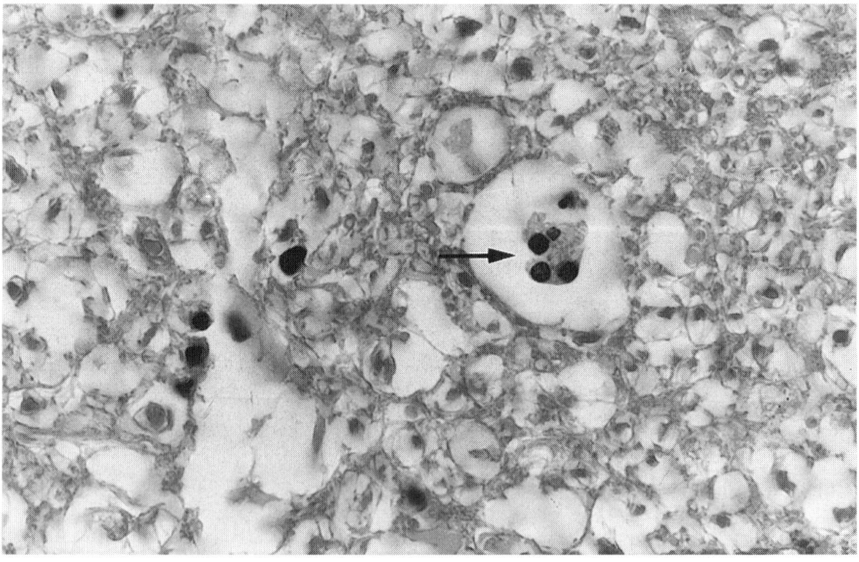

**Figure 5.2** Giant cells (arrow) in vacuoles located in the posterior column of a patient with vacuolar myelopathy. (Paraffin section; H&E; ×1650.)

columns throughout their length (Figure 5.1). The vacuoles are more extensive in the lateral column at the thoracic level. Some microglial nodules may be found in the grey matter. In demyelinated areas, macrophages are observed in myelin vacuoles (Goldstick *et al.*, 1985; Petito *et al.*, 1985; Weiser *et al.*, 1990). MGCs were occasionally seen in vacuolar lesions (Figure 5.2) (Budka *et al.*, 1988). In some series, immunolabelling demonstrated the presence of HIV p24, p17 and gp41 antigens in mononuclear or multinucleated cells in the areas with vacuolar damage. *In situ* hybridization demonstrated a correlation between HIV-1 expression and the extent of vacuolar myelopathy (Peress *et al.*, 1990). In another study, it was found that the presence of HIV DNA correlated with macrophage infiltration of the spinal cord but not with vacuolar myelopathy (Petito *et al.*, 1994). In most cases, vacuolar myelopathy was associated with HIV brain pathology (Petito *et al.*, 1985).

Some authors have identified a separate entity of HIV myelitis, in which multiple foci of inflammatory cells are associated with HIV-positive perivascular histiocytes/giant cells or microglia (Gray *et al.*, 1991; Hénin *et al.*, 1992). In a patient who died 1 month after the onset of a flaccid paraparesis, the gross pathology of the spinal cord was normal but a multifocal MGC myelitis was present at the microscopic level. HIV antigens were detected in macrophages, giant cells and microglia (Geny *et al.*, 1991). These lesions are similar to those observed in the brains of patients with the AIDS dementia complex (Rhodes, 1993). One of our patients with AIDS developed a Brown-Séquard syndrome within 2 weeks in association with a necrotic lesion of the spinal cord found at autopsy; MGCs containing HIV gp41 antigen were found in the necrotic lesions and the meninges around the spinal cord (Figures 5.3–5.5). Immunocytochemistry demonstrated the presence of viral antigens in some giant cells, indicating that this myelitis was caused directly by HIV.

Degeneration of the gracile tracts was observed in some patients with sensory neuropathy (Rance *et al.*, 1988; Scaravilli *et al.*, 1991). Study of the posterior dorsal root ganglia showed an increased number of nodules of Nageotte compared with control patients; a dying-back mechanism was suggested (Scaravilli *et al.*, 1991).

*Pathogenesis of vacuolar myelopathy*

The pathogenesis of vacuolar myelopathy has caused controversy. The pathological changes are similar to those of combined degeneration due to vitamin $B_{12}$ deficiency, suggesting a possible nutritional cause (Petito *et al.*, 1994); however, in most cases, blood vitamin $B_{12}$ and folate levels are normal and patients do not improve after treatment with vitamin $B_{12}$. Similar vacuolar changes have also been observed in non-HIV-infected patients with idiopathic myelopathy (Kamin and Petito, 1991). HIV production, detected by immunocytochemistry and *in situ* hybridization, was uncommon (3/39 cases) in spinal cords with vacuolar myelopathy (Rosenblum *et al.*, 1989). Using combined methods, Eilbott *et al.* (1989) demonstrated HIV expression in macrophages within vacuolar lesions and suggested a role for these infected

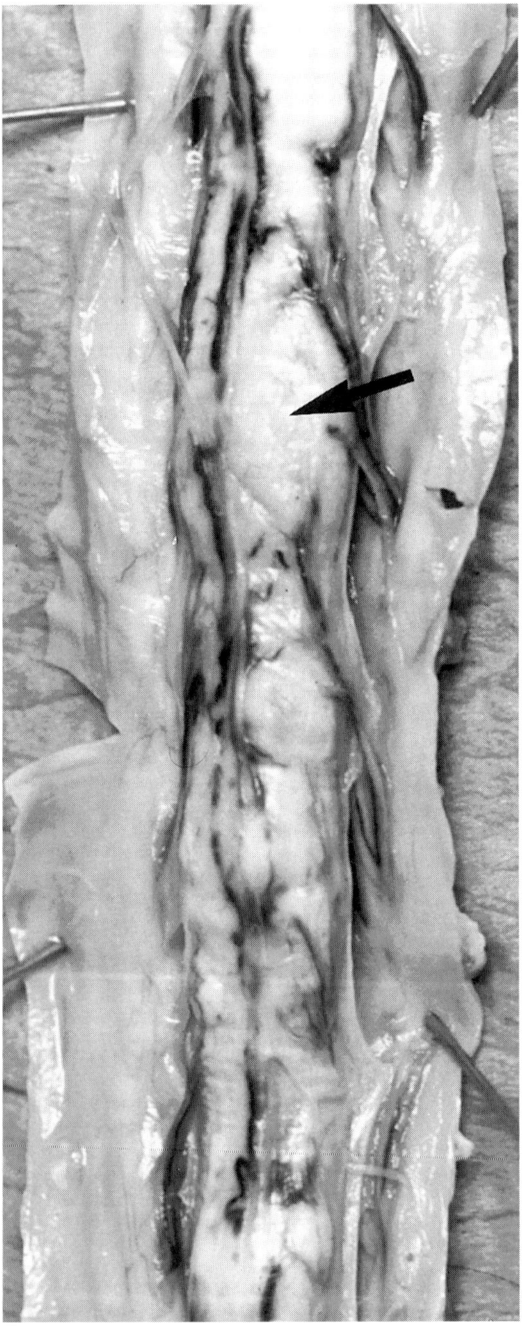

**Figure 5.3** Macroscopic aspect of the cervicodorsal spinal cord of a patient with subacute HIV myelitis showing swollen areas (arrow) corresponding to necrotic areas.

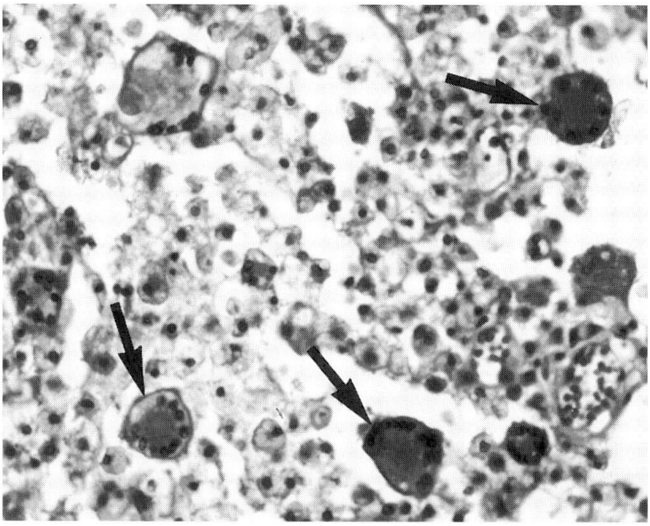

**Figure 5.4** Multinucleated giant cells (arrows) and macrophages in the necrotic cervical spinal cord of the same patient as in Figure 5.3. (Paraffin section; H&E; ×1160.)

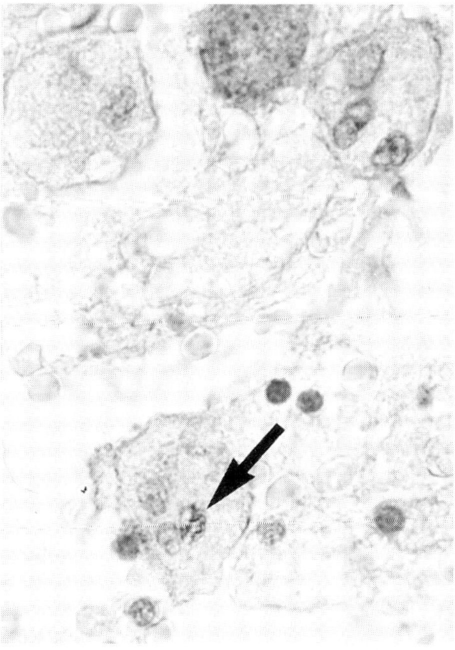

**Figure 5.5** Immunocytochemistry using an HIV gp41 antibody: HIV antigens are present in the cytoplasm of a multinucleated giant cell (arrow) in a patient with subacute necrotizing HIV myelitis. (Paraffin section; DAB; ×2080.)

macrophages in vacuolar myelopathy; however, most authors think that vacuolar myelopathy is not directly related to HIV infection (Brew *et al.*, 1989; Rosenblum *et al.*, 1989; Weiser *et al.*, 1990; Baumrind *et al.*, 1991; Kure *et al.*, 1991; Petito *et al.*, 1994). The absence of vacuolar myelopathy in children with AIDS, who do have viral DNA in MGCs in the spinal cord, also suggests that vacuolar myelopathy is not directly related to the infection (Sharer *et al.*, 1986). In the spinal cord of patients with AIDS, activated macrophages in vacuolar and non-vacuolar posterior and lateral funiculi were highly positive for the cytokines IL-1 and TNF-α, suggesting that these activated cells are present earlier than the vacuoles (Tyor *et al.*, 1993).

*Central spinal myelinolysis*, distinct from vacuolar myelopathy, has been found in some patients; lesions were non-specific and similar to pontine myelinolysis and possibly related to metabolic disturbances (Glass *et al.*, 1990; Rhodes, 1993).

## OPPORTUNISTIC INFECTIONS OF THE SPINAL CORD

Some opportunistic infections are amenable to therapy and must be detected as early as possible. These opportunistic infections include syphilis, cryptococcosis, tuberculosis, toxoplasmosis and HSV, VZV and CMV infection (see Chapter 4). We focus here on CMV myelitis and toxoplasmic abscesses, because in both instances the HIV-infected patient may present with an isolated lesion of the spinal cord and both conditions need early diagnosis and specific treatment (Chemouilli *et al.*, 1994).

### CMV infection

CMV myelitis is usually associated with radiculitis and/or peripheral neuropathy (see Chapter 7). Some patients can present with a subacute lesion of the spinal cord leading to complete paraplegia in a matter of days. On MRI the spinal cord may show focal enlargement. The CSF is abnormal with increased protein content and pleocytosis with polymorphonuclear cells. The glucose level may be low. The paraplegia responds poorly to treatment and the outcome is poor (Jacobson *et al.*, 1988; Mahieux *et al.*, 1989; Vinters *et al.*, 1989; Chemouilli *et al.*, 1994). The duration of the neurological illness in all cases with demonstrated symptomatic CMV infection of the CNS ranges from 3 weeks to 4 months. At autopsy in some cases, CMV encephalitis coexisted with CMV myeloradiculitis (Mahieux *et al.*, 1989; Bélec *et al.*, 1990; Chimelli *et al.*, 1990; Gray *et al.*, 1991). In several patients, we have observed multiple foci containing microglial nodules with cytomegalic cytopathology (Figure 5.6) in the lumbar grey matter or peripheral white matter of the spinal cord. The cells that contained cytomegalic inclusions comprised astrocytes, macrophages and a few endothelial cells. In addition to necrotic and inflammatory pathology, CMV may induce an ischaemic myelopathy due to vasculitis (Pattee *et al.*, 1990). In a patient with myelitis, immunocytochemistry demonstrated dual infection of the same giant cells by HIV and CMV (Bélec *et al.*, 1990). An ascending myelitis

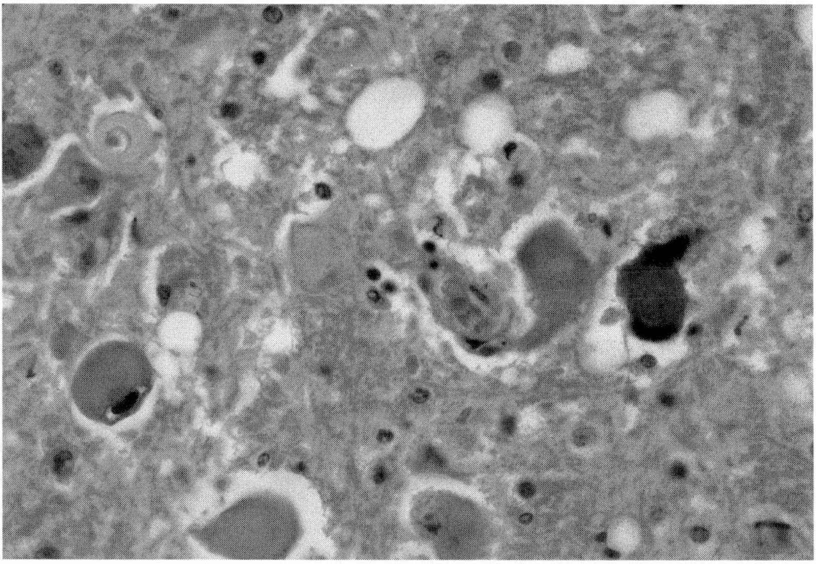

**(a)**

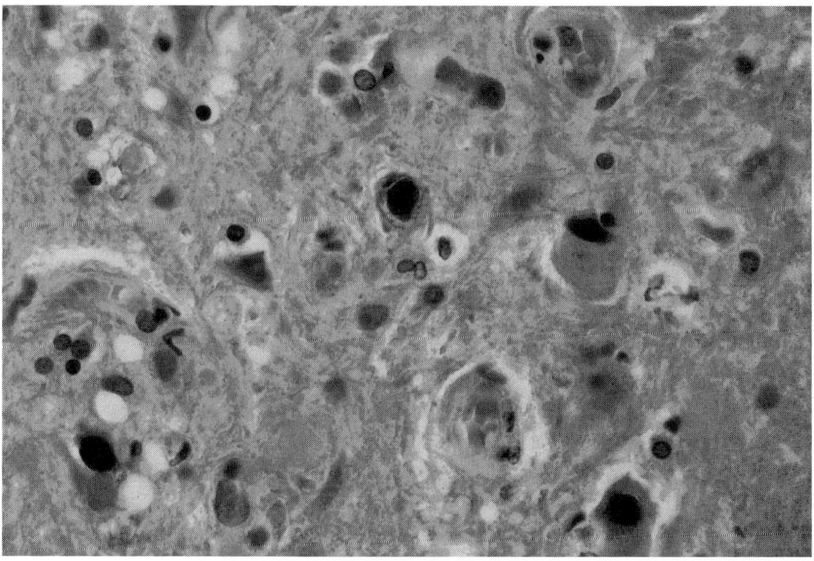

**(b)**

**Figure 5.6** (a) Several cytomegalic cells in the dorsal anterior horn of a patient with CMV myelitis. (Paraffin section; H&E; ×2740. (b) Immunocytochemistry of the same lesion: nuclear inclusions are stained by an early CMV antibody. (Paraffin section; DAB; ×2740.)

due to coinfection with CMV and herpes virus has also been reported (Tucker *et al.*, 1985). Despite therapy, a rapidly fatal course is the rule in all patients with CMV myelopathy.

**Spinal cord toxoplasmosis**

A focal lesion of the spinal cord is seldom due to development of an isolated toxoplasmic abscess, but this possibility should be considered because such lesions respond well to specific treatment (Herskovitz *et al.*, 1989; Chemouilli *et al.*, 1994). In one of our patients, MRI with gadolinium enhancement showed three enhancing lesions in the brain and one in the spinal cord (Figure 5.7).

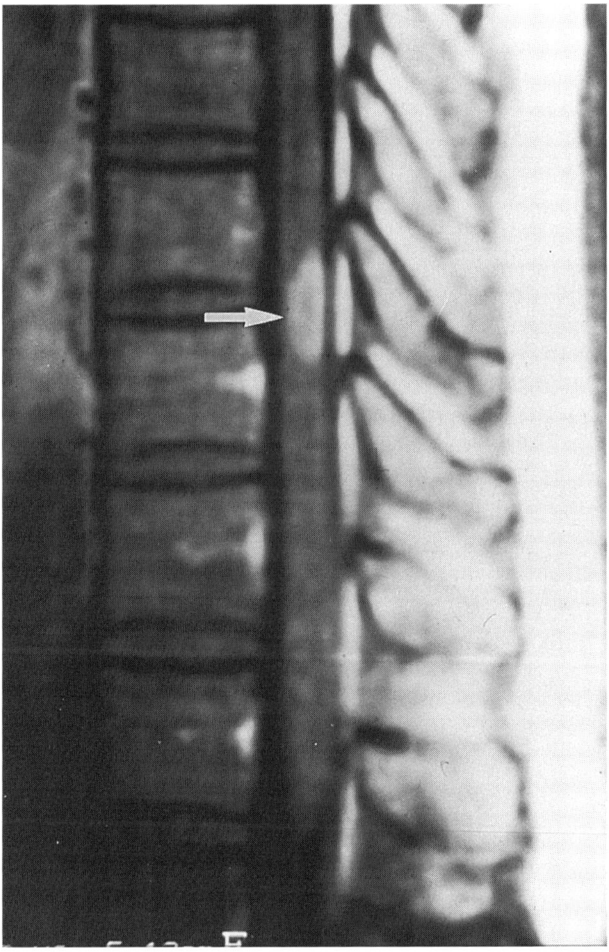

**Figure 5.7** $T_1$-weighted MRI, after gadolinium injection, showing a probable toxoplasmic abscess of the dorsal spinal cord (arrow) in a patient who recovered after antitoxoplasmic therapy.

Neurological signs and symptoms disappeared within a few weeks of treatment and the patient remained free of disease a year later (Chemouilli *et al.*, 1994). Toxoplasmic cysts may be observed in the spinal cord in systematic autopsies, sometimes associated with another infection such as CMV (Lacroix, 1991; Hénin *et al.*, 1992). Cerebral toxoplasmic abscesses were usually present when the spinal cord disorder occurred.

In HIV-infected patients with clinical manifestations suggesting spinal cord compression, antitoxoplasmic treatment should be undertaken in all patients with a focal spinal cord lesion if a toxoplasmic abscess cannot be excluded.

### Other infections

In tropical areas, some patients may suffer coinfection with HTLV-1 and HIV; paraparesis may be caused by HTLV-1 (Berger *et al.*, 1991).

Papovavirus infection of the spinal cord has been observed in a single patient (Hénin *et al.*, 1992); currently, no therapy for this infection is possible.

## SPINAL CORD LYMPHOMAS

Primary non-Hodgkin's lymphomas are common in the CNS of patients with AIDS (Ioachim *et al.*, 1991). A few cases of intraspinal cord (Ioachim *et al.*, 1991; Herida *et al.*, 1993) or epidural (Lang *et al.*, 1989; Gray *et al.*, 1991; Chemouilli *et al.*, 1994) lymphomas have been reported.

## ISCHAEMIC MYELOPATHY

Ischaemic myelopathy has been occasionally reported in the context of HIV infection. Brown-Séquard syndrome secondary to intravascular coagulation and ischaemic lesions of the spinal cord has been observed (Fénelon *et al.*, 1991). Necrotizing vasculitis of the CNS, predominating in the spinal cord, was responsible for a fatal outcome within 48 hours in a patient with ARC (Vinters *et al.*, 1988); this was later related to infection with VZV (Chrétien *et al.*, 1993).

## CONCLUSIONS

A wide range of lesions in the spinal cord can be responsible for an acute, subacute or chronic progressive sensorimotor deficit. The most common spinal cord disorder is the chronic variety, often associated with HIV-ADC. When the onset is subacute, focal treatable lesions caused by opportunistic infection must be considered, especially toxoplasmic abscess or CMV infection. The overall prognosis of spinal cord disease is extremely poor in HIV-infected patients.

## REFERENCES

Anders KH, Guerra WF, Tomiyasu U *et al.* (1986) The neuropathology of AIDS: UCLA experience and review. *American Journal of Pathology* **124**: 537–558.

Baumrind NL, Becker PS, Glass JD *et al.* (1991) Microglia and macrophages in HIV-associated myelopathy. *Journal of Neuropathology and Experimental Neurology* **50**: 343.

Bélec L, Gray F, Mikol J *et al.* (1990) Cytomegalovirus (CMV) encephalomyeloradiculitis and human immunodeficiency virus (HIV) encephalitis: presence of HIV and CMV coinfected multinucleated giant cells. *Acta Neuropathologica* **81**: 99–104.

Berger JR, Sheremata WA, Resnick L *et al.* (1989) Multiple sclerosis-like illness occurring with human immunodeficiency virus infection. *Neurology* **39**: 324–329.

Berger JR, Raffanti S, Svenningsson A *et al.* (1991) The role of HTLV in HIV-1 neurologic disease. *Neurology* **41**: 197–202.

Brew BJ, Hardy W, Zuckerman E *et al.* (1989) AIDS-related vacuolar myelopathy is not associated with coinfection by human T-lymphotropic virus type 1. *Annals of Neurology* **26**: 679–681.

Budka H, Maier H and Pohl P (1988) Human immunodeficiency virus in vacuolar myelopathy of the acquired immunodeficiency syndrome. *New England Journal of Medicine* **319**: 1667–1668.

Budka H, Wiley CA, Kleihues P *et al.* (1991) HIV-associated disease of the nervous system: review of nomenclature and proposal for neuropathology-based terminology. *Brain Pathology* **1**: 143–152.

Chemouilli P, Taussig D, Lacroix C and Gasnault (1994) Atteinte de la moëlle épinière et virus de l'immunodéficience humaine. *Presse Medicale* **23**: 1646–1650.

Chimelli L, de Freitas MRG, Bazin AR *et al.* (1990) Encéphalo-myéloradiculite à cytomégalovirus au cours du syndrome d'immuno-déficience acquise. *Rev Neurol (Paris)* **146**: 354–360.

Chrétien F, Gray F, Lescs MC *et al.* (1993) Acute varicella-zoster virus ventriculitis and meningo-myelo-radiculitis in acquired immunodeficiency syndrome. *Acta Neuropathologica* **86**: 659–665.

Denning DW, Anderson D, Rudge P and Smith H (1987) Acute myelopathy associated with primary infection with human immunodeficiency virus. *British Medical Journal* **294**: 143–144.

Eilbott DJ, Peress N, Burger H *et al.* (1989) Human immunodeficiency virus hyper 1 in spiral cord of acquired immunodeficiency syndrome patients with myelopathy: expression and replication of macrophages. *Proceedings of the National Academy of Science USA* **86**: 3337–3341.

Fénelon G, Gray F, Scaravilli F *et al.* (1991) Ischemic myelopathy secondary to disseminated intravascular coagulation in AIDS. *Journal of Neurology* **238**: 51–54.

Geny C, Gherardi R, Boudes P *et al.* (1991) Multifocal multinucleated giant cell myelitis in an AIDS patient. *Neuropathology and Applied Neurobiology* **17**: 157–162.

Glass JD, Becker PS and Price DL (1990) Central spinal myelinolysis in AIDS. *Journal of Neuropathology and Experimental Neurology* **49**: 348.

Goldstick L, Mandybur TI and Bode R (1985) Spinal cord degeneration in AIDS. *Neurology* **35**: 103–106.

Gray F and Gherardi R (1990) Les lésions médullaires et radiculaires au cours de l'infection par le virus de l'immunodéficience humaine. *Revue Neurologique* **146**: 655–664.

Gray F, Geny C, Lionnet F *et al.* (1991) Etude neuropathologique de 135 cas adultes de syndrome d'immuno-deficience acquise (SIDA). *Annales de Pathologie* **11**: 236–247.

Hénin D, Smith TW, De Girolami U *et al.* (1992) Neuropathology of the spinal cord in the acquired immunodeficiency syndrome. *Human Pathology* **23**: 1106–1114.

Herida M, Khuong MA, De Broucker T *et al.* (1993) Lymphome primitif du système nerveux central à localisation médullaire révélatrice chez un patient infecté par le virus de l'immunodéficience humaine. *Annals of Medicine Internelle* **144**: 64–66.

Herskovitz S, Siegel SE, Schneider AT *et al.* (1989) Spinal cord toxoplasmosis in AIDS. *Neurology* **39**: 1552–1553.

Ioachim HL, Dorsett B, Cronin W *et al.* (1991) Acquired immunodeficiency syndrome-associated lymphomas: clinical, pathologic, immunologic, and viral characteristics of 111 cases. *Human Pathology* **22**: 659–673.

Jacobson MA, Mills J, Rush J *et al.* (1988) Failure of antiviral therapy for acquired immunodeficiency syndrome-related cytomegalovirus myelitis. *Archives of Neurology* **45**: 1090–1092.

Kamin SS and Petito CK (1991) Idiopathic myelopathies with white matter vacuolation in non-acquired immunodeficiency syndrome patients. *Human Pathology* **22**: 816–824.

Kure K, Llena JF, Lyman WD *et al.* (1991). Human immunodeficiency virus-1 infection of the nervous system: an autopsy study of 268 adult, pediatric, and fetal brains. *Human Pathology* **22**: 700–710.

Lacroix C (1991) Aspects anatomopathologiques du système nerveux central. In: *Manifestations Neurologiques et Infections Rétrovirales* (eds G. Said and AG Saimot), pp. 99–109. Paris: Pradel.

Lang W, Miklossy J, Dernaz JP *et al.* (1989) Neuropathology of the acquired immune deficiency syndrome (AIDS): a report of 135 consecutive autopsy cases from Switzerland. *Acta Neuropathologica* **77**: 379–390.

Mahieux F, Gray F, Fénelon G *et al.* (1989) Acute myeloradiculitis due to cytomegalovirus as the initial manifestation of AIDS. *Journal of Neurology, Neurosurgery and Psychiatry* **52**: 270–274.

Pattee GL, Kleinschmidt-De Masters BK, Sandberg EJ *et al.* (1990) CMV arteritis with acute necrotic thoracic myelitis in an AIDS patient. *Neurology* **40**: 235 (Suppl. 1).

Peress N, Burger H, La Neve D *et al.* (1990) HIV-1 expression: AIDS vacuolar myelopathy correlates with extent of disease. *Journal of Neuropathology and Experimental Neurology* **49**: 351.

Petito CK, Navia BA, Cho E-S *et al.* (1985) Vacuolar myelopathy pathologically resembling subacute combined degeneration in patients with acquired immune deficiency syndrome (AIDS). *New England Journal of Medicine* **312**: 874–879.

Petito CK, Vecchio D and Chen YT (1994) HIV antigen and DNA in AIDS spinal cords correlate with macrophage infiltration but not with vacuolar myelopathy. *Journal of Neuropathology and Experimental Neurology* **53**: 86–94.

Rance NE, McArthur JC, Cornblath DR *et al.* (1988) Gracile tract degeneration in patients with sensory neuropathy and AIDS. *Neurology* **38**: 265–271.

Rhodes RH (1993) Histopathologic features in the central nervous system of 400 acquired immunodeficiency syndrome cases: implications of rates of occurrence. *Human Pathology* **24**: 1189–1198.

Rosenblum M, Scheck AC, Cronin K *et al.* (1989) Dissociation of AIDS-related vacuolar myelopathy and productive HIV-1 infection of the spinal cord. *Neurology* **39**: 892–896.

Scaravilli F, Sinclair E, Arango JC *et al.* (1991) The pathology of the posterior root ganglia in AIDS and its relationship to the pallor of the gracile tract. *Acta Neuropathologica* **84**: 163–170.

Sharer LR, Epstein LG, Cho E-S and Petito CK (1986) HTLV-III and vacuolar myelopathy. *New England Journal of Medicine* **315**: 62–63.

Singh BM, Levine S, Yarrish RL *et al.* (1986) Spinal cord syndromes in the acquired immune deficiency syndrome. *Acta Neurologica Scandinavica* **73**: 590–598.

Smith T, Jakobsen J and Trojaborg W (1990) Myelopathy and HIV infection. *AIDS* **4**: 589–591.

Tucker T, Dix RD, Katzen C *et al.* (1985) Cytomegalovirus and herpes virus ascending myelitis in a patient with acquired immune deficiency syndrome. *Annals of Neurology* **18**: 74–79.

Tyor WR, Glass JD, Baumrid N *et al.* (1993) Cytokine expression of macrophages in HIV-1-associated vacuolar myelopathy. *Neurology* **43**: 1002–1009.

Vinters HV, Guerra WF, Eppolito L and Reith PE (1988) Necrotizing vasculitis of the nervous system in a patient with AIDS-related complex. *Neuropathology and Applied Neurobiology* **14**: 417–424.

Vinters HV, Kwock MK, Ho H *et al.* (1989) Cytomegalovirus in the nervous system of patients with the acquired immune deficiency syndrome. *Brain* **112**: 270–274.

Weiser B, Peress N, La Neve *et al.* (1990) Human immunodeficiency virus type 1 expression in the central nervous system correlates directly with extent of disease. *Proceedings of the National Academy of Sciences USA* **87**: 3997–4001.

# 6

# *Neurological Aspects of HIV-1 Infection in Children*

## INTRODUCTION AND GENERAL BACKGROUND

HIV infection in children represents 1–3% of declared AIDS cases in industrialized countries, and 20% in sub-Saharan Africa (Delfraissy *et al.*, 1992).

Children can be infected by HIV-1 after transmission of the virus from the mother, after transfusion with contaminated blood or during treatment of haemophilia, or as sexually active or intravenous drug-using adolescents. This chapter considers only the consequences of HIV-1 infection in children born to HIV-1-infected mothers. The clinical consequences of HIV-1 infection after contaminated blood transfusion in the neonatal period are similar to those observed after maternofetal transmission of the virus, but the initial viral load is potentially different (and so might be the ability of the virus to penetrate the blood–brain barrier). HIV-1 infection in patients with haemophilia or in adolescents seems to follow a course similar to that of adult patients.

### Rate and time of HIV-1 transmission from mother to child

The rate of transmission of the virus from HIV-1-infected mothers to offspring has recently been clarified. Studies from developed countries agree on a rate of transmission between 15 and 25% (Blanche *et al.*, 1989; European Collaborative Study, 1991; Delfraissy *et al.*, 1992), which is reduced by zidovudine treatment during pregnancy (Connor *et al.*, 1994). In developing countries this rate might be higher, although the results are highly variable from one study to another due to technical difficulties in conducting large epidemiological studies in impoverished countries (Hira *et al.*, 1989; Lallemant *et al.*, 1989; Ryder *et al.*, 1989; Dabis *et al.*, 1993; Lepage *et al.*, 1993).

The time of HIV-1 transmission probably differs among patients (discussed in Delfraissy *et al.*, 1992). Early passage of the virus (before the twentieth week) has been reported but seems infrequent (Lyman *et al.*, 1990; Ehrnst *et al.*, 1991; Pizzo and Butler, 1991). Passage during the last weeks of pregnancy or during delivery is probably more frequent and is supported by two series of arguments.

(1) The number of circulating infected cells increases during the first weeks of life: viral isolation in blood is less frequent during the neonatal period of HIV-infected children compared with later on, including during the asymptomatic period (Ehrnst *et al.*, 1991; Burgard *et al.*, 1992; Strugo *et al.*, 1992). Moreover, in some cases, cultures that were initially negative become positive during the first 3 months of life and the concentration of p24 antigen increases during the same period.
(2) No signs of early perturbation of structural brain development (gyral abnormalities or neuronal migration disorders) have been observed in HIV-1-infected children, in contrast with what is observed after early transmission of rubella virus or CMV.

**Modes of contamination of mothers**

Modes of contamination of mothers are highly variable in different countries. In Africa, the West Indies and parts of Asia, most of the women have been contaminated after heterosexual contact. In Europe and most parts of America, intravenous drug use is an important cause of contamination, either directly (the mother using or having used intravenous drugs) or indirectly (heterosexual contact with an intravenous drug user). In the ongoing French cohort, 47.5% of the mothers are intravenous drug users, 47.5% have been infected after heterosexual contact (half infected while living in France and half while living in Central Africa or Haiti) and less than 5% received a contaminated blood transfusion before the pregnancy.

**Consequences of intravenous drug use on neurological development of the offspring**

Since most of the studies on the long-term evolution of HIV-1-infected children come from developed countries, it is important to consider the long-term consequences of intravenous drug use by the mother on the development of the child before implying a role of HIV-1 infection itself. Zagon and Slotkin (1992) have recently reviewed the effects of different toxins on brain development, but in fact the factors are highly interlinked since drug use increases the rate of prematurity and is often associated with maternal nutritional problems. Moreover, it is difficult to know the actual types of intoxication that occurred during the pregnancy: in our experience in France, the majority of women infected after intravenous drug use stopped taking drugs before the pregnancy (25% of the children had a withdrawal syndrome at birth; Blanche *et al.*, 1989), whereas some other mothers were still using more than five different toxins during pregnancy, including alcohol and cigarettes, which have known deleterious effects on brain development.

## HIV-1-RELATED CNS DISEASE

### Clinical variations in the expression of neurological disease after HIV-1 infection

*Nomenclature and classification*

The wide variation in the symptoms induced by HIV infection in children was recognized very early (Scott *et al.*, 1984, 1989; Blanche *et al.*, 1990) and two successive classification systems for HIV-infected children less than 13 years of age was established by the CDC. The last one distinguished three mutually exclusive clinical categories: N, no signs/symptoms; A, mild signs/symptoms; B, moderate signs/symptoms; C, severe signs/symptoms.

Neurological symptoms are included in clinical category C:

> Encephalopathy (at least one of the following progressive findings present for at least 2 months in the absence of a concurrent illness other than HIV infection that could explain the findings): a) failure to attain or loss of developmental milestones or loss of intellectual ability, verified by standard developmental scale or neuropsychological tests; b) impaired brain growth or acquired microcephaly demonstrated by head circumference measurements or brain atrophy demonstrated by computerized tomography or magnetic resonance imaging (serial imaging is required for children <2 years of age); c) acquired symmetric motor deficit manifested by two or more of the following: paresis, pathologic reflexes, ataxia, gait disturbance (Centers for Disease Control, 1994).

Other classifications of neurological symptoms have been used in parallel, mostly based on the rate of progression of the encephalopathy (Belman *et al.*, 1985; Epstein *et al.*, 1985, 1986). This classification turned out to be difficult to use since a given patient can often have an initially progressive encephalopathy followed by a stable phase that can last for several months or years, followed by another progressive phase: nothing suggests that these different patterns correspond to different types of pathogenesis. The static encephalopathy initially described is infrequent in our experience and might not be due to HIV-1 infection but to other maternal factors. Indeed, we have followed five HIV-1-negative patients born to HIV-1-infected drug addict mothers who suffered from such a static encephalopathy.

A consensus report on nomenclature in 1991 proposed that the term *HIV-associated progressive encephalopathy of childhood* replace the various other terms found in the literature (American Academy of Neurology AIDS Task Force, 1991). One limitation with this term is that not all the neurological and neuropsychological symptoms observed during HIV-1 infection fit and, furthermore, it does not refer to either the age of onset or the general evolution of the disease.

*Two modes of evolution of HIV infection*

Neurological symptoms should not be viewed in isolation: associations between clinical symptoms, their age of occurrence and that of severe immunodeficiency allowed the definition of at least two modes of evolution.

Firstly, 20% of reports of infantile AIDS cases occurred during the first 7 months of life, while AIDS in other patients was reported regularly up to the age of 10 years (Auger *et al.*, 1988).

Secondly, one-third of the 94 patients we followed suffered from early onset of opportunistic infections and of severe encephalopathy and had a survival rate of 48 ± 24% at 3 years. In contrast, patients without severe encephalopathy or opportunistic infections had a probability of survival of 97±3% at 3 years (Blanche *et al.*, 1989). Moreover, the occurrence of severe encephalopathy was correlated with the intensity of immune deficiency and viral replication during the first year of life (Duliège *et al.*, 1992). This is confirmed in our ongoing cohort following the babies of more than 1000 HIV-1-infected women, although the percentage of patients suffering from the early and severe symptoms is closer to 20%.

More recently, a correlation was demonstrated between the development of early and severe symptoms (including encephalopathy) and the detection of p24 antigen at birth (Burgard *et al.*, 1992) and between the development of these symptoms and the maternal status at delivery (Blanche *et al.*, 1994).

In the remaining part of this chapter, a two-part classification is used that corresponds to the bimodal expression of the disease (Blanche *et al.*, 1990).

(1) A severe infantile disease defined as the onset of an 'HIV-associated progressive encephalopathy of childhood' and/or opportunistic infections during the first 3 years of life (without clear-cut limit in terms of age). This is associated with an early and severe immune deficit and with a higher rate of positive viral cultures in blood during the first 2 months of life. It occurs in 15–20% of infected children, at least in developed countries, with neurological symptoms in the majority of them (Blanche *et al.*, 1990; Belman, 1992; Lobato *et al.*, 1995).

(2) A slowly progressive disease during which, for several years, children either remain asymptomatic or have reversible symptoms. Similarly, no severe immune deficiency can be detected for several years. Whether these patients might have HIV-related neurological or neuropsychological symptoms or even suffer from 'HIV-associated progressive encephalopathy of childhood' of late onset is discussed later. This mode of evolution is by far the most frequent (close to 80% of HIV-infected children in our experience).

It is clear, however, that as a better understanding of the pathophysiology of the disease develops, such a classification might have to be reconsidered. Moreover, the epidemiology and natural history of HIV-1 infection may be modified by the introduction of antiviral therapy.

*Neurological symptoms during the severe infantile form of the disease*

The first abnormal neurological signs are usually observed between the age of 4 and 18 months, and mostly between 4 and 12 months. In our own cohort of patients followed at a single neurology clinic, the first symptom was noted before 12 months in 70% of these patients but was delayed between 24 and 36 months in 15% (Figure 6.1).

Increasingly patent motor symptoms are initially noted with both abnormal rigidity of limbs and abnormal postural tone, not very different from what is observed in cerebral palsy due to other causes. Over time, these symptoms result in spastic paraparesis or quadriparesis, sometimes associated with dystonic posturing, and in loss of motor milestones. In 30–50% of the children, buccolingual dyspraxia develops: the mouth stays open with abnormal and permanent drooling and difficulties (at appropriate age) with chewing small pieces of food. Stagnation of cognitive, behavioural and socially adaptive skills usually occurs later and initially they appear comparatively less affected (Belman *et al.*, 1985; Epstein *et al.*, 1985, 1986; Tardieu *et al.*, 1987; Blanche *et al.*, 1990; European Collaborative Study, 1990; Belman, 1992). Subsequently, the pattern of regression is quite variable from one child to another, although most decline in a stepwise manner with long periods of plateau over 2–4 years. After 3 years the children are usually clearly mentally retarded with small head circumference and severe spastic tetraparesis (Belman, 1992). It is not unusual for the children to make some cognitive or even motor acquisitions during the plateau periods. Death usually occurs before the age of 5 years; the estimated median survival time after diagnosis was 22 months in a recent study (Lobato *et al.*, 1995).

Symptoms seem to be slightly different when they first occur between 24 months and 3 years (Tardieu *et al.*, unpublished observations; Belman *et al.*, 1988). In the patients we followed prospectively, no motor or cognitive symptoms were noted before the age of 2 years. Signs of severe spastic diplegia appeared within a few weeks and remained relatively stable thereafter, whereas cognitive development slowed down over subsequent months. Biological signs of immune deficiency were first observed 6–9 months previous. This slightly less active neurological disease could correspond to a lower viral infection during the perinatal period or to a modification of early symptoms by antiviral

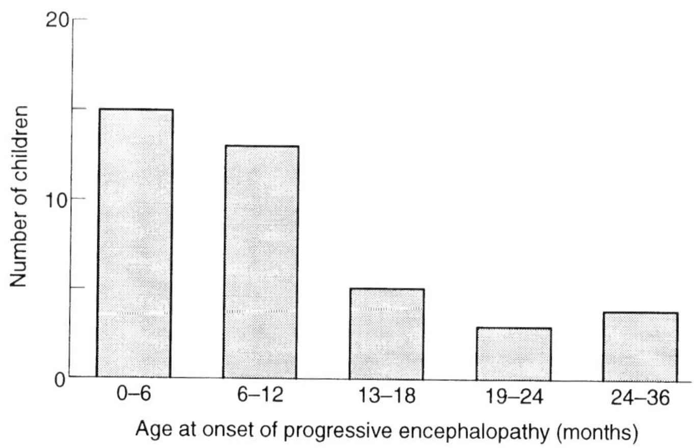


**Figure 6.1** Time of occurrence of early signs of progressive encephalopathy (CDC class P2B) during the first 3 years of life, in a personal series of 40 vertically infected patients.

treatment (however, one of our patients had not received AZT before the onset of neurological symptoms). The late appearance of these symptoms in a previously neurologically normal child could also suggest the possibility of CNS infection with other viruses such as CMV. In our patients, no opportunistic infection was demonstrated, despite several attempts being made during the 6–34 months (median 12 months) preceding death.

*Neurological symptoms during the slowly progressive form of the disease*
In this mode of evolution of the disease, which is observed in 80–85% of infected children, no permanent neurological symptoms are present during the first years of life. However, it is not unusual to observe slight and non-permanent delay in the acquisition of motor tone during the first 6 months (AL Belman, personal communication; Belman, 1992; Msellati *et al.*, 1993). However, at 6 years of age most children have a normal general appearance and a normal neurological examination, including head circumference.

Two questions arise: (1) what are the cognitive abilities, neuropsychological behaviour and overall school performances at school age in these children and (2) could an 'HIV-associated progressive encephalopathy of childhood' have a very late onset?

*Cognitive abilities and school performances in school-age children.* This is important because most HIV-1-infected children will reach school age, at least in developed countries. Very few results are available at present and future results might concern mostly patients under antiviral therapy. Moreover, methodological problems complicate the approach.

(1) A large group of patients has to be followed from birth (to avoid biased selection).
(2) Children should be tested after the age of 6 years, when well-standardized and selective tests are available.
(3) A control group is difficult to obtain for both technical and ethical considerations (it is difficult and may be unethical to require tests from a 6-year-old HIV-1-reverter child born to a seropositive intravenous drug-using woman). By using standardized tests, HIV-1-infected children can at least be compared with children of the same age in the general population.
(4) A comparison between evaluations from different countries is important because of large differences in the psychosocial status of infected mothers, but is difficult because of differences in the tests.

Several recent data corrected the initial results, suggesting a high frequency of mental retardation and school failure (Ultmann *et al.*, 1985, 1987; Belman *et al.*, 1988; Diamond, 1989; Diamond *et al.*, 1990). For example, Levenson *et al.* (1992) recently reported that 44% of HIV-1-infected children (age 5 years ± 20 months) scored in the mentally retarded range but also observed that neurologically normal HIV-infected children had results similar to those of seroreverters. In the patients we are following, we observed that most have normal development at the age of 9.5 years and that 67% were following regular school at a normal pace, 15% performed in the borderline range and 18% were considered to have failed (Tardieu *et al.*, 1995). However, selective deficit in visuospatial organization and in temporal orientation was frequent. Very similar results were observed in children infected through neonatal blood transfusion (Cohen *et al.*, 1991). Interestingly, we also observed that school achievements and results at cognitive tests were not related to the mode of infection of the mothers (meaning that children born to intravenous drug users had results similar to those of others) and that children with normal school achievement had a higher percentage of circulating $CD4^+$ T cells during the course of infection (Tardieu *et al.*, 1995). This last result suggests that the percentage of circulating $CD4^+$ T cells during the first years of life are predictive of future school adaptation or cognitive abilities.

Hyperactivity, attention deficit and anxiety are probably more frequent among HIV-infected children, although there is a paucity of data in this area.

*Could an 'HIV-associated progressive encephalopathy of childhood' have a very late onset?* By analogy with the occurrence of HIV-1-related encephalopathy in adults with AIDS, one could expect that such an encephalopathy could happen in children at any age. In fact, the onset of a progressive encephalopathy is very infrequent after the age of 3 years. However, it does occur: patient 3 described by Epstein *et al.* 1985) had symptoms of progressive encephalopathy at the age of 6 years; among the 400 patients we are following, one patient had very similar symptoms (including pseudobulbar palsy) beginning at the age of 10 years, and a 13-year-old boy suffered from progressive encephalopathy with acute psychiatric symptoms persisting until his death 6 months later. In a collaborative study with M. Mintz, we observed that some of these children have extrapyramidal symptoms, which can be improved by levodopa therapy (Mintz *et al.*, 1996).

*Unusual neurological symptoms during the course of HIV infection*

(1) Seizures are very infrequent and are usually an early symptom of secondary complications.
(2) Isolated spinal cord symptoms are also unusual but spinal cord symptoms are one of the most frequent signs of progressive encephalopathy (Dickson *et al.*, 1989a; Sharer *et al.*, 1990).
(3) Peripheral nerve lesions: in contrast to what is observed in adults, both acute and chronic peripheral nerve diseases are very infrequent. One case of polyradiculoneuritis has been reported (Raphael *et al.*, 1991).
(4) Myopathy: no HIV-related polymyositis has been reported. In two children a myopathy probably related to the use of zidovudine has been reported (Dickson *et al.*, 1990; Walter *et al.*, 1991).

## CSF studies

Cellularity and protein content are usually normal in CSF but oligoclonal bands are frequent on protein electrophoresis (Epstein *et al.*, 1987a; Blanche *et al.*,

1990). Several cytokines have also been detected, such as interferon α, IL-6 and IL-1β (Mintz *et al.*, 1989; Gallo *et al.*, 1991).

HIV p24 antigen can be detected in CSF, usually at a titre lower than in matched serum. Its detection is more frequent, although still relatively rare, in patients with neurological symptoms (Epstein *et al.*, 1987a; Blanche *et al.*, 1990; Gallo *et al.*, 1991). Anti-HIV antibody titres, as detected by ELISA, are high in the CSF of most patients with the slowly progressive mode of evolution, whereas they become low or undetectable in the CSF of children with severe neurological symptoms (Tardieu *et al.*, 1987; Blanche *et al.*, 1990).

Altogether, CSF studies are not necessary in the usual management of HIV-infected children: several of the biological results that can be obtained in CSF are indeed linked with the occurrence of neurological lesions, but they are also highly correlated to similar biological results obtained in serum, which are sufficie~t to establysh a prognosis (Duliège *et al.*, 1992). CSF studies, however, are mandatory when unexpected new neurological symptoms are observed and this is discussed below.

## Brain imaging

### *CT*

Three abnormalities on CT were described soon after the initial description of the disease (Belman *et al.*, 1986; Epstein *et al.*, 1987b; Price *et al.*, 1988):

(1) enlargement of the subarachnoid space and ventricles, which is not always associated with brain atrophy (as defined by a pathologically small head circumference); (2) It calcifications of basal ganglia and subcortical area – calcifications are usually punctiform and numerous within a small area; and (3) hypodensity of the white matter.

The frequency of detection of these different pathological aspects is difficult to establish. In a recent large study of 100 consecutive patients (50% in CDC stage C and 58% of the patients having acquired the disease through vertical transmission), it was reported that calcifications were detected in 22% of the total study population (DeCarli *et al.*, 1993). They were found only, but not always, in patients in CDC stage C. Other CT abnormalities could be observed in non-encephalopathic children but were usually mild.

CT is not helpful enough in the care of HIV-1-infected children to still be routinely performed in our institution. However, it is required if unexpected neurological symptoms occur.

### *MRI*

Very few studies of MRI in HIV-infected children have been published, although several centres, including our own, now have extensive experience (Figure 6.2).

In 91 consecutive HIV-1-infected children we followed (18% in CDC stage C),

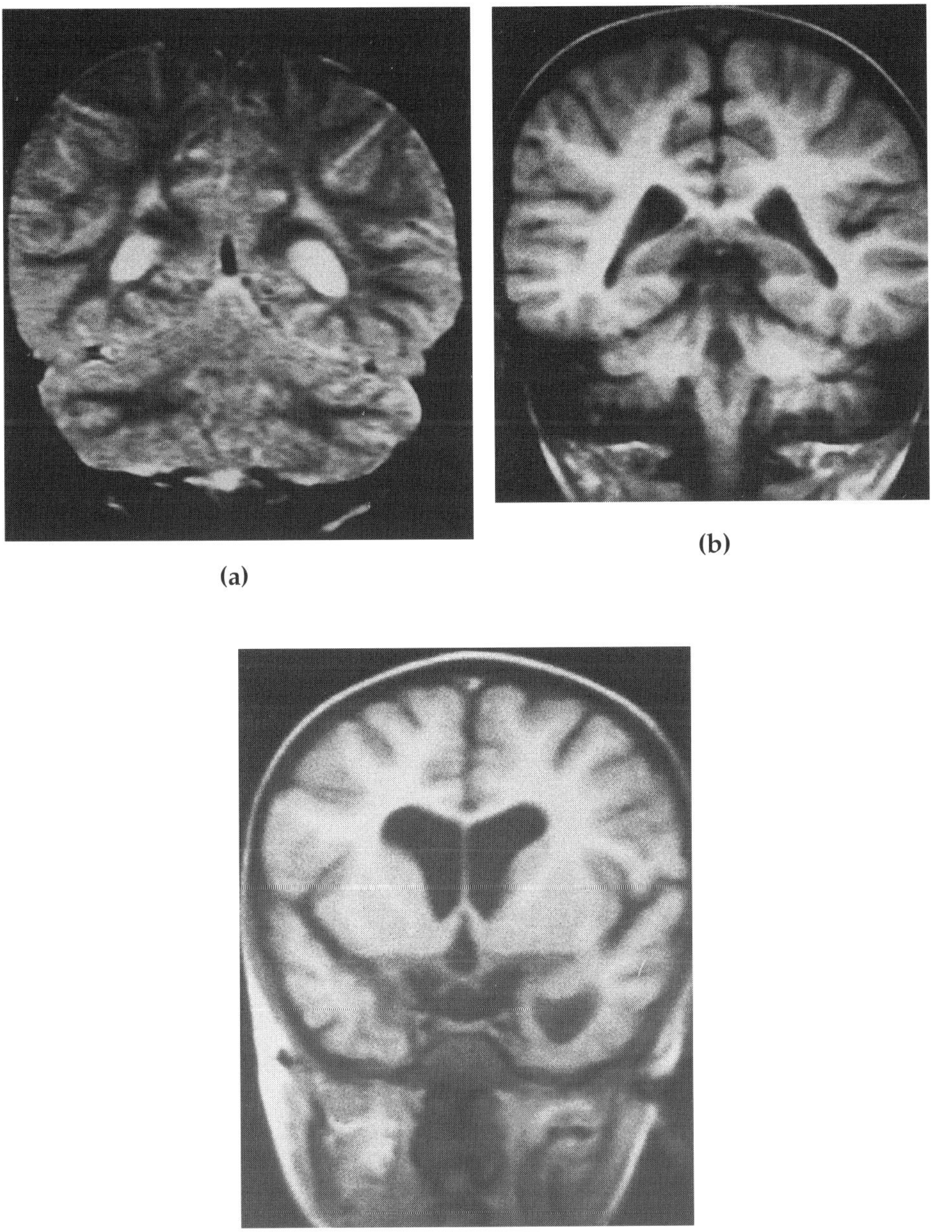

(a) (b) (c)

**Figure 6.2** Coronal $T_1$- (b, c) and $T_2$- (a) weighted MRI. Moderate atrophy is observed with enlargement of ventricles and pericerebral sulci (c). In the occipital region, no abnormality is seen on the $T_1$-weighted sequence (b) whereas the $T_2$-weighted sequence (a) shows an abnormal high-intensity signal in the white matter.

cerebral MRI was abnormal in 40% (Tardieu *et al.*, 1991). The most frequent abnormalities were found in the white matter and consisted of large areas of hypersignal on $T_2$-weighted images (25% of studied patients) or, less frequently, of plaque-like lesions (3%) (Berger *et al.*, 1989). Areas of hyposignals on $T_1$-weighted images and hypersignals on $T_2$-weighted images, suggestive of leucomalacia, were observed in 8% of the patients and signs of CNS atrophy in 8%. Studies of the relationships between the MRI findings and the clinical course of the disease indicated that brain atrophy was significantly more frequent in patients with a severe encephalopathy, although 41% of patients from this group had normal MRI. On the other hand, 26% of patients without neurological symptoms had CNS lesions detected by MRI. Finally, the white matter lesions detected by MRI appeared early during the course of the infection and seemed to remain rather stable thereafter.

*Positron emission tomography*
We had the opportunity to study children by positron emission tomography with $^{18}$F-labelled fluorodeoxyglucose and found diffuse hypometabolism and subcortical hypermetabolism in the three children in stage C. The other five children, who had no neurological symptoms, had temporo-occipital cortical hypometabolism, mainly on the right side (Depas *et al.*, 1995). Improvement of these lesions after antiviral treatment has been reported in one case (Pizzo *et al.*, 1988).

## Treatment

*Effect of antiviral drugs on HIV-1-induced neurological symptoms*
Two antiviral drugs, AZT and dideoxyinosine, have so far been tested but it is still difficult to get a general view of their neurological effects, mostly because different clinical situations have been evaluated within the same protocol (including young children with existing severe encephalopathy and permanent brain lesions).

*Effect of AZT on neuropsychological functioning.* An initial study evaluated the effect of continuous intravenous infusion of zidovudine in a small group of 13 children with symptomatic infection and suggested an increase of IQ score over a 6-month period, even in patients who had appeared normal at their initial pretreatment evaluation or were older than 6 years of age (Pizzo *et al.*, 1988; Brouwers *et al.*, 1990; DeCarli *et al.*, 1991). A larger multicentre study was subsequently published testing the effect, over the same follow-up period, of oral zidovudine on cognitive functions of 55 children (from a group of 88 patients aged 4 months to 11 years, 77% vertically infected) (McKinney *et al.*, 1991). A significant increase in cognitive test scores was observed in the 25 youngest patients (less than 30 months of age, 15 of whom had severe encephalopathy) but not in the oldest patients (13 patients older than 6 years of age, none of whom had neurological symptoms). As the authors discussed, it was difficult in the infant patients to determine if the improvement was related to the direct effect of zidovudine on HIV infection of the CNS or to its effect on general physical well-being (Blanche *et al.*, 1991; McKinney *et al.*, 1991).

In conclusion, it is certainly possible that zidovudine may help prevent deterioration of cognitive functions. Several factors, such as the age of patients at initiation of antiviral treatment and their clinical condition at that time or the mode of administration of zidovudine, might be found in the future to influence subsequent cognitive functions.

*Effect of dideoxyinosine or dideoxycytidine on cognitive functions.* Very few studies have been published. In a phase I/II study in 43 children (aged 7 months to 19 years) with symptomatic HIV infection of different origin, some improvement in IQ score was noted after 24 weeks of dideoxyinosine but individual results were difficult to interpret (Butler *et al.*, 1991). Finally, in another phase I/II study in 15 children treated with dideoxycytidine, no modification of IQ score was detected (Pizzo *et al.*, 1990).

*Non-specific therapeutic approach*

In patients suffering from HIV-related progressive encephalopathy occurring early in life, general supportive measures including physical therapy, posture devices and an adapted educational programme are helpful. It has been our policy in France to rely upon existing structures already specializing in the care of handicapped children instead of upon newly created structures specializing in the care of HIV-1-infected children, but other policies have been used in other countries with good results.

In our experience, children with no clinical neurological symptoms are able to follow normal nursery and elementary school with good success. Less than 10% of the patients we are following who are older than 6 years of age require schools with specifically adapted programmes.

### Neuropathological lesions

The different types of neuropathological lesions observed after HIV infection have long been described but their respective frequency and relationship with the evolution of the disease are still poorly defined (Figure 6.3). (Sharer *et al.*, 1985; Epstein *et al.*, 1988; Dickson *et al.*, 1989b; Cho and Sharer, 1990; Wiley *et al.*, 1990; Kure *et al.*, 1991; Vazeux *et al.*, 1992; Lacroix *et al.*, 1993). It is generally accepted that, at time of death, the vast majority of children have neuropathological abnormalities (Kozlowski *et al.*, 1990).

Multinucleated cells are the hallmark of HIV encephalitis (Sharer *et al.*, 1985; Budka, 1986) but seem to be detected in less than half of the patients (Kozlowski *et al.*, 1990; Vazeux *et al.*, 1992; Lacroix *et al.*, 1993). They are of variable size and can be found isolated or close to microglial nodules. Their number is quite variable from one patient to another but, in the series of patients we studied, there was no direct correlation between the number of giant cells and the severity of the encephalopathy (Vazeux *et al.*, 1992). Finally, they can be detected

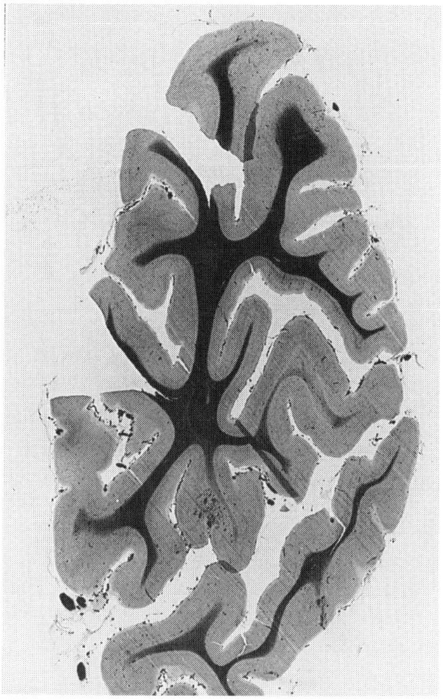

(a)

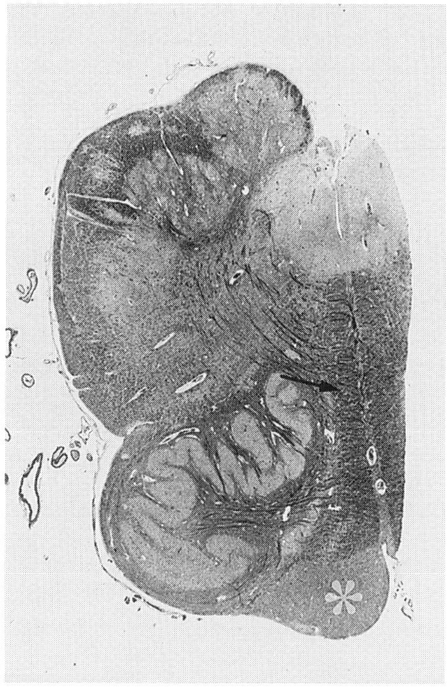

(b)

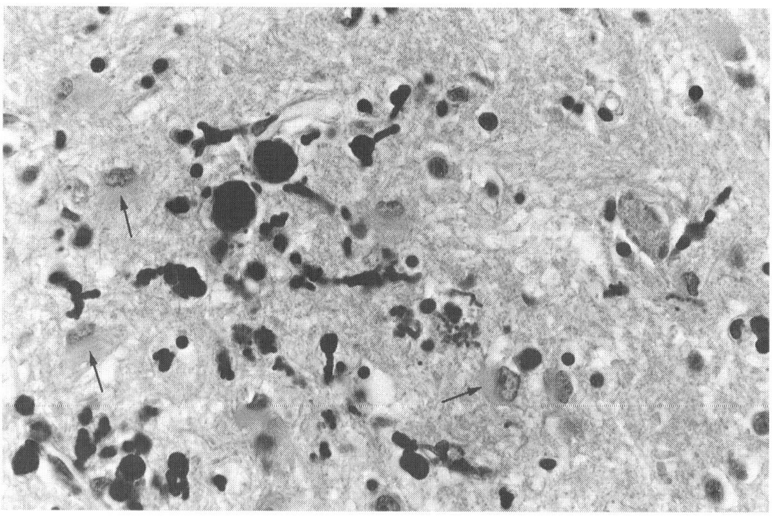

(c)

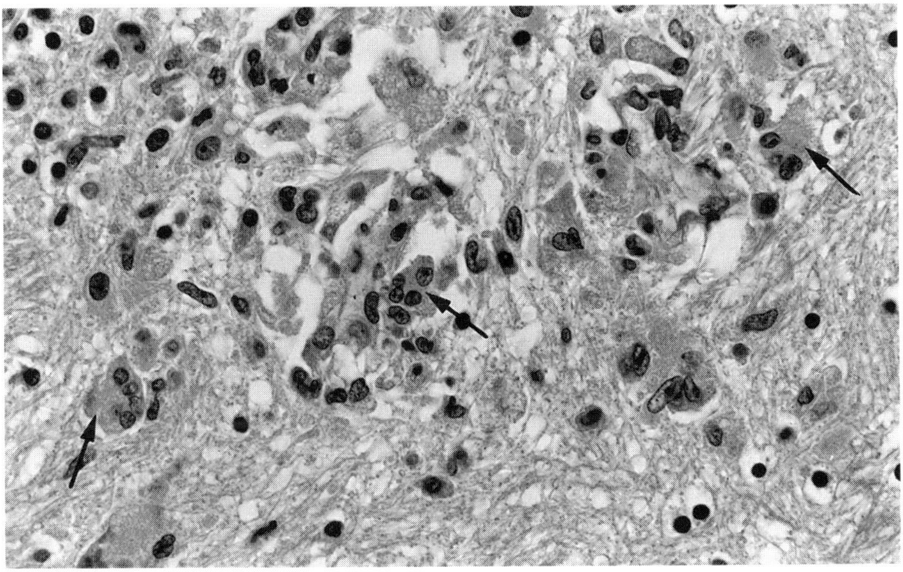

**(d)**

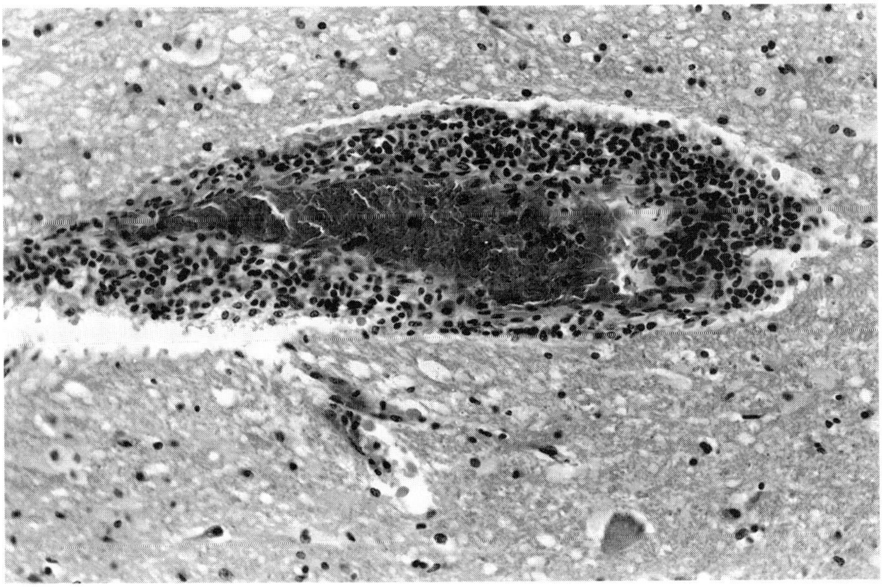

**(e)**

**Figure 6.3** HIV-1-related neuropathological lesions. (a) Cortical atrophy. (Celloidin section; Wolcke stain.) (b) Pallor of the pyramidal tracts (arrow). (c) Calcifications and glial cells (arrows) in basal ganglia. (H&E; ×930.) (d) Microglial nodules and multinucleated cells (arrows). (H&E; ×1000.) (e) Vasculitis. (H&E; ×500.)

very early in life, since we found some giant cells and microglial nodules in the white matter and cerebral cortex of a 2-month-old boy.

Microglial nodules can be found as microscopic foci of macrophages/ microglia (CD68 or *Ricinus* lectin positive by immunocytochemistry), associated with few $CD4^+$ T lymphocytes, astrocytes and occasionally polymorphonuclear cells. Microglial nodules can be located in the basal ganglia, white matter, brainstem, temporal lobe and internal capsule and are frequently associated with giant cells.

Detection of HIV p24, p17 or gp41 antigens by immunocytochemistry or HIV nucleic acid by *in situ* hybridization is possible on brain frozen sections but is also inconsistent (Shaw *et al.*, 1985; Sharer *et al.*, 1986, 1990; de la Monte *et al.*, 1987; Brüstle *et al.*, 1992; Vazeux *et al.*, 1992). In our series, the intensity of detection of HIV products in brain sections is not related to the severity of clinical neurological symptoms at time of death (Vazeux *et al.*, 1992).

Inflammatory cells or infiltration by inflammatory cells are frequently observed in the white matter, basal ganglia and leptomeninges. The perivascular cells comprise $CD4^+$ T lymphocytes and macrophages, whereas infiltration by $CD8^+$ T-lymphocyte can be located far from the vessels.

Perivascular calcifications are frequently observed in the basal ganglia, cerebral and cerebellar white matter and the cortex. They are present in all age groups, but are more frequent before 3 years of age (Kozlowski *et al.*, 1990).

Two lesions are detected in the white matter: an atrophy that is more pronounced than in the grey matter, and a diffuse pallor after myelin-specific staining. Moreover, selective pallor of the pyramidal tracts (and not of the sensory tracts) with inconsistent preservation of axons can be detected on Bodian staining in the spinal cord, medulla and corpus callosum (Belman, 1992)

Proliferation of reactive astrocytes is frequently present, large gemistocytes being located preferentially in the white matter and to a lesser degree in the cortex or basal ganglia. In most cases, the gliosis was associated with diffuse demyelination (Anders *et al.*, 1986; Belman, 1992).

Spongiosis, either extended or as multiple small foci in the basal ganglia, is probably secondary to ischaemic processes.

Microscopic infarcts and coagulation necrosis can also be observed, sometimes without inflammatory infiltration.

An important question is to consider whether there is evidence of neuronal death in the brains of the children. Although no studies have directly addressed this question, most report a reduction in brain weight and cerebral and cortical atrophy on gross examination. A morphometric study on five brains showed a reduction in the volume and surface of total grey and white matter (Kraszpulski *et al.*, 1991).

## SECONDARY CNS COMPLICATIONS ASSOCIATED WITH HIV-1 INFECTION

### Clinical observations

During the course of HIV-1 infection, several secondary lesions of the CNS can be clinically observed. In our experience, all of them occurred after the onset of severe immune deficiency (at least on a biological background, i.e. when $CD4^+$ T-cell counts were less than 200 $ml^{-1}$).

The frequency of secondary lesions is not clearly determined and might depend on the age of the children. It has been evaluated at 8% for patients followed in Paris (occurring at a median age of 6 years) and 15% for patients followed in New York City.

Several types of secondary lesion have been described and four clinical situations can be delineated (excluding bacterial meningitis which has no specific feature but can be of severe evolution, the secondary lesions described only on a neuropathological background and those associated with congenital CNS infection which are very unusual (Tardieu *et al.*, 1991b; Mitchell *et al.*, 1992).

*Acute retinitis and encephalitis*

The most frequent aetiological agent is CMV (Auger *et al.*, 1988; Belman, 1992; Butler *et al.*, 1992). Clinical symptoms include acute loss of vision in one or both eyes or acute onset of strabismus. Signs of CMV retinitis are usually easily observed at fundus examination. Progressive neurological symptoms include fever, seizures, confusion or sometimes isolated tetraparesis. These symptoms usually occur at the same time as symptoms of CMV infection in lung, liver or blood. On the electroencephalogram slow waves are observed. CT is of little help, whereas MRI shows large areas of hypersignal in the white matter on $T_2$-weighted images, which cannot be distinguished from what is observed during HIV infection.

A diagnosis is difficult to establish but can be made by isolation of the virus from blood or CSF and by observation of intra-blood–brain barrier production of antibodies against the suspected virus. PCR techniques will probably be very helpful.

Treatment with ganciclovir has been used occasionally but no formal study has established its benefits (Tardieu, unpublished observation; Butler *et al.*, 1992).

Other viruses such as measles (Mustafa *et al.*, 1993; Lacroix *et al.*, 1995) or VZV (Frank *et al.*, 1989) can also be encountered. One of the patients we followed had a bacillary angiomatosis (unpublished observation).

*Tumour-like lesions*

The most frequent aetiologies are toxoplasmosis, lymphoma and sarcoma (Shank *et al.*, 1987; Belman *et al.*, 1988; Epstein *et al.*, 1988; Dickson *et al.*, 1989b; Goldstein *et al.*, 1990; Keohane *et al.*, 1991; Belman, 1992). Clinical symptoms include signs of intracranial hypertension associated with focal symptoms or seizures. Toxoplasmosis is frequently, but not always, associated with high fever.

Brain imaging is of great help and usually shows several lesions of variable location. Each lesion on CT usually has a hyperdense centre surrounded by a hypodense halo, suggesting oedema.

A final diagnosis is difficult to establish and the titration of antibody titres against *Toxoplasma* in blood or even in CSF is usually of no help. Treatment with antitoxoplasmic agents is usually instituted for 3 months. If the lesions remain unchanged, the diagnosis of toxoplasmosis is unlikely and it is our practice to propose stereotactic biopsy of the lesions in order to establish a definitive diagnosis.

*Acute focal lesions*

This complication is one of the most frequently encountered (Belman *et al.*, 1988; Park *et al.*, 1988; Frank *et al.*, 1989; Kure *et al.*, 1989; Kugler *et al.*, 1991; Husson *et al.*, 1992; Phillipet *et al.*, 1994). The symptoms are acute hemiplegia, associated with aphasia or other focal symptoms or seizures.

Four different aetiologies have been observed with different appearances on brain imaging:

(1) intracerebral haemorrhage, usually associated with thrombocytopenia (Dickson *et al.*, 1990; Kozlowski *et al.*, 1990);
(2) multiple brain infarcts with aneurysmal lesions of large vessels, associated with multiple areas of vascular obstruction of small cortical vessels;
(3) isolated obstruction of a middle cerebral artery;
(4) isolated or multiple zones of necrosis without permanent abnormalities of brain vessels as determined by arteriography, which might be related to acute parenchymal necrosis.

Several mechanisms are probably involved, including vasculitis due to VZV infection, mycotic aneurysm, infiltration of the arterial wall by HIV-1-infected cells (Kure *et al.*, 1989) or, in the latter situation, vasculitis of very small vessels or suffusion of neurotoxic factors or HIV-infected monocytes or lymphocytes into the parenchyma, as described *in vitro* (Tardieu *et al.*, 1992).

*Progressive encephalopathy with abnormal appearance of white matter on MRI*

This is less common and very difficult to analyse. It is defined clinically by a change in mental status, sometimes associated with tetraparesis. Protein and cellular contents in the CSF are normal; hyperintensity signals on $T_2$-weighted MRI are observed. The two most frequent aetiologies seem to be secondary infection with a papovavirus leading to progressive multifocal encephalitis (Berger *et al.*, 1992; Van der Steenhoven *et al.*, 1992), or progressive HIV-1-related encephalopathy. Both diagnoses are very difficult to establish firmly. CSF studies using PCR with an SV40 probe might be very helpful, although the validity of the test has not yet been established. Brain biopsy might also be of help, although difficult to perform in patients in poor general condition.

Infection with mycobacteria, mycoplasma and viruses such as CMV and VZV can probably also induce an acute leucoencephalopathy.

## Neuropathological lesions

*Opportunistic infections*

CMV encephalitis has been detected in roughly 7% of anatomical cases (Kozlowski *et al.*, 1990). Most lesions are located in the periventricular areas with necrosis of the ependymal surface (Belec *et al.*, 1990). Typical nuclear and cytoplasmic inclusions, which can be labelled by a specific early CMV antibody, are detected in ependymal cells and in giant cells (macrophages). In one case we have also observed microglial nodules located in the basal ganglia, thalamus and hippocampus that contained cytomegalic cells but no HIV antigen, as detected by immunocytochemistry on frozen sections.

Measles encephalitis has been observed in three infants (LR Sharer, H Budka and PGE Kennedy, personal communications). We followed a 5-year-old girl who developed an acute necrotizing measles encephalitis reminiscent of the delayed type described in immunosuppressed children (Figure 6.4a) (Lacroix *et al.*, 1995). Gross examination showed necrosis of both frontal lobes with relative preservation of the white matter. We found many positive cells (macrophages) in frozen sections of the frontal cortex and basal ganglia. Immunocytochemistry for HIV antibodies was negative.

In the few reported cases of papovavirus infection, neuropathological lesions were similar to those previously described (Berger *et al.*, 1992; Van der Steenhoven *et al.*, 1992).

A few cases of congenital toxoplasmosis have been described in children with AIDS (Mitchell *et al.*, 1992; Taccone *et al.*, 1992); a 7-year-old child we followed had acquired acute cerebellar toxoplasmosis diagnosed with stereotactic biopsy (Figure 6.4b, c).

We have observed *Aspergillus* haemorrhagic abscesses located in the left frontal and parietal cortex of a 2-year-old child with severe progressive encephalopathy (Figure 6.4d). Another case of pseudotumoral aspergilloma of a hemisphere extending through the bone and skin has been reported by Kozlowski *et al.* (1990).

Two cases of cerebral abscesses with *Candida albicans* infection have been reported (Kozlowski *et al.*, 1990) and we have observed one such case.

A single observation of *Cryptococcus* infection has been reported (Kozlowski *et al.*, 1990).

Dickson *et al.* (1990) reported a miniscule 6-year-old child who had disseminated associated CNS infection with *Mycobacterium avium-intracellulare*.

Multiple microabscesses were present in a 24-month-old child (Lacroix *et al.*, 1993). Numerous small clusters of polymorphonuclear cells were present in the thalamus, pons and white matter; some microglial nodules contained polymorphonuclear cells and microglia. No organism was detected with histological techniques. Cerebral microabscesses have not been observed in

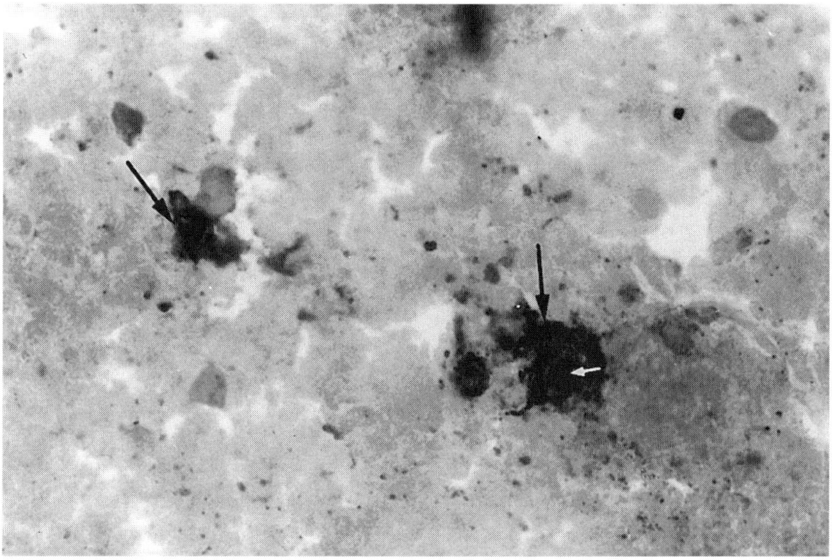

**(a)**

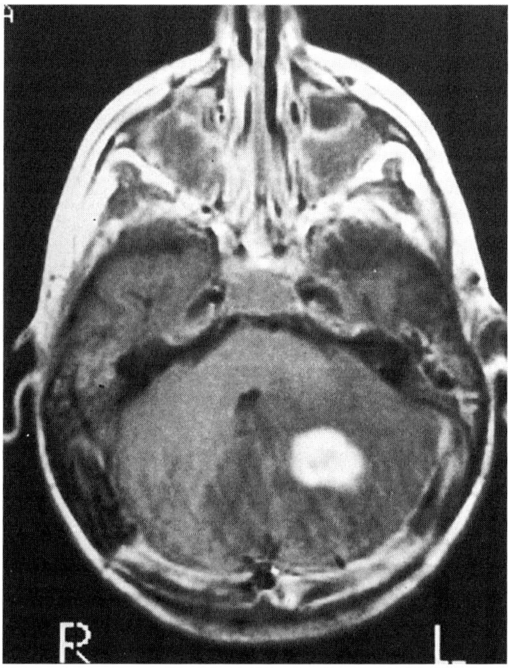


**(b)**

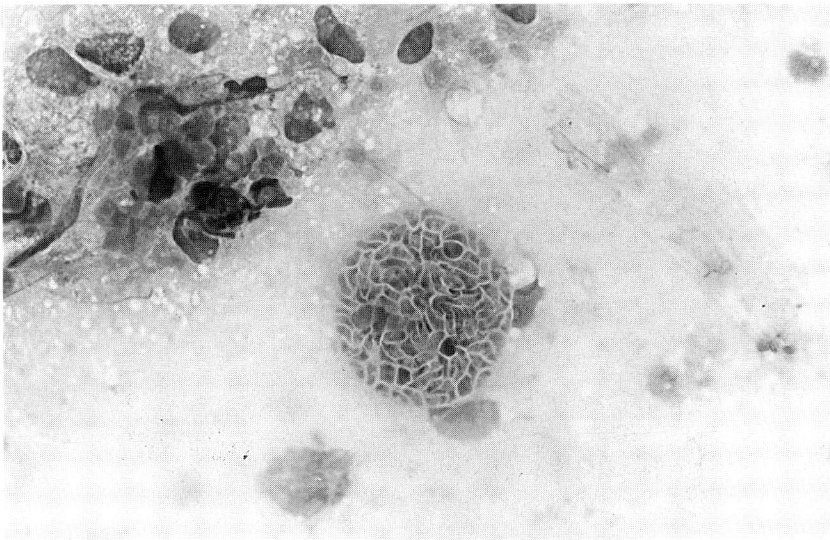

**(c)**

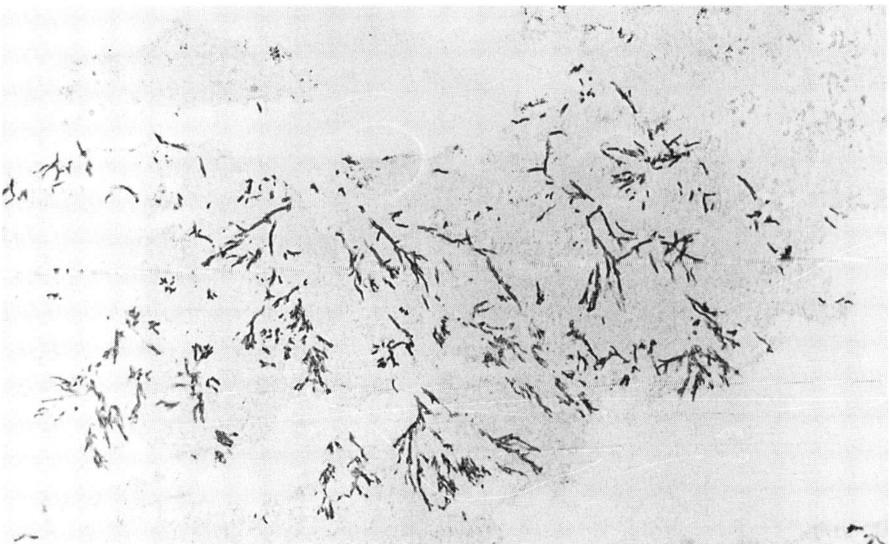

**(d)**

**Figure 6.4** Different neuropathological aspects of opportunistic infections of the CNS. (a) Acute necrotizing measles encephalitis: immunocytochemistry showing immunolabelling of cells (black arrows: cytoplasm; white arrows: nucleus) with an anti-measles antibody. (Congelation; ×1600.) (b, c) Cerebellar toxoplasmosis in a 7-year-old boy: (b) CT image (Courtesy E. Vilmer, Paris.); (c) neuropathology of a stereotactic biopsy, Smear (H&E; ×1600). (d) *Aspergillus* abscess in the frontal cortex of a 2-year-old child. (Grocott; ×250.)

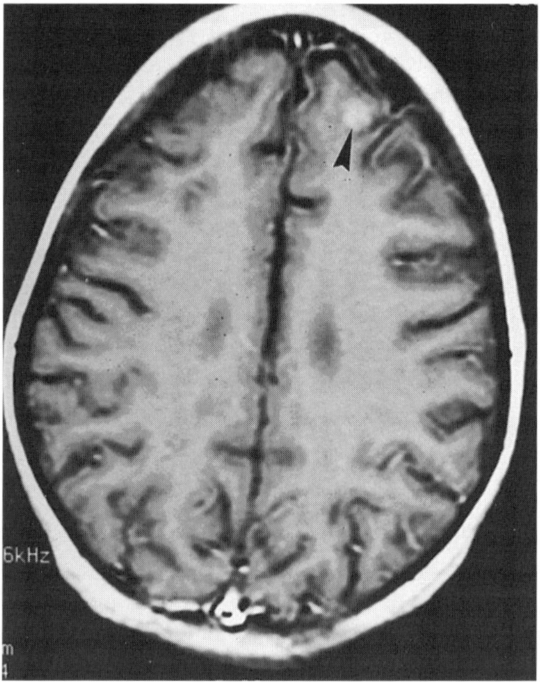


**(a)**

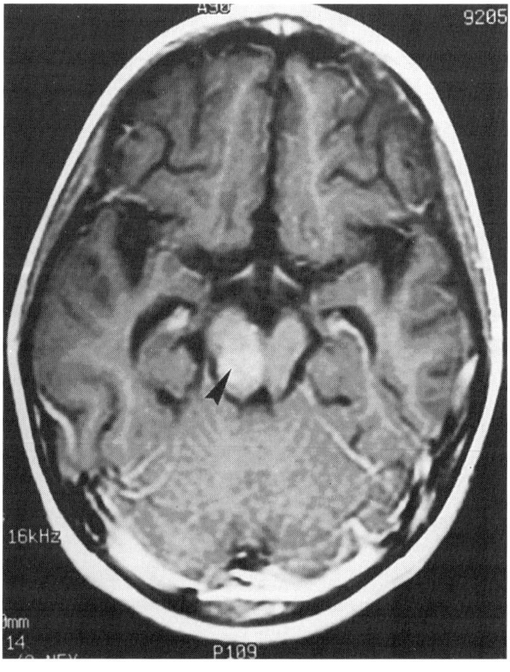


**(b)**

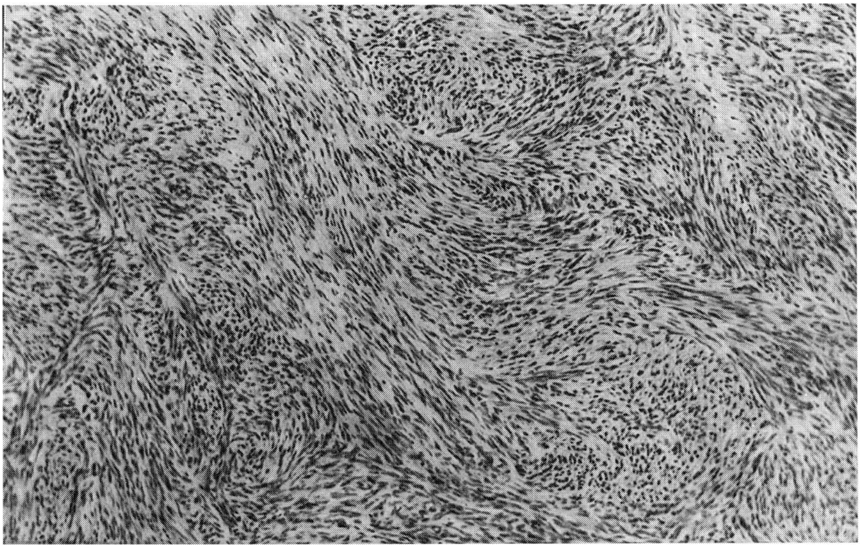

**(c)**

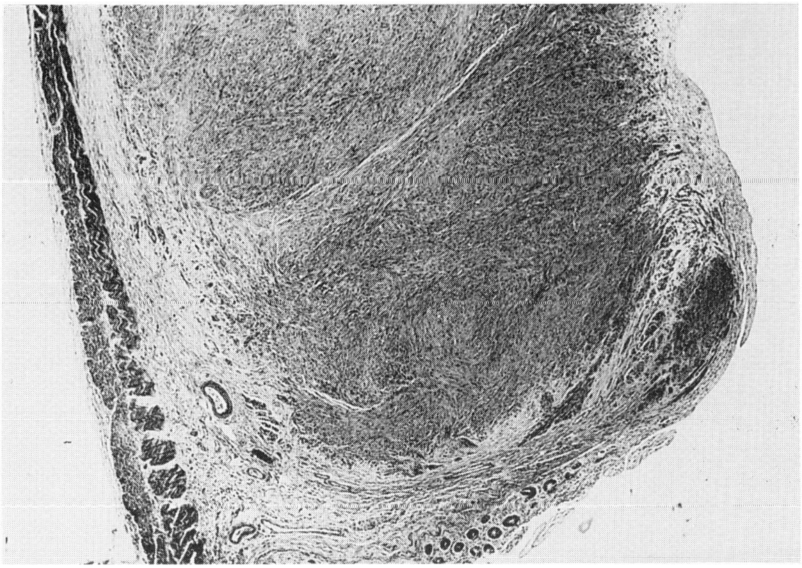

**(d)**

**Figure 6.5** Leiomyosarcoma in a 9-year-old child. (a, b) CT images of the frontal and brainstem lesions (arrowheads). (c) Neuropathology of a stereotactic biopsy of the frontal lesion (H&E; ×250.) (d) Leiomyosarcoma of the intestinal tract found at autopsy.

other series. This has also been described in the muscles of one child (Raphael *et al.*, 1989).

*Tumours*

Lymphomas are located in the periventricular region and are high grade with B-cell proliferation. Persistent EBV infection was present in one case (Andiman *et al.*, 1985).

One case of leiomyosarcoma has been reported and we followed a 9-year-old child with multiple brain tumours (Figure 6.5). The frontal lesion contained fusiform neoplastic cells, labelled by anti-smooth muscle actin antibodies, and calcifications. This was associated with massive astrocytic gliosis in the white matter. A small (5 mm) tumour in the intestinal tract was found at autopsy.

*Vascular and ischaemic lesions*

Perivascular lymphocytic infiltrates are frequently observed in the brains of children with AIDS, and were associated with fibrinoid necrosis of the vessel walls in one case (Epstein *et al.*, 1988). We have also observed numerous perivascular infiltrates comprising B cells and $CD4^+$ T cells and macrophages around capillaries in an 18-month-old patient. Similar cases of granulomatous angiitis in adults with AIDS have been described (Yankner *et al.*, 1986). Ischaemic lesions can be observed as large cerebral infarcts or as multiple cerebral microinfarcts and can be associated with aneurysmal arteriopathy as already discussed.

## CONCLUSION

The neurological aspects of HIV-1 infection in children will probably change: antiviral treatments will be used more extensively, allowing longer and better survival but introducing their own complications, as has been observed in oncology. There also might be differences between tropical and subtropical countries and this needs to be more carefully evaluated.

## REFERENCES

American Academy of Neurology AIDS Task Force (1991) Report of a working group. *Neurology* **41**: 778–785.

Anders KH, Guerra WF, Tomiyasu U *et al.* (1986) The neuropathology of AIDS: UCLA experience and review. *American Journal of Pathology* **124**: 537–558.

Andiman WA, Martin K, Rubinstein A *et al.* (1985) Opportunistic lymphoproliferations associated with Epstein–Barr viral DNA in infants and children with AIDS. *Lancet* **21**: 1390–1393.

Auger I, Thomas P, de Gruttola V *et al.* (1988) Incubation period for paediatric AIDS patients. *Nature* **336**: 575–577.

Belec L, Tayot J, Tron P *et al.* (1990) Cytomegalovirus encephalopathy in an infant with congenital acquired immuno-deficiency syndrome. *Neuropediatrics* **21**: 124–129.

Belman AL (1992) AIDS and the child's central nervous system. Pediatric neurology. *Pediatric Clinics of North America* **39**: 691–714.

Belman AL, Ultmann MH, Horoupian D *et al.* (1985) Neurologic complications in infants and children with acquired immune deficiency syndrome. *Annals of Neurology* **18**: 560–566.

Belman AL, Lantos G, Houroupian D *et al.* (1986) AIDS: calcifications of the basal ganglia in infants and children. *Neurology* **36**: 1192–1199.

Belman AL, Diamond G, Dickson D *et al.* (1988) Pediatric AIDS: neurologic syndromes. *American Journal of Diseases of Children* **142**: 29–35.

Berger JR, Sheremata WA, Resnick L *et al.* (1989) Multiple sclerosis-like illness occurring with human immunodeficiency infection. *Neurology* **39**: 324–329.

Berger J, Albrecht J, Belman AL *et al.* (1992) Progressive multifocal leukoencephalopathy in children with HIV infection. *AIDS* **6**: 837–841.

Blanche S, Rouzioux C, Guihard-Moscato ML *et al.* (1989) A prospective study of infants born to women seropositive for human immunodeficiency virus type 1. *New England Journal of Medicine* **320**: 1643–1648.

Blanche S, Tardieu M, Duliège AM *et al.* (1990) Longitudinal study of 94 symptomatic infants with materno-foetal HIV infection: evidence for a bimodal expression of clinical and biological symptoms. *American Journal of Diseases of Children* **144**: 1210–1215.

Blanche S, Duliège AM, Navarette M *et al.* (1991) Zidovudine in children with an HIV infection acquired in the perinatal period. *Pediatrics* **88**: 364–370.

Blanche S, Mayaux MJ, Rouzioux C *et al.* (1994) Relationship between maternal status at delivery and disease progression in vertically HIV-1-infected children. *New England Journal of Medicine* **330**: 308–312.

Brouwers P, Moss H, Wolters P *et al.* (1990) Effect of continuous-infusion zidovudine therapy on neuropsychologic functioning in children with symptomatic human immunodeficiency virus infection. *Journal of Pediatrics* **117**: 980–985.

Brüstle O, Spiegel H, Leib SL *et al.* (1992) Distribution of human immunodeficiency virus (HIV) in the CNS of children with severe HIV encephalomyelopathy. *Acta Neuropathologica* **84**: 24–31.

Budka H (1986) Multinucleated giant cell in brain: a hallmark of the acquired immune deficiency syndrome (AIDS). *Acta Neuropathologica* **69**: 253–258.

Burgard M, Mayaux MJ, Blanche S *et al.* (1992) The use of viral culture and p24 antigen testing to diagnose human immunodeficiency virus infection in neonates. *New England Journal of Medicine* **327**: 1192–1197.

Butler KM, Husson RN, Balis F *et al.* (1991) Dideoxyinosine in children with symptomatic human immunodeficiency virus infection. *New England Journal of Medicine* **324**: 137–144.

Butler KM, De Smet MC, Husson RN *et al.* (1992) Treatment of aggressive cytomegalovirus retinitis with ganciclovir in combination with foscarnet in a child infected with human immunodeficiency virus. *Journal of Pediatrics* **120**: 483–486.

Centers for Disease Control (1994) Classification system for human immunodeficiency virus (HIV) infection in children under 13 years of age. *Morbidity and Mortality Weekly Report* **43/RR-12**: 1–19.

Cho E-S and Sharer LR (1990) HIV encephalopathy in children. In: *Brain in Pediatric AIDS* (eds PB Kozlowski, DA Snider, PM Vietze and HM Wisniewski), pp. 158–164. Basel: Karger.

Cohen SE, Mundy T, Karassik B *et al.* (1991) Neuropsychological functioning in human immunodeficiency virus type 1 seropositive children infected through neonatal blood transfusion. *Pediatrics* **88**: 58–68.

Connor EM, Sperling RS, Gelber R *et al.* (1994) Reduction of maternal–fetal transmission of human immunodeficiency virus type 1 with zidovudine treatment. *New England Journal of Medicine* **331**: 1173–1180.

Dabis F, Msellati P, Dunn D *et al.* (1993) Estimating the rate of mother to child transmissions of HIV. Report of a workshop on methodological issues, Ghent (Belgium). *AIDS* **7**: 1139–1148.

DeCarli C, Fugate L, Falloon J *et al.* (1991) Brain growth and cognitive improvement in children with HIV induced encephalopathy after 6 months of continuous infusion therapy. *AIDS* **4**: 585–592.

DeCarli C, Civitello LA, Brouwers P *et al.* (1993) The prevalence of computed tomographic abnormalities of the cerebrum in 100 consecutive children symptomatic with the human immune deficiency virus. *Annals of Neurology* **34**: 198–205.

de la Monte SM, Ho DD, Schooley RT *et al.* (1987) Subacute encephalomyelitis of AIDS and its relation to HTLV-III infection. *Neurology* **37**: 562–569.

Delfraissy JF, Blanche S, Rouzioux C *et al.* (1992) Perinatal HIV transmission facts and controversies. *Immunodeficiency Reviews* **3**: 305–327.

Depas G, Chiron C, Tardieu M *et al.* (1995) Functional brain imaging in HIV-1-infected children born to seropositive mothers. *Journal of Nuclear Medicine* **36**: 2169–2174.

Diamond GW (1989) Developmental problems in children with HIV infection. *Mental Retardation* **4**: 213–217.

Diamond GW, Gurdin P, Wiznia AA *et al.* (1990) Effects of congenital HIV infection on neurodevelopmental status of babies in foster care. *Developmental Medicine and Child Neurology* **32**: 999–1005.

Dickson DW, Belman AL, Kim TS *et al.* (1989a) Spinal cord pathology in pediatric acquired immunodeficiency syndrome. *Neurology* **39**: 227–235.

Dickson DW, Belman AL, Park YD *et al.* (1989b) Central nervous system pathology in pediatric AIDS: an autopsy study. *APMIS* Suppl. 8: 40–57.

Dickson DW, Llena JF, Weidenheim KM *et al.* (1990) Central nervous system pathology in children with AIDS and focal neurologic signs – stroke and lymphomas. In: *Brain in Pediatric AIDS* (eds PB Kozlowski, DA Snider, PM Vietze and HM Wisniewski), pp. 147–157. Basel: Karger.

Duliège AM, Messiah A, Blanche S *et al.* (1992) Natural history of HIV1 infection in children: prognostic value of the laboratory parameters on the bimodal progression of the disease. *Pediatric Infectious Disease Journal* **11**: 630–635.

Ehrnst A, Lindgren S, Dictor M *et al.* (1991) HIV in pregnant women and their offspring: evidence for late transmission. *Lancet* **338**: 203–207.

Epstein LG and Sharer LR (1988) Neurology of human immunodeficiency virus infection in children. In: *AIDS and the Nervous System* (ed Rosenblum ML, pp. 79–101. New York: Raven Press.

Epstein LG, Sharer LR, Joshi VV *et al.* (1985) Progressive encephalopathy in children with acquired immune deficiency syndrome. *Annals of Neurology* **17**: 488–496.

Epstein LG, Sharer LR, Oleske JM *et al.* (1986) Neurologic manifestations of human immunodeficiency virus infection in children. *Pediatrics* **78**: 678–687.

Epstein LG, Goudsmit J, Paul DA *et al.* (1987a) Expression of human immunodeficiency virus in cerebrospinal fluid of children with progressive encephalopathy. *Annals of Neurology* **21**: 397–401.

Epstein LG, Berman CZ, Shareer LR *et al.* (1987b). Unilateral calcification and contrast enhancement of the basal ganglia in a child with AIDS encephalopathy. *American Journal of Neuroradiology* **8**: 163–165.

Epstein LG, Dicarlo F, Joshi V *et al.* (1988) Primary lymphoma of the central nervous system in children with acquired immunodeficiency syndrome. *Pediatrics* **82**: 355–363.

European Collaborative Study (1990) Neurologic signs in young children with human immunodeficiency virus infection. *Pediatric Infectious Disease Journal* **9**: 402–406.

European Collaborative Study (1991) Children born to women with HIV-1 infection: natural history and risk of transmission. *Lancet* **347**: 253–260.

Frank Y, Lim W, Kahn E *et al.* (1989) Multiple ischemic infarcts in a child with AIDS, varicella zoster infection and cerebral vasculitis. *Pediatric Neurology* **5**: 64–67.

Gallo P, Laverda AM, DeRossi A *et al.* (1991) Immunological markers in the cerebrospinal fluid of HIV-1 infected children. *Acta Paediatrica Scandinavica* **80**: 659–666.

Goldstein J, Dickson DW, Rubinstein A *et al.* (1990) Primary CNS lymphoma in a pediatric patient with acquired immunodeficiency syndrome treated with radiation. *Cancer* **66**: 2503–2508.

Hira SK, Kamanga J, Bhat GJ *et al.* (1989) Perinatal transmission of HIV1 in Zambia. *British Medical Journal* **299**: 1250–1252.

Husson RN, Saini R, Lewis LL *et al.* (1992) Cerebral artery aneurysms in children infected with human immunodeficiency virus. *Journal of Pediatrics* **121**: 927–930.

Keohane C, Robain O, Ponsot G *et al.* (1991) Cerebral lymphoma and HIV encephalitis in a case of paediatric AIDS, with pre-existing multicystic encephalomalacia. *Irish Journal of Medical Science* **160**: 179–182.

Kozlowski PB, Sher JH, Dickson DW *et al.* (1990) Central nervous system in pediatric HIV infection: a multicenter study. In: *Brain in Pediatric AIDS* (eds PB Kozlowski, DA Snider, PM Viutzu and0HM Wisniewski), pp. 132–146. Basel: Karger.

Kraszpulski M, Kozlowski PB, Sersen EA *et al.* (1991) Morphometric study of 28 brain structures in pediatric AIDS (abstract). *Journal of Neuropathology and Experimental Neurology* **50**: 325.

Kugler SL, Barzilai A, Hodes DS *et al.* (1991) Acute hemiplegia associated with HIV infection. *Pediatric Neurology* **7**: 207–210.

Kure K, Park YD, Kim TS *et al.* (1989) Immunohistochemical localization of an HIV epitope in cerebral aneurysmal arteriopathy in pediatric AIDS. *Pediatric Pathology* **9**: 655–662.

Kure K, Liena JF, Lyman WD *et al.* (1991) Human immunodeficiency virus-1 infection of the nervous system: an autopsy study of 268 adult, pediatric and fetal brains. *Human Pathology* **22**: 700–710.

Lacroix C, Vazeux R, Brousse N *et al.* (1993) Etude neuropathologique de 10 enfants infectés par le VIH. *Revue Neurologique* **149**: 37–45.

Lacroix C, Blanche S, Dussaix E *et al.* (1995) Acute necrotizing measles encephalitis in a child with AIDS. *Journal of Neurology* **242**: 249–256.

Lallemant M, Lallemant-Lecoeur S, Cheynier D *et al.* (1989) Mother-to-child transmission of HIV1 and infant survival in Brazzaville, Congo. *AIDS* **3**: 643–646.

Lepage P, Van de Perre P, Msellati P *et al.* (1993) Mother-to-child transmission of human immunodeficiency virus type 1 (HIV1) and its determinants: a cohort study in Kigali, Rwanda. *American Journal of Epidemiology* **137**: 589–599.

Levenson Jr RL, Mellins CA, Zawadzki R *et al.* (1992) Cognitive assessment of human immunodeficiency virus exposed children. *American Journal of Diseases of Children* **146**: 1479–1483.

Lobato MN, Caldwell B, Ng P *et al.* (1995). Encephalopathy in children with perinatally acquired human immunodeficiency virus infection. *Journal of Pediatrics* **126**: 710–715.

Lyman WD, Kressy Y, Kure K *et al.* (1990) Detection of HIV in fetal central nervous system tissue. *AIDS* **4**: 917–920.

McKinney Jr RE, Maha MA, Connor EM *et al.* (1991) A multicenter trial of oral zidovudine in children with advanced human immunodeficiency virus disease. *New England Journal of Medicine* **324**: 1018–1025.

Mintz M, Rapaport R, Oleske M *et al.* (1989) Elevated serum levels of tumor necrosis factor are associated with progressive encephalopathy in children with acquired immunodeficiency syndrome. *American Journal of Diseases of Children* **143**: 771–774.

Mintz M, Tardieu M, Hoyt L *et al.* (1996) Levodopa therapy improves motor function in HIV-infected children with extrapyramidal syndromes. *Neurology* **47**: 1583–1585.

Mitchell CD, Erlich SS, Mastrucci MT *et al.* (1992) Congenital toxoplasmosis occurring in infants perinatally infected with HIV-1. *Pediatric Infectious Disease Journal* **11**: 232–237.

Msellati M, Lepage P, Hitimana D-G *et al.* (1993) Neurodevelopmental testing of children born to human immunodeficiency virus type 1 seropositive and seronegative mothers: a prospective cohort study in Kigali, Rwanda. *Pediatrics* **92**: 843–848.

Mustafa MM, Weitman SD, Winick NJ *et al.* (1993) Subacute measles encephalitis in the young immunocompromised host: report of two cases diagnosed by polymerase chain reaction and treated with ribavirin and review of the literature. *Clinical Infectious Diseases* **16**: 654–660.

Park Y, Belman AL, Dickson DW *et al.* (1988) Stroke in pediatric acquired immunodeficiency syndrome. *Annals of Neurology* **24**: 359–363.

Phillipet P, Blanche S, Sebag G *et al.* (1994) Stroke and cerebral infarcts in children infected with human immunodeficiency virus. *Archives of Pediatric and Adolescent Medicine* **148**: 965–970.

Pizzo PA and Butler KM (1991) In the vertical transmission of HIV, timing may be everything (Editorial). *New England Journal of Medicine* **325**: 652–654.

Pizzo PA, Eddy J, Balis FM *et al.* (1988) Effect of continuous intravenous infusion of zidovudine (AZT) in children with symptomatic HIV infection. *New England Journal of Medicine* **319**: 889–896.

Pizzo PA, Butler K, Balis F *et al.* (1990) Dideoxycytidine alone and in an alternating schedule with zidovudine in children with symptomatic human immunodeficiency virus infection. *Journal of Pediatrics* **117**: 799–808.

Price DB, Inglese CM, Jacobs J *et al.* (1988) Pediatrics AIDS. Neuroradiologic and neurodevelopmental findings. *Pediatric Radiology* **18**: 445–448.

Raphael SA, Wolfson BJ, Parker P *et al.* (1989) Pyomyositis in a child with acquired immunodeficiency syndrome. *American Journal of Diseases of Children* **143**: 779–781.

Raphael SA, Price ML, Lischner HW *et al.* (1991) Inflammatory demyelinating polyneuropathy in a child with symptomatic human immunodeficiency virus infection. *Journal of Pediatrics* **118**: 242–245.

Ryder RW, Nsa W, Hassig SE *et al.* (1989) Perinatal transmission of the human immunodeficiency virus type 1 to infants of seropositive women in Zaire. *New England Journal of Medicine* **320**: 1637–1642.

Scott GB, Buck BE, Leterman JC *et al.* (1984) Acquired immunodeficiency in infants. *New England Journal of Medicine* **310**: 76–80.

Scott G, Hutto C, Makuch RW *et al.* (1989) Survival in children with perinatally acquired human immunodeficiency virus type 1 infection. *New England Journal of Medicine* **321**: 1791–1796.

Shank GD, Redfield RR and Fischer GW (1987) *Toxoplasma* encephalitis in an infant with acquired immunodeficiency syndrome. *Pediatric Infectious Disease Journal* **6**: 70–71.

Sharer LR, Cho ES and Epstein LG (1985) Multinucleated giant cells and HTLV-III in AIDS encephalopathy. *Human Pathology* **16**: 760.

Sharer LR, Epstein LG, Cho ES *et al.* (1986) Pathologic features of AIDS encephalopathy in children: evidence for LAV/HTL VIII infection in brain. *Human Pathology* **17**: 271–284.

Sharer LR, Dowling PC, Michaels J *et al.* (1990) Spinal cord disease in children with HIV-1 infection: a combined molecular and neuropathological study. *Neuropathology and Applied Neurobiology* **16**: 317–331.

Shaw GM, Harper ME, Hahn BH *et al.* (1985) HTLV-III infection in brains of children and adults with AIDS encephalopathy. *Science* **227**: 177–182.

Strugo I, Wittek AE, Israele V *et al.* (1992) Meningoencephalitis in a neonate congenitally infected with human immunodeficiency virus type 1. *Journal of Pediatrics* **120**: 93–95.

Taccone A, Fondelli MP, Ferrea G *et al.* (1992) An unusual CT presentation of congenital cerebral toxoplasmosis in an 8 month-old boy with AIDS. *Pediatric Radiology* **22**: 68–69.

Tardieu M, Blanche S, Rouzioux C *et al.* (1987) Atteintes du système nerveux au cours des infections à HIV1 du nourrisson. *Archives Francaises de Pediatrie* **44**: 495–499.

Tardieu M, Blanche S and Brunelle F (1991a) Cerebral magnetic resonance imaging studies in HIV-1 infected children born to seropositive mothers (abstract). Presented at Neuroscience of HIV-1 infection, a satellite conference of the VII International Conference on AIDS, Padova, Italy, 1991, p. 60.

Tardieu M, Blanche S and Lacroix C (1991b) Atteinte neurologique au cours de l'infection par le VIH chez l'enfant. In: *Manifestations Neurologiques et Infections Rétrovirales. SIDA et Autres Rétroviroses* (eds G. Said and AG Saimot), pp. 169–182. Paris: Pradd.

Tardieu M, Héry C, Peudenier S *et al.* (1992) Human immunodeficiency virus type 1-infected monocytic cells can destroy human neural cells after cell-to-cell adhesion. *Annals of Neurology* **31**: 689–695.

Tardieu M, Mayaux MJ, Seibel N *et al.* (1995) Cognitive assessment of school age children infected with maternally transmitted human immunodeficiency virus type 1. *Journal of Pediatrics* **126**: 375–379.

Ultmann MH, Belman AL, Ruff HA *et al.* (1985) Developmental abnormalities in infants and children with acquired immune deficiency syndrome (AIDS) and AIDS-related complex. *Developmental Medicine and Child Neurology* **27**: 563–571.

Ultmann MH, Diamond GW, Ruff HA *et al.* (1987) Developmental abnormalities in children with acquired immunodeficiency syndrome (AIDS): a follow-up study. *International Journal of Neuroscience* **32**: 661–667.

Van der Steenhoven JJ, Dbaibo G, Boyko OB *et al.* (1992) Progressive multifocal leukoencephalopathy in pediatric acquired immunodeficiency syndrome. *Pediatric Infectious Disease Journal* **11**: 232–237.

Vazeux R, Lacroix-Claudo C, Blanche S *et al.* (1992) Low levels of human immunodeficiency virus replication in the brain tissue of children with severe acquired immunodeficiency syndrome encephalopathy. *American Journal of Pathology* **140**: 137–144.

Walter EB, Drucker RP, McKinney ER *et al.* (1991) Myopathy in human immunodeficiency virus-infected children receiving long-term zidovudine therapy. *Journal of Pediatrics* **119**: 152–155.

Wiley CA, Belman AL, Dickson DW *et al.* (1990) Human immunodeficiency virus within the brains of children with AIDS. *Clinical Neuropathology* **9**: 1–6.

Yankner BA, Skolnick PR, Shoukimas GM *et al.* (1986) Cerebral granulomatosis angiitis associated with isolation of human T-lymphotrophic virus type III from the central nervous system. *Annals of Neurology* **20**: 362–364.

Zagon IS and Slotkin TA (eds) (1992) *Maternal Substance Abuse and the Developing Nervous System.* San Diego: Academic Press.

# 7

## *Peripheral Nerve Disease in HIV-infected Patients*

Lesions of the peripheral nervous system (PNS) occur at different stages of the progressive immunosuppression that characterizes HIV infection, yet the frequency and patterns of PNS involvement vary with both the stage of the disease and the criteria used to determine the presence of neuropathy (Eidelberg *et al.*, 1986; Bailey *et al.*, 1988; Miller *et al.*, 1988; Léger *et al.*, 1989; Barohn *et al.*, 1993). In this chapter we review and illustrate the different aspects of peripheral nerve involvement and discuss the practical problems posed by the occurrence of neuropathy in this setting. The mechanisms of alteration of the PNS also vary with the stage of the disease. Nerve lesions may be secondary to the inflammatory–immune response subsequent to HIV infection and to vasculitis in the early stages of HIV infection. Later on, as the immunosuppression progresses, the incidence of opportunistic infections and, less commonly, malignant lymphoma increases.

### EPIDEMIOLOGY

#### Subclinical involvement of peripheral nerves

Minor electrophysiological abnormalities of the peripheral nerves are common in asymptomatic HIV-infected patients. Subclinical neuropathy, as detected by electromyogram–nerve conduction studies, was found in 73% of patients by Comi *et al.* (1986) and in 59% of asymptomatic patients by Chavanet *et al.* (1989). In contrast, no nerve conduction abnormality was found in another prospective study of 15 patients with AIDS (Mah *et al.*, 1988). In another study of 28 asymptomatic HIV-positive patients, reduction of nerve conduction velocity was found in 11 and abnormal vibratory threshold in 10, but the correlation between patients with reduced conduction velocity and those with abnormal vibratory threshold was poor (Gulevich *et al.*, 1992).

The epidemiology of peripheral neuropathy has been the subject of several interesting studies. PNS involvement is much more common in immunologically compromised HIV-infected persons as shown in a long-term follow-up of a cohort of 817 individuals (Barohn *et al.*, 1993). Of the 798 HIV-positive subjects 12 had symptoms or signs of peripheral neuropathy; all patients with peripheral neuropathy had $CD4^+$ T-cell counts of less than 300 $mm^{-3}$. The authors found that a lower $CD4^+$ T-cell count correlated with worsening electrophysiological parameters of peripheral nerve function, even in neurologically asymptomatic individuals. Of the 300 HIV-infected subjects without clinical evidence of peripheral neuropathy who had nerve conduction studies performed, 296 had normal nerve conduction study parameters. Subjects in the group with $CD4^+$ T-cell counts less than 200 $mm^{-3}$ had significantly lower nerve conduction study parameters compared with subjects in groups with higher $CD4^+$ T-cell counts ($P < 0.05$). In another cohort study, 94 patients infected with HIV were evaluated clinically and electrophysiologically for the presence of peripheral neuropathy and the results compared with evaluations of CNS function (Hall *et al.*, 1991): 34% had some degree of peripheral neuropathy; 12% of the 49 asymptomatic patients, 45% of the 11 patients with AIDS, and 21% of the 34 patients with ARC had neuropathy on clinical examination; and 23% had neuropathy on electrophysiological evaluation. The authors found a significant correlation between the presence of neuropathy and evidence of CNS dysfunction. The discrepancy between these two studies is only apparent because one study (Barohn *et al.*, 1993) focused on the $CD4^+$ T-cell count, while the other one (Hall *et al.*, 1991), which was clinically oriented, showed that peripheral neuropathy was fairly common in patients with symptomatic HIV infection. In another study, Ronchi *et al.* (1992) found a progressive decline in motor and sensory nerve conduction velocities in 124 patients at different stages of immunodepression, without clinical neuropathy. All studies confirm that symptomatic neuropathy is rare in patients with a relatively preserved $CD4^+$ T-cell count (Bozzette *et al.*, 1991).

The conclusions suggested by the epidemiological studies in cohorts of HIV-infected patients and by our own experience are: (1) minor electrophysiological abnormalities are more common in immunodepressed patients compared with the early stages of HIV infection; (2) the minor, early-onset, electrophysiological abnormalities detected in asymptomatic HIV-infected subjects are not predictive of the occurrence of symptomatic peripheral neuropathy; and (3) electrophysiological testing is not useful in the management of asymptomatic patients.

**Incidence of symptomatic peripheral neuropathy in HIV-infected patients**

Earlier studies on peripheral neuropathy in HIV-infected patients found incidences of symptomatic peripheral neuropathy of 5% (Snider *et al.*, 1983), 6% (Lange *et al.*, 1988) and 8% (Leport *et al.*, 1987). Interestingly, peripheral neuropathy is virtually unknown in HIV-positive children (Raphaël *et al.*, 1991; Lacroix *et al.*, 1993). In an interesting prospective study performed on 40 patients with AIDS, So *et al.* (1988) found clinical and electrophysiological signs of distal symmetrical neuropathy in 35%. The diagnosis of neuropathy was based on the presence of distal paraesthesiae with hypoaesthesia and decreased, or loss of, ankle reflexes. Signs of peripheral neuropathy were associated with marked reduction of the sensory action potential of the sural nerve, but the conduction velocity in the patients with neuropathy was not significantly different from that in patients without neuropathy, a finding in favour of axonal nerve lesions. More recently, Hall *et al.* (1991) found peripheral neuropathy on clinical examination in 21% (7/34) of their patients with ARC and in 45% of those with AIDS (5/11) in a prospective evaluation of a cohort of patients without neurological complaints. Interestingly, electrophysiological evidence for peripheral neuropathy was found in 26% (9/34) of ARC and 36% (4/11) of AIDS patients in this cohort. In other words, performing nerve conduction studies did not significantly increase the finding of peripheral neuropathy in their ARC and AIDS patients. Gulevich *et al.* (1992) found clinical evidence for peripheral neuropathy, confirmed by nerve conduction studies, in 10% (3/31) of ARC/AIDS outpatient volunteers. In qnother study on patients with ARC or AIDS, Vishnubhakat and Beresford (1988) found clinical evidence of neuropathy in 44% and electrophysiological signs in 71% of the patients. In contrast, Gastaut *et al.* (1989) found clinical and laboratory evidence of peripheral neuropathy in 93% of the 29 patients in their series. These discrepancies between studies result from the different criteria used by investigators for the diagnosis of neuropathy.

### Occurrence of peripheral neuropathy in patients with asymptomatic HIV infection

This is an important issue to neurologists because the neuropathy may be the presenting and only manifestation of HIV infection (Janssen *et al.*, 1988). Widely divergent figures have been found, reflecting the stage of HIV infection and the method used to assess the evidence for peripheral neuropathy. In a personal retrospective series of 40 patients referred for evaluation of a peripheral neuropathy that occurred in the context of HIV infection, 57% of the patients had AIDS, 31% had ARC, 10% were asymptomatic seropositive and 2% manifested an inflammatory neuropathy at the time of seroconversion for HIV-1. Thus, in 12% of the patients with HIV-related peripheral neuropathy seen in a neurological unit, the neuropathy was the first and revealing clinical manifestation of HIV infection. Obviously this figure does not reflect the actual incidence of peripheral neuropathy in the general population of HIV-infected patients. It shows, rather, that neurologists may have to deal with patients presenting with neuropathy, or with other neurological manifestations, without knowing that they are seropositive for HIV.

## HIV-RELATED PERIPHERAL NEUROPATHY

The remarkable variety of peripheral neuropathies seen in HIV-infected patients is well established (Mishra *et al.*, 1985; Bailey *et al.*, 1988; Lange *et al.*,

1988; Barohn *et al.*, 1993). HIV-associated peripheral neuropathies may have a number of presentations, including focal or multifocal peripheral neuropathies, with radicular, plexus or nerve trunk involvement, distal symmetrical sensory or sensorimotor polyneuropathy, inflammatory polyneuritis of the Guillain–Barré type, unilateral or bilateral facial palsy, and autonomic neuropathy. The diversity of clinical manifestations reflects the complexity and possibly the summation of various mechanisms, including the inflammatory reaction of the host to the presence of HIV-infected cells in the endoneurium, benign or malignant lymphocytic proliferation, necrotizing and infective vasculitis and, at the stage of immunosuppression, the occurrence of neuropathies due to opportunistic infection of endoneurial cells, especially by CMV.

## Clinical aspects

### *Guillain–Barré-like inflammatory polyneuritis*

The course of HIV infection varies among individual patients, but there is usually a period of latency of approximately 10 years that follows primary infection and development of detectable humoral and cellular immune responses. In 50–70% of patients with primary HIV infection, an acute illness develops approximately 3–6 weeks after initial infection with high fever, diarrhoea, rash, adenopathy and mononucleosis. This period is associated with high levels of viraemia, and within 1 week to 3 months there is an immune response to HIV (review in Pantaleo *et al.*, 1993). During this period or later in the course of HIV infection, but usually in patients with a normal or near-normal $CD4^{+}$ T-cell count, a Guillain–Barré syndrome with mild to severe motor deficit, facial diplegia, areflexia and distal sensory symptoms can develop within a few days (Hagberg *et al.*, 1986; Piette *et al.*, 1987; Vendrell *et al.*, 1987; Beytout *et al.*, 1989). In a review of 139 published cases of symptomatic primary HIV-1 infection, Clark *et al.* (1991) found that 8% of the patients presented with peripheral neuropathy and another 8% manifested encephalopathy. Respiratory failure occurs, as in non-HIV-related Guillain–Barré syndrome. CSF abnormalities include an increased protein content that contrasts with a low cell count; however, the cell count is often more elevated than in classical Guillain–Barré syndrome. The outcome of HIV-related Guillain–Barré syndrome is no different from that in non-HIV-related Guillain–Barré syndrome. Facial nerve palsy, which likely represents minor forms of Guillain–Barré syndrome, may also reveal HIV infection (Follezou *et al.*, 1987; Brown *et al.*, 1988; Belec *et al.*, 1989; Wechsler and Ho, 1989). Occasionally an acute Guillain–Barré-like syndrome can be associated with massive rhabdomyolysis (Mahé *et al.*, 1989; Del Rio *et al.*, 1990). Variants of Guillain–Barré syndrome also occur, including axonal forms (Goldstein *et al.*, 1993), the Miller–Fisher syndrome with ataxia, ophthalmoplegia and areflexia (Sillevis Smith and Portegies, 1990), and relapsing forms (Gibbels and Diederich, 1988).

*Subacute multifocal neuropathies*

If not the most common presentation, subacute multifocal neuropathies represent the most original form of peripheral neuropathy seen in HIV-infected patients before the onset of immunosuppression (Lipkin *et al.*, 1985; Eidelberg *et al.*, 1986; de la Monte *et al.*, 1988; Barohn *et al.*, 1989). Inaugural manifestations of the neuropathy, which can reveal both the neuropathy and HIV infection, include numbness, tingling or pains in one limb extremity. The sensory symptoms usually progress towards more proximal parts of the limb in a matter of days and then often affect another limb, usually the opposite. Motor deficit follows the onset of sensory symptoms within a few days. The patient may become severely handicapped within a few days or weeks. Sphincter disturbances are uncommon in this form. Examination reveals a variable degree of motor deficit, usually asymmetrical, occasionally in the distribution of one or several nerve trunks. The deficit is reminiscent of a more proximal involvement of plexus and/or spinal roots. The sensory deficit predominantly affects light touch and position sense. CSF protein content may remain normal. In some cases, the neuropathy is predominantly motor. Tendon reflexes may be increased due to simultaneous inflammatory lesions of the CNS. This may look like a motor neurone disease.

The course of multifocal neuropathy is usually subacute and often spontaneously favourable. The patient may recover normal or near-normal sensorimotor functions within a few months. On occasion, when nerve biopsy has shown prominent inflammatory infiltration and vasculitis, we treat the patient with corticosteroids for a few weeks or months, depending on the degree of disability. Relapsing demyelinating neuropathy has been observed. Mild to moderate mental deterioration and signs of pyramidal irritation may accompany peripheral neuropathy, especially late in the course of HIV infection. Multifocal neuropathies may also occur in immunodepressed patients, but at this stage the diagnosis must consider the possibility of infiltration of nerve trunks or spinal roots by malignant lymphomas or, more often, the development of CMV neuropathy.

*Distal symmetrical polyneuropathy*

Originally described by Snider *et al.* (1983), distal symmetrical polyneuropathy is the most common pattern of neuropathy in HIV-positive patients. It occurs mainly during the late stages of HIV infection and was found to affect 11.5% of AIDS patients in a cohort of 1500 HIV-infected patients (Fuller *et al.*, 1993). In a recent multicentre study of a cohort of patients with AIDS, it was found that there seemed to be an increasing incidence rate of sensory neuropathy among HIV-infected individuals: 2.81 per 100 person-years in 1992 versus 0.45 in 1988 (Bacellar *et al.*, 1994). This increased incidence rate may be due to different factors, including increased life expectancy and longer duration of HIV infection, but the use of potentially neurotoxic antiretroviral treatments may also play a role.

Distal symmetrical polyneuropathy is often very painful and patients often consult for unbearable burning pains of the feet, made worse by contact with bed sheets or by examination. Motor deficit is often minor or absent, at least at the onset during the first weeks or months, but painful retraction of the tendon of the triceps suralis muscle is common, preventing patients from walking normally, even when muscle strength is preserved. Attempts at foot dorsiflexion are sometimes unbearable. Ankle jerks may be decreased, normal or exaggerated; patellar reflexes are often increased. Stocking, non-dissociated sensory loss is a common finding. Position sense and vibratory sensation may be impaired. Babinski's sign is often present, indicating simultaneous lesions of the CNS, as seen in cases with vacuolar myelopathy (Petito *et al.*, 1985). The prognosis of late-onset distal symmetrical polyneuropathy is invariably poor. This disorder does not improve spontaneously, 40–70% of such patients dying within 6 months after the first manifestations (Cornblath and McArthur, 1988).

*Autonomic disturbances*
In HIV-infected patients, autonomic disturbances occur during the course of a Guillain–Barré syndrome or as an isolated manifestation. However, symptomatic autonomic disturbances remain uncommon in HIV-infected patients and only isolated cases have been reported in this context. These manifestations include postural hypotension with syncope, paroxysmal hypertension, sphincter disturbances, pupillary abnormalities, cardiac arrhythmia, syncope, abnormal sweating and variations of body temperature (Craddock *et al.*, 1987; Evenhouse *et al.*, 1987; Lin-Greenberger and Taneja-Uppal, 1987; Miller and Semple, 1987; Villa *et al.*, 1987; Harle *et al.*, 1988). In one of our patients, dysautonomic manifestations lasted only a few weeks and spontaneously improved, as happens in acute pandysautonomia, a manifestation that shares features with Guillain–Barré syndrome. In a systematic evaluation of autonomic function in 26 HIV-positive patients (8 ARC/18 AIDS), Freeman *et al.* (1990) found that parameters such as heart rate variation, orthostatic fall in blood pressure and blood pressure response to isometric exercise were significantly different from those in control patients. Five patients also had a distal symmetrical sensory polyneuropathy, and there was a correlation between the presence of other neurological disease, including dementia, myelopathy and distal neuropathy, and the abnormalities in autonomic testing. Here again, the results show that there may be some subclinical involvement of the autonomic nervous system; however, systematic testing of autonomic function is not necessary in asymptomatic patients.

*Less common HIV peripheral neuropathies*
Patients with HIV infection may develop sensory ataxia attributed by some to a sensory neuronopathy, sometimes associated with spinal cord involvement (Singh *et al.*, 1986). Bilateral eighth cranial nerve involvement has been observed on a single occasion (Grimaldi *et al.*, 1993). The optic nerve is not a peripheral nerve, but patients with AIDS may develop optic neuropathy from a variety of causes, mainly opportunistic infection or lymphomas. However,

there is some clinical and histological evidence that HIV-1 can be responsible for optic neuropathy (Newman and Lessell, 1992; Sadun *et al.*, 1995). So and Olney (1994) found that in 6 of 23 patients with AIDS who developed an acute lumbosacral polyradiculopathy, with rapidly progressive flaccid paraparesis and areflexia that was frequently associated with sphincter disturbances, the neuropathy was due to HIV infection and not to an opportunistic infection by CMV or to infiltration by a malignant lymphoma. In the authors' opinion, the neurological deficits in the polyradiculopathy due to HIV seemed less severe than those due to infection with CMV or to malignant lymphoma.

**Electrophysiological studies in patients with symptomatic HIV neuropathy**

The results of electrophysiological studies performed in patients with symptomatic neuropathy associated with HIV infection reflect the diversity of underlying nerve lesions (Cornblath *et al.*, 1987; Miller *et al.*, 1988; Gastaut *et al.*, 1989; Léger *et al.*, 1989). When axonal lesions predominate, as in late-onset distal symmetrical polyneuropathy, electrophysiological tests show decreased sensory action potentials in distal nerves, associated with mild reduction of the conduction velocity in the same nerve. Sensory nerve may become unexcitable eventually. In multifocal demyelinating neuropathy, conduction velocity is decreased, sometimes in association with conduction blocks, which characterize focal demyelination of nerve trunks. Prolonged F-wave latency results from demyelination of motor roots.

**CSF abnormalities**

CSF abnormalities are common in HIV-infected patients who have no signs or symptoms of neuropathy or of CNS involvement, but a marked increase in CSF protein also occurs in patients with HIV-associated Guillain Barré like syndrome. In this context, however, pleocytosis is often associated with high CSF protein content. In the other patterns of neuropathy, CSF examination often shows a mild increase in protein and cell content. In a large HIV-positive, mostly asymptomatic, population of patients who underwent CSF evaluation, at least one of the following CSF abnormalities (elevated protein, elevated cell count, elevated IgG index or synthesis, oligoclonal bands) was found in 63% and three or four CSF abnormalities occurred in 25% (Marshall *et al.*, 1988). There was no correlation between CSF abnormalities and the stage of the disease. In a follow-up study of patients who had three CSF examinations over 3 years of follow-up, there was an increase in nucleated cells and IgG over time (Collier *et al.*, 1990). This was independent of neurological complications or the CD4$^+$ T-cell count. Thus, CSF abnormalities observed in patients with neuropathy may not be directly related to the neuropathy. In another study performed in asymptomatic HIV-positive patients, the mean density of nucleated cells in the CSF was 10.7 ± 3.4/ml, but the protein content was normal in 20/22 asymptomatic HIV-positive subjects (Soubeyrand *et al.*, 1989). Thus mild abnormalities of the CSF are common in asymptomatic HIV-positive subjects whilst major CSF changes are encountered only in patients who present with neurological manifestations. The virus has been detected in the CSF of patients with neurological manifestations (Ho *et al.*, 1985), but this test is not done routinely.

**Pathology**

In nerve biopsy specimens from patients with HIV-related Guillain–Barré syndrome, the whole range of lesions seen in non-HIV-related Guillain–Barré syndrome can be encountered, including characteristic macrophage-mediated demyelination (Figure 7.1), mixed axonal and demyelinating lesions, or predominantly axonal lesions. In this context the intensity of inflammatory infiltrates varies, but is usually more pronounced in biopsy samples of distal nerves in HIV-related Guillain–Barré syndrome compared with non-HIV-related Guillain–Barré syndrome. Also, the presence of inflammatory lesions of muscle fibres is more frequent in this setting than in non-HIV-infected patients, indicating the presence of latent myositis. In multifocal demyelinating neuropathy, asymmetrical predominantly demyelinating nerve lesions comparable to those found in HIV-related Guillain–Barré syndrome are present in peripheral nerves and can be visualized in nerve biopsy specimens (Figure 7.2). In some cases, the nerve lesions seen on biopsy specimens are scarce, suggesting that proximal demyelinating lesions, likely of nerve roots, have induced deficit secondary to conduction block with little or no secondary axonal degeneration. Several papers have focused on sural nerve pathology in HIV-positive patients (Mah *et al.*, 1988; Chaunu *et al.*, 1989; Fuller *et al.*, 1990). De la Monte *et al.* (1988) studied 21 AIDS/ARC patients and found that 11 (52%) had symptoms of polyneuropathy, mainly distal symmetrical polyneuropathy. However, in 19/20 (95%) of these patients in whom the sural nerve was examined, there was histological evidence of neuropathy, with both demyelinating and axonal changes. This rather high frequency of pathological evidence of peripheral neuropathy was not found by Mah *et al.* (1988), who detected abnormalities in the sural nerve of only 12 of 25 (48%) AIDS patients at autopsy.

Different patterns of vasculitis have been encountered in this setting, ranging from lymphocytic cuffing of endoneurial and epineurial blood vessels to massive destruction of epineurial arteries with the characteristic features of necrotizing arteritis (Said *et al.*, 1987, 1988; Calabrese, 1991). These lesions, like those of classical polyarteritis nodosa, are associated with fibrinoid necrosis, transmural infiltration and sparing of adjacent venules, but lack the presence of polymorphonuclear cells (Figure 7.3). Replication of HIV has been found in nerves from patients with vasculitis (Gherardi *et al.*, 1989). In patients with relapsing demyelinating polyneuropathy, the classical patterns of acquired chronic inflammatory polyneuropathy can be found, including demyelinated and remyelinated fibres sometimes with onion bulb formations (Gibbels and Diederich, 1988). In some patients with multifocal demyelinating neuropathy, there is an intense lymphocytic proliferation of $CD8^+$ and B lymphocytes with

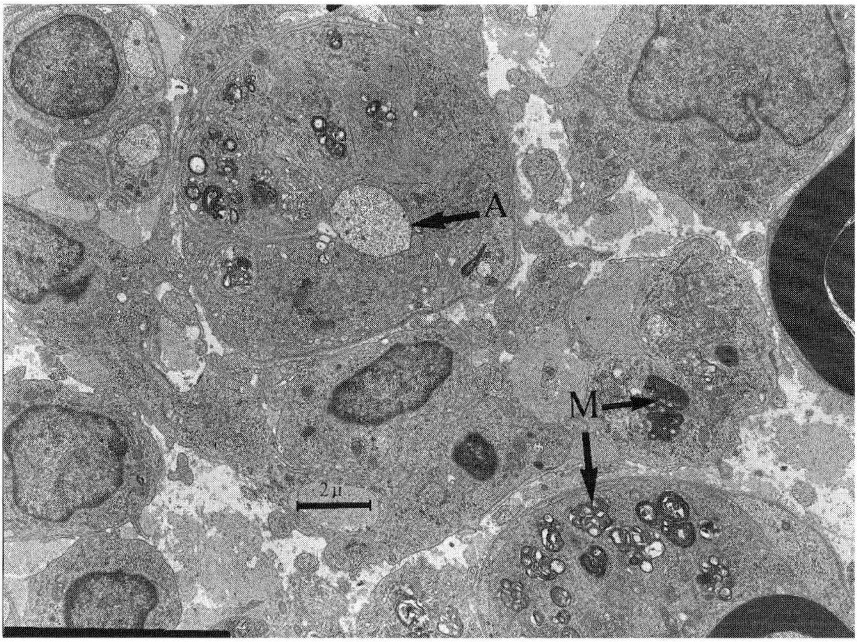


**Figure 7.1** Electron micrograph of a nerve biopsy specimen from a patient with a normal CD4⁺ T-cell count and severe Guillain–Barré syndrome, which did not respond to plasma exchange or intravenous immunoglobulins. The patient remained on a respirator for 3 months before starting to recover. Note the demyelinated axon (A) and the presence of myelin debris in macrophages (M). (Uranyl acetate and lead citrate.)

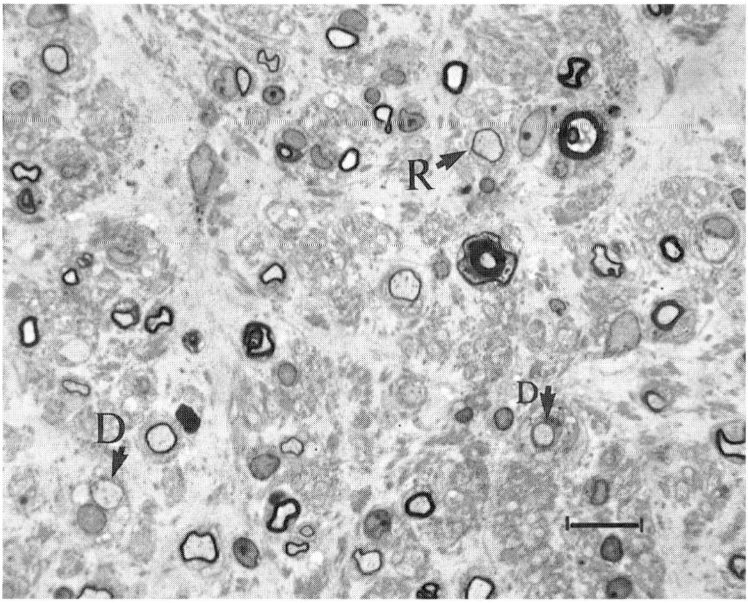


**Figure 7.2** Cross-section of a nerve biopsy from a patient with relapsing inflammatory demyelinating polyneuropathy. The biopsy was performed during the third relapse. The patient, who had a $CD4^+$ T-cell count of 300 $mm^{-3}$, recovered spontaneously. Note the presence of many demyelinated (D) or thinly remyelinated (R) axons. (Thionin blue; Bar: 13 µm.)

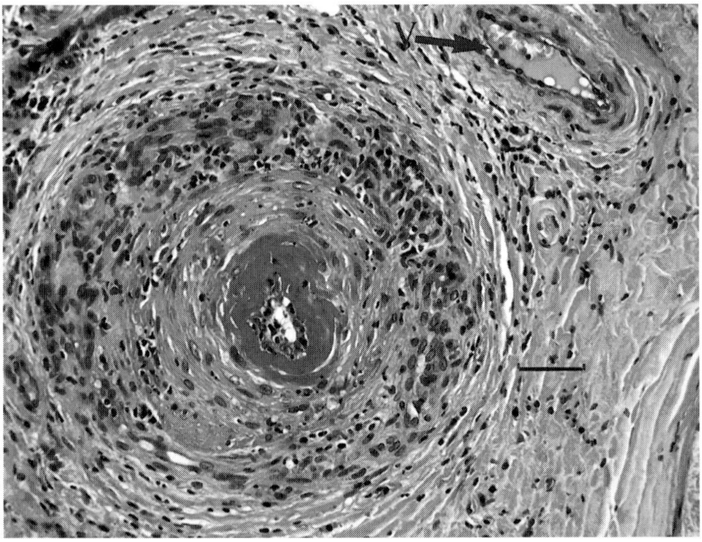


**Figure 7.3** Necrotizing arteritis and neuropathy: a lesion of necrotizing arteritis affecting an epineurial artery in a nerve biopsy specimen from a patient with multifocal inflammatory neuropathy. Note the presence of fibrinoid necrosis and transmural inflammatory infiltration of the artery, leucocytoclasia and sparing of the adjacent venule (V) as observed in polyarteritis nodosa. (H&E; bar: 14 μm.)

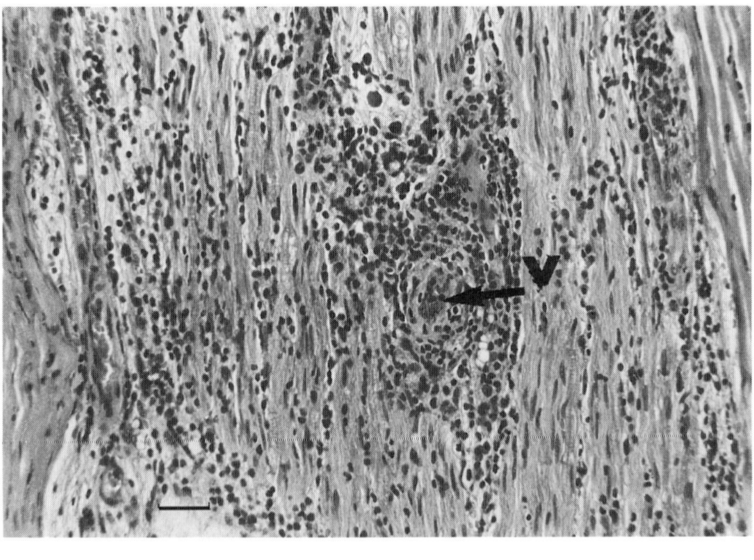


**Figure 7.4** Inflammatory multifocal demyelinating neuropathy of early onset in a patient with a high $CD4^+$ T-cell count and polyclonal hypergammaglobulinaemia. The conspicuous cellular infiltrate seen around the endoneurial blood vessel comprised B and T lymphocytes and macrophages, v: vessel. (H&E; bar: 13 μm.)

massive infiltration of the different nerve compartments, muscle and other organs, in association with increased secretion of immunoglobulins (Figure 7.4).

In patients with distal symmetrical sensory polyneuropathy that occurs when the $CD4^+$ T-cell count is very low, nerve biopsy specimens show only axonal lesions with little inflammatory infiltrate in most instances (Figures 7.5 and 7.6). Demyelinating lesions are uncommon at this stage. At autopsy, in addition to the peripheral nerve changes, there is degeneration of axons and myelin in the fasciculus gracilis, presumably as a result of both central and peripheral degeneration from a dorsal root ganglion lesion (Rance *et al.*, 1988). Massive axonal degeneration of nerve fibres, although less common in the early stages of HIV infection, can be observed in patients with subnormal $CD4^+$ T-cell counts. The prognosis for recovery is poor when axonal lesions predominate. The presence of retroviruses has not been convincingly demonstrated in Schwann cells or in peripheral neurones and axons. Nerve cells and glial cells do not express the CD4 receptor on their surface and are unlikely to be infected by HIV. In contrast, when there is an inflammatory infiltrate with $CD4^+$ T cells and macrophages, the natural refuges of HIV, the presence of retroviruses in these recruited cells is not surprising (Gibbels & Diederich, 1988).

## CYTOMEGALOVIRUS NEUROPATHY

CMV neuropathy is the only neuropathy for which a specific treatment exists in patients with AIDS. The importance of early diagnosis and treatment of CMV neuropathy is thus obvious. Additionally, CMV is the most common viral opportunistic agent in AIDS (Selik *et al.*, 1987).

### Virus and epidemiology

Human CMV belongs to the Herpesviridae. The complete enveloped virion ranges in size from 180 to 250 nm in diameter, making it one of the largest human viral pathogens (Roizman and Batterson, 1985). Human CMV is morphologically indistinguishable from the other herpesviruses but shares no cross-reactive antigens with any of them, and causes *in vivo* infection only in humans and *in vitro* infection only in human fibroblasts. The characteristic features of infected cells are enlargement and the formation of nuclear and cytoplasmic inclusion bodies. Although these inclusions largely consist of virions and aggregates of viral proteins, much of the cytomegaly results from the stimulation of host-cell nucleic acid and protein synthesis that accompanies CMV infection (review in Yarrish, 1987). The virus, as other herpesviruses, persists indefinitely in the infected host in a quiescent form, subject to reactivation by appropriate stimuli. Cell-mediated immunity seems to be the host's major defence against the virus, since the presence of antibodies to CMV do not prevent the development of clinical manifestations due to reactivation of the virus.

CMV infection is exceedingly common throughout the world. The

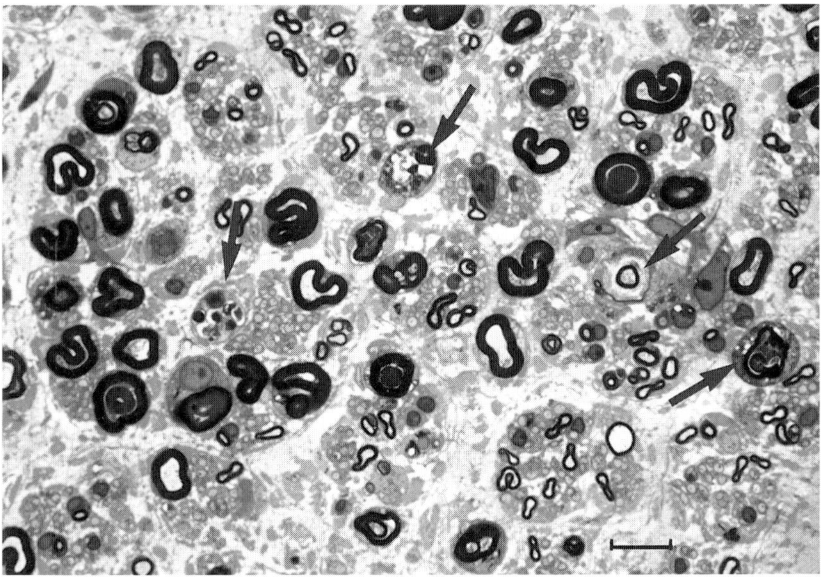

**Figure 7.5** Late-onset distal symmetrical sensory neuropathy: irreversible axonal lesions encountered in this type of polyneuropathy, which occurs in patients with a low CD4+ T-cell count. Note the presence of many fibres undergoing axonal degeneration (arrows). (Thionin blue staining; 1-μm thick section; bar: 7.5 μm.)

**Figure 7.6** Groups of teased fibre preparations. (A) Fibres at different stages of axonal degeneration from a nerve biopsy of a patient with late-onset polyneuropathy. (B) Group of teased fibres from a patient with early-onset multifocal demyelinating neuropathy and polyclonal hypergammaglobulinaemia, showing segmental demyelination of the fibres. In this patient the demyelinating neuropathy was associated with a striking proliferation of lymphocytes (see Figure 7.4).

seropositivity rates ranges from 40–60% in industrialized countries to 80–100% in developing countries (Krech, 1973). Actually, by using more sensitive immunofluorescence tests, virtually all adults are seropositive to CMV. Blood and sexual transmission of the virus are among the many routes of transmission. In addition, sexually active homosexuals not already infected are likely to become so in a very short time. Thus, latent infection with CMV is virtually universal. In immunocompetent individuals CMV may cause a form of mononucleosis, but is most often asymptomatic.

In subjects with normal immunological status, CMV has been suggested as the aetiology only in occasional cases of Guillain–Barré syndrome (Leonard and Tobin, 1971; Dowling *et al.*, 1977; Bishopric *et al.*, 1985). Conversely, in patients with impaired cell-mediated immunity, especially in patients with AIDS and in transplant recipients, CMV infection is the most common opportunistic infection and one of the most frequent causes of death, especially in AIDS patients. Manifestations include interstitial pneumonitis, necrotizing adrenalitis, gastrointestinal ulceration, encephalomyelitis and retinitis. Peripheral neuropathy has only been reported in AIDS. In such patients, lesions of the PNS are often associated with other determinants of CMV infection, but in some cases peripheral neuropathy is the only and presenting manifestation of AIDS.

**Clinical aspects**

Focal or multifocal neuropathy and lumbosacral polyradiculoneuropathy are the two main patterns of neuropathy observed, sometimes concurrently, in the context of CMV infection in AIDS (Behar *et al.*, 1987; Said *et al.*, 1991; Fuller *et al.*, 1993; Roullet *et al.*, 1994). Both types of manifestation can be associated with lesions of the CNS (Jeantils *et al.*, 1986; Vinters *et al.*, 1989; Said *et al.*, 1991). The neuropathy is often painful at onset. Sensory and motor deficit are often severe, due to the necrotic pattern of the lesions found in the nervous system. Virtually any nerve can be involved including oculomotor, optic and other cranial nerves, laryngeal nerve with hoarseness (Small *et al.*, 1989) and nerve trunks of the limbs (Snider *et al.*, 1983; Said *et al.*, 1991). The occurrence of severe subacute multifocal neuropathy in patients with low $CD4^+$ T-cell counts, especially when associated with fever and cachexia, is highly suggestive of the diagnosis of CMV neuropathy. In several reports on the clinical patterns or prognosis of CMV neuropathy, the evidence for CMV as the aetiology is often only indirect, based on the results from serological, culture or PCR methods, which may not be sufficient to incriminate this agent (Cohen *et al.*, 1993). The diagnosis of CMV-related neuropathy is made difficult by the ubiquity of the virus, which can be found in blood, secretory products and even tissues without being responsible for significant pathological changes. Additionally, serological reactions are not reliable in this context to incriminate CMV. The use of PCR to detect CMV DNA in the CSF may identify more patients with neurological manifestations associated with CMV infection (Gozlan *et al.*, 1992; Simpson and Morgello, 1992; Wolf and Spector, 1992; Clifford *et al.*, 1993; Cohen *et al.*, 1993).

The association of CMV retinitis, colitis or pulmonary lesions with progressive peripheral neuropathy suggests that the virus is responsible for the neuropathy too. In fact, the best evidence for CMV as the cause of the neuropathy is the demonstration of specific pathology in nerve biopsy specimens, with characteristic viral inclusions and lesions of surrounding tissue; however, the lesions may be proximal to the site of the nerve biopsy, in spinal roots or even in the spinal cord, or the nerve biopsy may not be demonstrative. Thus, a normal nerve biopsy does not exclude the diagnosis of peripheral neuropathy due to CMV. Obviously, patients with simultaneous manifestations of specific involvement of other organs including retinitis, colitis, etc., usually in association with fever and cachexia, are already being treated. When the neuropathy is the only manifestation of CMV infection, characteristic abnormalities of the CSF associated with detection of CMV in culture or of CMV DNA are very helpful. The most specific sign is the presence of a large number of polymorphonuclear cells in the CSF (de Gans *et al.*, 1990), which is more common in the polyradiculopathic form of the disease than in the multifocal type. Nerve biopsy is useful in patients with subacute multifocal neuropathy, especially when the electromyogram shows unequivocal signs of involvement of distal nerves in patients with no sign of involvement of other organs. In such cases, nerve biopsy can be the only way to reach the diagnosis, by revealing specific nerve lesions.

The overall prognosis of CMV neuropathy is poor, due to late diagnosis and the necrotic lesions of the nervous system. When treatment is started in patients in relatively good condition the prognosis is better, and some of our patients have survived more than 2 years with histologically proven symptomatic CMV neuropathy (Said *et al.*, 1991; Kim and Hollander, 1993; Roullet *et al.*, 1994).

Treatment of CMV infection rests on daily intravenous infusion of ganciclovir or foscarnet, which must be maintained indefinitely to avoid relapses. The decision to treat is sometimes difficult to make when there is no pathological evidence for CMV as the aetiology in patients who have no simultaneous lesions of other organs. Under such circumstances, the decision to treat rests on evaluation by the clinician of the likelihood of CMV being responsible. In this context, CSF examination is one of the most important diagnostic tools in CMV neuropathy, especially when the patient presents with a rapidly progressive cauda equina syndrome or with a more diffuse polyradiculopathy that predominates in the lumbosacral roots. CSF examination frequently shows increased protein content with pleocytosis (de Gans *et al.*, 1990), but the most characteristic feature is the presence of a large proportion of polymorphonuclear cells associated with decreased glucose content and the presence of CMV in cultures. The CSF may remain normal as in some of our cases, which were confirmed by peripheral nerve biopsy or at autopsy. Also, the CSF content can vary very quickly, within a few days, from normal values to high protein with marked pleocytosis, as in one of our patients. Thus, it may be necessary to repeat the CSF examination to detect diagnostic abnormalities. Electromyography will show non-specific signs of axonal neuropathy or a mixture of axonal and demyelinating neuropathy when nerve trunks are involved.

**Other causes of acute lumbosacral polyradiculopathy**

CMV is not the only cause of acute lumbosacral polyradiculopathy. In a series of 23 patients with AIDS who had acute lumbosacral polyradiculopathy, with rapidly progressive flaccid paraparesis and areflexia that was frequently associated with sphincter disturbances (So and Olney, 1994), persuasive laboratory evidence of CMV polyradiculopathy (polymorphonuclear pleocytosis or confirmatory CSF culture) was found in 15. Treatment with ganciclovir in these patients led to clinical stabilization, although worsening during the first 2 weeks of treatment was common. Most patients with CMV polyradiculopathy had severe residual deficits.

**Pathology** (Figures 7.7–7.11)

Pathology caused by CMV ranges from occasional scattered cytomegalic cells with little or no surrounding inflammation to large areas of necrosis with a prominent neutrophilic, mononuclear or mixed response. The pattern, site and severity of nerve lesions greatly vary from patient to patient; lesions are multifocal and asymmetrical, destroying a nerve fascicle in part or totally while neighbouring ones are spared. The lesions often predominate on lower spinal roots, but may also affect nerve trunks, cranial nerves and the CNS (Vinters *et al.*, 1989; Kalayjian *et al.*, 1993). In one report, multiple foci of endoneurial necrosis were associated with inflammatory infiltrates in nerve specimens sampled by biopsy (Said *et al.*, 1991). The inflammatory and necrotic endoneurial lesions disseminated in the endoneurium are found predominantly around endoneurial capillaries. Mononuclear and neutrophilic polymorphonuclear cells predominate in the inflammatory infiltrates. Gigantic cells of 30–50 μm diameter with their typical owl-eye appearance, containing the intranuclear and intracytoplasmic inclusions characteristic of CMV infection, are present in foci of dense inflammation. Similar cells can be found in the CSF or blood smears (Glass and Erozan, 1993). Some CMV-infected cells are not surrounded by inflammatory infiltrates. Hypertrophic cells bulging into the lumen are also present in the wall of endoneurial capillaries. Such cells can be recovered in blood smears. Immunostaining of paraffin or frozen sections with an anti-CMV monoclonal antibody can be useful to detect specific inclusions. Fibroblasts and cells of the monocyte–macrophage lineage infected with CMV can undergo mitosis in the endoneurium. The number of cells containing specific inclusions vary greatly: from case to case, within the same specimen, from one fascicle to another, and from one microscopic section to another. The arsence of CMV inclusions in a nerve biopsy specimen obviously does not rule out the diagnosis, since specific lesions may be located in the spinal roots. A prominent neutrophilic cell response is often associated with mixed, axonal and demyelinating multifocal lesions of neighbouring nerve fibres. Because of this wide range of abnormality and because of the ubiquity of CMV in patients with

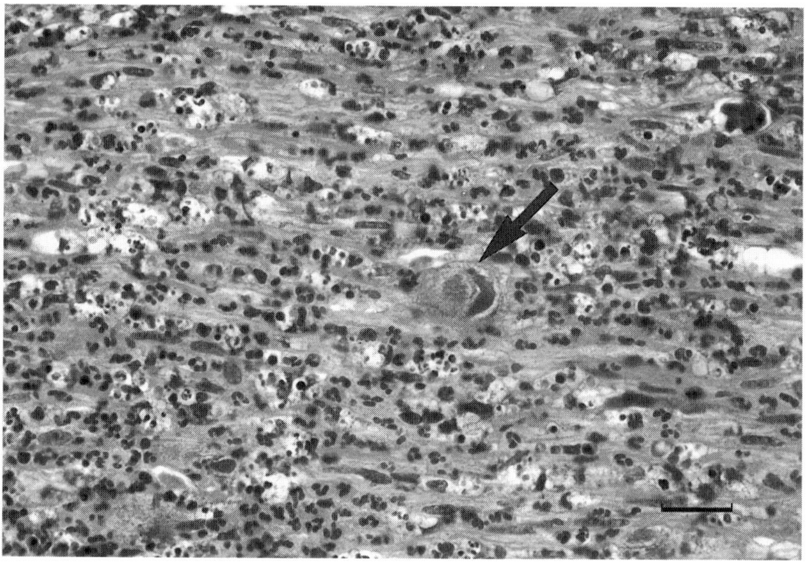

**Figure 7.7** Cytomegalovirus neuropathy: nerve biopsy specimen from a patient with multifocal sensorimotor neuropathy and a CD4$^{+}$ T-cell count of 150 mm$^{-3}$. There is massive destruction of axons associated with a conspicuous inflammatory infiltrate predominantly composed of polymorphonuclear cells. Note the presence of a giant cell with typical owl-eye inclusion (arrow), characteristic of CMV infection. (H&E; bar: 83 μm.)

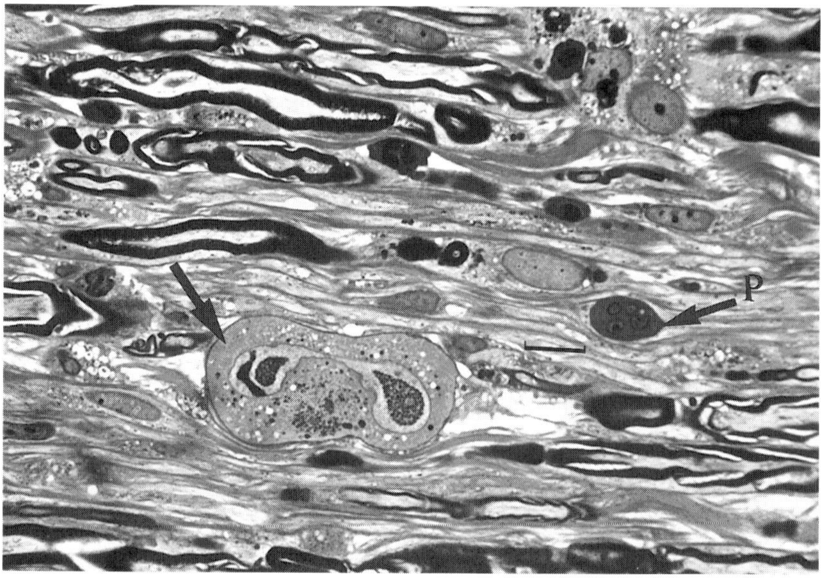


**Figure 7.8** Cytomegalovirus neuropathy: nerve biopsy specimen from a patient with severe multifocal sensorimotor neuropathy and a low CD4$^{+}$ T-cell count. Note the presence of a large dividing cell (arrow), which contains nuclear and cytoplasmic inclusions characteristic of CMV infection. Note also the presence of a polymorphonuclear cell (P). CMV attracts polymorphonuclear cells in affected tissues and in the CSF. (Thionin blue; 1-μm thick section; bar: 7.5 μm.)

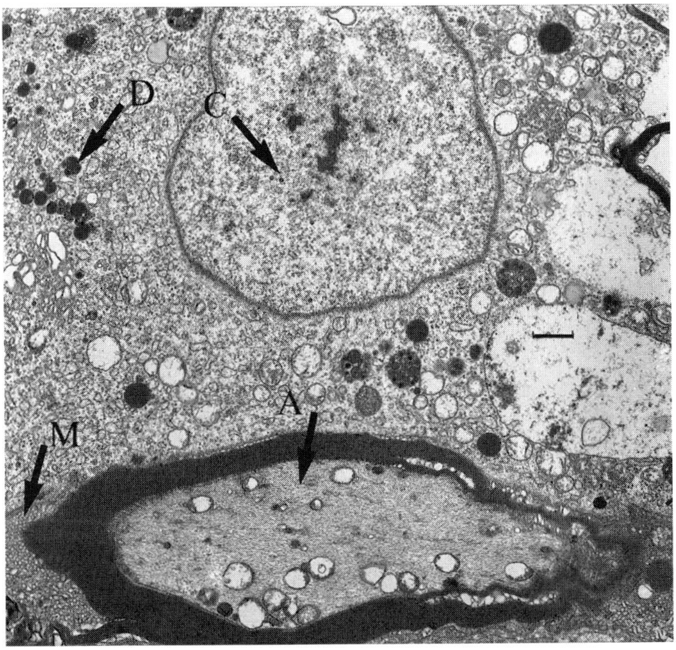


**Figure 7.9** Cytomegalovirus neuropathy: electron micrograph of a nerve biopsy specimen from a patient with multifocal neuropathy and HIV infection with a low $CD4^+$ T-cell count, showing the presence of herpes-type viral particles characteristic of cytomegalovirus (C) in the nucleus and cytoplasm of a Schwann cell. Note that the axon (A) is well preserved, while the myelin sheath is undergoing microvesicular degeneration (M). Dense osmiophilic bodies (D), which contain proviral DNA, are commonly encountered in infected cells. (Uranyl acetate and lead citrate; bar: 0.7 μm.)

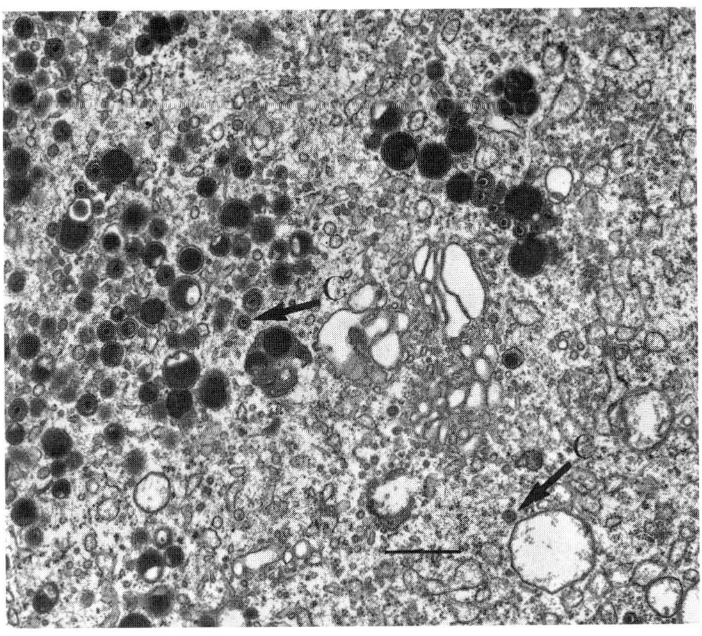


**Figure 7.10** Cytomegalovirus neuropathy: dense osmiophilic cytoplasmic inclusions from the Schwann cell shown in Figure 7.9, illustrating the replication of CMV in the cytoplasm. Dense osmiophilic inclusions and CMV particles (C) were present in the cytoplasm of this Schwann cell. (Uranyl acetate and lead citrate; bar: 0.68 μm.)

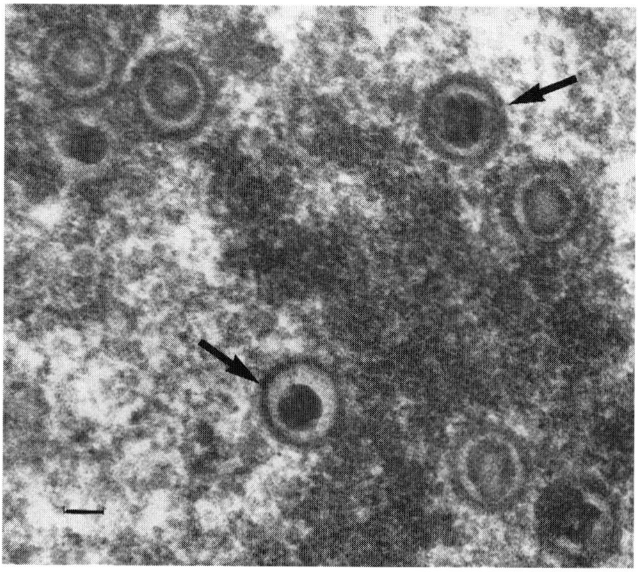

**Figure 7.11** Cytomegalovirus neuropathy: details of the nucleus of an endoneurial cell infected with CMV (arrows). (Uranyl acetate and lead citrate; bar: 0.07 μm.)

AIDS, only cytopathology showing CMV associated with inflammatory reaction and with lesions of surrounding nerve fibres can account for the neuropathy. Endothelial cells of endoneurial capillaries are often infected with CMV and inflammatory infiltrates predominate around blood vessels; however, vessels remain permeable to blood, making an ischaemic mechanism unlikely. Vasculitis with necrosis of the vessel wall occurs.

The multifocal necrotic endoneurial lesions with neutrophilic cell response, which may look like multiple endoneurial microabscesses, seem unique to this agent and differ markedly from the lesions observed in other types of neuropathy associated with HIV infection. Endoneurial polymorphonuclear cell reaction is very uncommon in inflammatory or infectious neuropathies of other origin.

In CMV-proven neuropathy, teased fibre preparations show a mixture of fibres undergoing axonal degeneration and fibres with segmental abnormalities of the myelin sheath. In most cases axonal degeneration predominates. Many demyelinated–remyelinated fibres exhibit marked irregularity of the thickness of the myelin sheath, reminiscent of those observed in 'tomaculous' neuropathy. Abnormal fibres are often clustered, with bunches of demyelinated or degenerating fibres observed in the vicinity of endoneurial inflammatory infiltrates. In some of our patients with CMV-related neuropathy who presented with weakness of peripheral origin, specific lesions were found at post-mortem examination in the spinal cord and motor deficit was related to degeneration of anterior horn cells that occurred in the vicinity of foci of inflammation and necrosis. CMV was present in glial and endothelial cells but not neurones within the CNS. CMV-infected cells could not be detected in the dorsal root ganglia.

Electron microscopic examination of nerve specimens shows herpes-type virions at different stages of maturation. The virions, approximately 170 nm diameter, are present in the nuclei and cytoplasm of cells of the monocyte–macrophage lineage, endoneurial fibroblasts, endothelial cells and, less often, Schwann cells, sometimes associated with secondary, microvesicular changes of the myelin sheath. Osmiophilic inclusions surrounded by either a single or double membrane are present in the cytoplasm of infected cells. These inclusions, which have the same electron density as the core of the virions, contain proviral DNA.

## PERIPHERAL NERVE LESIONS AND MALIGNANT LYMPHOMA IN HIV-INFECTED PATIENTS

Malignant lymphoma infiltrating spinal roots, plexuses or cranial nerves (Figure 7.12) can also complicate the course of AIDS (Gold *et al.*, 1988; Léger *et al.*, 1992; Berger JR *et al.*, 1993). Gold *et al.* (1988) reported on four patients with

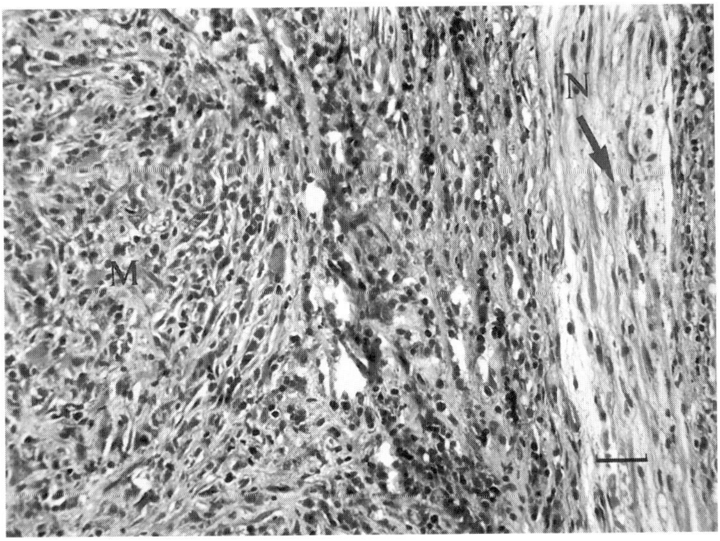


**Figure 7.12** Malignant lymphoma infiltrating cranial nerves: biopsy specimen of the temporal muscle from a patient with a low CD4$^+$ T-cell count who developed progressive facial palsy with involvement of the fifth cranial nerve. CT showed thickening of the temporal muscle, which was biopsied and found to be infiltrated with malignant lymphocytes. Note the massive infiltration of the muscle (M) by lymphocytes. N, nerve bundle. (H&E; bar: 70 μm.)

AIDS who manifested focal or multifocal peripheral neurological deficit due to infiltration by lymphoma, including one with a Hodgkin-type and another with a Burkitt-type lymphoma. All patients had elevated serum lactate dehydrogenase levels, an indicator of disease activity in patients with lymphoma. In their patients abnormalities of the CSF were common, including the presence of lymphoblasts. Metastasis from systemic lymphoma accounted for the polyradiculopathy in 2 of 23 patients included in a series of patients with lumbosacral polyradiculopathy (So & Olney, 1994). Berger JR *et al.* (1993) reported on three HIV-infected patients who developed cranial neuropathy as the initial manifestation of an AIDS-related large cell lymphoma. At the time of presentation for neurological disease, the $CD4^{+}$ T-cell count was below 400 $ml^{-1}$ in these patients. Initial manifestations were retro-orbital headache and oculomotor nerve palsy in two patients and an abducens nerve palsy in the other. Repeatedly negative CSF cytology and recovery from the cranial neuropathy obscured the diagnosis. The authors observed spontaneous and corticosteroid-associated improvement of the cranial neuropathy and concluded that absence of abnormalities on brain-imaging studies and negative CSF cytology did not exclude this diagnosis.

## PATHOPHYSIOLOGY OF NERVE LESIONS

After the initial invasion with HIV, an acute inflammatory peripheral neuropathy similar to that observed in Guillain–Barré syndrome may occur, sometimes in association with signs of involvement of the CNS, including cerebellar ataxia and mental confusion. Their pathogenesis is not clear, but most of the early manifestations are spontaneously reversible, although sometimes incompletely. In response to penetration of HIV intense activation of the immune system occurs and a complex inflammatory immune response results from entry of HIV with macrophages into the nervous system. The intense secretion of immunoglobulins and the presence of helper T cells probably manage to control the effects of viral invasion. Guillain–Barré-like syndrome, which is observed early in the course of HIV infection as well as after a number of other viral infections, probably results from a cross-reaction of the polyclonal antibody response to HIV infection with components of the myelin sheath.

Vasculitis also plays a role in HIV neuropathy. Necrotizing arteritis, sometimes observed in association with inflammatory neuropathy occurring during the course of HIV infection, may result from local complement activation in the vicinity of foci of inflammation. Occlusion of epineurial inflammatory nerve vessels can add ischaemic lesions to the inflammatory lesions already present in HIV neuropathies. When the inflammatory lesions of nerve vessels are restricted to endoneurial capillaries, they are milder and usually associated with predominantly demyelinating lesions of nerve fibres, presumably due to release of cytokines and products of macrophage activation. A role for cryoglobulinaemia has been suggested in patients with multifocal neuropathy (Stricker *et al.*, 1992). Cross-reaction between the gp120 glycoprotein of the virus and MAG, a common component of the myelin of the CNS but not the PNS, is suspected by some authors (Van-den-Berg *et al.*, 1992). Release of excessive amounts of TNF has been incriminated in the occurrence of AIDS dementia complex as well as in peripheral neuropathy (Tyor *et al.*, 1992), but convincing data have yet to be provided.

As the immunosuppression progresses because of the gradual loss of $CD4^+$ T cells, the lesions of the PNS become increasingly destructive, with more axonal lesions and less cellular infiltration. The reason why late nerve lesions are more destructive and more axonal compared with early lesions is not clear. This may be related to the progressive weakness of the phagocytic cell response. In CMV neuropathy, loss of specific CD4+ T cells and reactivation of latent CMV infection leads to infection of endothelial cell and then of neighbouring endoneurial cells. Necrosis in foci of CMV infection leads to the destruction of neighbouring fibres, more often via a bystander mechanism rather than infection of Schwann cells, which is an uncommon phenomenon. A role for nutritional factors or vitamin $B_{12}$ deficiency has been suggested. It is true that some patients with late distal symmetrical sensory neuropathy also have signs of spinal cord involvement reminiscent of those seen in vitamin $B_{12}$ deficiency. It is interesting that vitamin $B_{12}$ metabolism has been shown to be abnormal in HIV-positive patients (Kieburtz *et al.*, 1991); in this study HIV-positive patients had either low serum $B_{12}$ or an abnormal Schilling's test. In such patients, however, supplementation with vitamin $B_{12}$ does not appear to be effective.

## DRUG-INDUCED NEUROPATHY IN HIV-POSITIVE PATIENTS

The antiretroviral drugs dideoxyinosine (Kieburtz *et al.*, 1992) and dideoxycytidine (Dubinsky *et al.*, 1989; Berger AR *et al.*, 1993) have been shown to cause a painful sensory–motor neuropathy indistinguishable from distal sensory polyneuropathy (DSPN). However, the symptoms and signs generally resolve on withdrawal of these drugs within a few weeks. AZT does not cause peripheral neuropathy (Bozzette *et al.*, 1991). In a controlled study, the incidence of peripheral neuropathy was 23/118 patients treated with dideoxyinosine compared with 22/127 patients treated with AZT (Montaner *et al.*, 1995). Lamivudine triphosphate, a recently introduced nucleoside analogue structurally related to zalcitibine, seems less neurotoxic than dideoxyinosine and dideoxycytidine, to which it is now often added to treat HIV infection. However, it may induce a mild axonal, reversible, distal symmetrical polyneuropathy in a small proportion of patients.

In patients taking antiretroviral drugs attention should be given to the occurrence of distal paraesthesiae and the drug should be withdrawn, at least for a few weeks, if the patient has sensory loss. Electrophysiological tests, especially nerve conduction velocity, can remain normal in spite of the presence of signs and symptoms of neuropathy because distal axonopathy often modifies nerve action potentials and conduction velocity long after the onset symptoms.

## TREATMENT OF NEUROPATHY

There is not much choice about the treatment available in neuropathies associated with HIV infection. In patients with acute or subacute inflammatory demyelinating neuropathy, which occurs mostly in non-immunodepressed patients, the same treatments can be used as for non-HIV-infected patients with Guillain–Barré syndrome or acquired chronic demyelinating neuropathy. In non-immunodepressed patients with subacute or demyelinating neuropathy, we favour the use of corticosteroids for a few weeks, especially when the nerve biopsy has documented the presence of dense inflammatory infiltrates and/or vasculitis. Improvement of neurological deficit occurs within a few weeks or months. Since spontaneous improvement also occurs at that stage, it is wiser to treat only patients with disabling or progressive neurological deficit. Plasma exchange (Cornblath, 1988) or intravenous immunoglobulins (Chimowitz *et al.*, 1992) have been successfully used by some in acute demyelinating neuropathy associated with HIV infection, but spontaneous improvement of demyelinating neuropathies (Persuy *et al.*, 1988) is common in non-immunodepressed patients, and failure of these treatments is also common. No controlled study is presently available.

Occasional improvement of distal symmetrical sensory polyneuropathy after AZT therapy has been reported (Yarchoan *et al.*, 1987; Giala *et al.*, 1988). Treatment is symptomatic for the dysaesthesias (tricyclic antidepressants, carbamazepine, phenytoin). Capsaicin cream (0.25%) can be useful in some patients when applied to dysaesthetic feet four times daily. However, a beneficial response may be delayed for 3 or 4 weeks. Administration of opiates may be necessary in some cases. In all cases, psychological support and physiotherapy must be associated with drug treatment.

CMV infection of the nervous system responds well to treatment with ganciclovir when treated early (Miller *et al.*, 1990; Said *et al.*, 1991; Roullet *et al.*, 1994) (see treatment of CMV infection in Chapter 4).

## REFERENCES

Bacellar H, Munoz A, Miller EN *et al.* (1994) Temporal trends in the incidence of HIV-1 related neurologic diseases: multicenter cohort study, 1985–1992. *Neurology* **44**: 1892–1900.

Bailey RO, Baltch AL, Venkatesh R *et al.* (1988) Sensory motor neuropathy associated with AIDS. *Neurology* **38**: 886–891.

Barohn RJ, Kissel JT, Warmolts JR and Mendell JR (1989) Chronic inflammatory demyelinating polyradiculoneuropathy: clinical characteristics, course, and recommendations for diagnostic criteria. *Archives of Neurology* **46**: 878–884.

Barohn RJ, Gronseth GS, LeForce B *et al.* (1993) Peripheral nervous system involvement in a large cohort of human immunodeficiency virus-infected individuals. *Archives of Neurology* **50**: 167–171.

Behar R, Wiley C and McCutchan JA (1987) Cytomegalovirus polyradiculoneuropathy in acquired immune deficiency syndrome. *Neurology* **37**: 557–561.

Belec L, Gherardi R, Georges AJ *et al.* (1989) Peripheral facial paralysis and HIV infection: report of four African cases and review of the literature. *Journal of Neurology* **236**: 411–414.

Berger AR, Arezzo JC, Schaumburg HH *et al.* (1993) 2′,3′-Dideoxycytidine (ddC) toxic neuropathy: a study of 52 patients. *Neurology* **43**: 358–362.

Berger JR, Flaster M, Schatz N *et al.* (1993) Cranial neuropathy heralding otherwise occult AIDS-related large cell lymphoma. *Journal of Clinical Neuro-ophthalmology* **13**: 113–118.

Beytout J, Llory JF, Clavelou P *et al.* (1989) Méningoradiculite à la phase de primo-infection à VIH. Intérêt de la plasmaphérèse. *Presse Medicale* **18**: 1031–1032.

Bishopric G, Bruner J and Butler J (1985) Guillain–Barré syndrome with cytomegalovirus infection of peripheral nerves. *Archives of Pathology and Laboratory Medicine* **109**: 1106–1110.

Bozzette SA, Santangelo J, Villasana D *et al.* (1991) Peripheral nerve function in persons with asymptomatic or minimally symptomatic HIV disease: absence of zidovudine neurotoxicity. *Journal of Acquired Immune Deficiency Syndromes* **4**: 851–855.

Brown MM, Thompson A, Goh BT, Forster GE and Swash M (1988) Bell's palsy and HIV infection. *Journal of Neurology, Neurosurgery and Psychiatry* **51**: 425–426.

Calabrese LH (1991) Vasculitis and infection with the human immunodeficiency virus. *Rheumatic Disease Clinics of North America* **17**: 131–147.

Chaunu MP, Ratinahirana H, Raphael M *et al.* (1989) The spectrum of changes on 20 nerve biopsies in patients with HIV infection. *Muscle and Nerve* **12**: 452–459.

Chavanet P, Solary E, Giroud M *et al.* (1989) Infraclinical neuropathies related to immunodeficiency virus infection associated with higher T-helper cell count. *Journal of Acquired Immune Deficiency Syndromes* **2**: 564–565.

Chimowitz MI, Audet AM, Hallet A and Kelly JJ (1992) The treatment of HIV associated chronic inflammatory demyelinating polyneuropathy (HIV CIDP) with intravenous immunoglobulin (IVIG). *Neurology* **42** (Suppl. 3): 335.

Cinque P, Vago L, Brytting M *et al.* (1992) Cytomegalovirus infection of the central nervous system in patients with AIDS. Diagnosis by DNA amplification from cerebrospinal fluid. *Journal of Infectious Diseases* **166**: 1408–1411.

Clark SJ, Saag MS, Hahn BH *et al.* (1991) Primary HIV-1 infection. *New England Journal of Medicine* **325**: 734–735.

Clifford DB, Buller RS, Mohamed S *et al.* (1993) Use of polymerase chain reaction to demonstrate cytomegalovirus DNA in CSF of patients with human immunodeficiency virus infection. *Neurology* **43**: 75–79.

Cohen BA, McArthur JC, Grohman S *et al.* (1993) Neurologic prognosis of cytomegalovirus polyradiculomyelopathy in AIDS. *Neurology* **43**: 493–499.

Collier AC, Bozzette S, Coombs RW *et al.* (1990) A pilot study of low dose zidovudine in human immunodeficiency virus infection. *New England Journal of Medicine* **323**: 1015–1021.

Comi G, Medaglini S, Galardi G *et al.* (1986) Subclinical neuromuscular involvement in acquired immune deficiency syndrome. *Muscle and Nerve* **9**: 665.

Cornblath DR (1988) Treatment of the neuromuscular complications of human immunodeficiency virus infection. *Annals of Neurology* **23** (Suppl.).

Cornblath DR, McArthur JC (1988) Predominantly sensory neuropathy in patients with AIDS and AIDS related complex. *Neurology* **38**: 794–796.

Cornblath DR, McArthur JC, Kennedy PGE, Witte AS and Griffin JW (1987) Inflammatory demyelinating peripheral neuropathies associated with human T-cell lymphotropic virus type III infection. *Annals of Neurology* **21**: 32–40.

Craddock C, Pasvol G, Bull R, Protheroe A and Hopkin J (1987) Cardiorespiratory arrest and autonomic neuropathy in AIDS. *Lancet* **ii**: 16–18.

de Gans J, Tiessens G, Portegies P, Tutuarima JA and Troost D (1990) Predominance of polymorphonuclear leukocytes in cerebrospinal fluid of AIDS patients with cytomegalovirus polyradiculomyelitis. *AIDS* **3**: 1155–1158.

de la Monte SM, Gabuzda DH, Ho DD *et al.* (1988) Peripheral neuropathy in the acquired immunodeficiency syndrome. *Annals of Neurology* **23**: 485–492.

Del Rio C, Soffer O, Widell JL *et al.* (1990) Acute human immunodeficiency virus infection temporally associated with rhabdomyolysis, acute renal failure, and nephrosis. *Reviews of Infectious Diseases* **12**: 282–285.

Dowling P, Menonna J and Cook S (1977) Cytomegalovirus complement fixation antibody in Guillain–Barré syndrome. *Neurology* **27**: 1153–1156.

Dubinsky RM, Yarchoan R, Dalakas M *et al.* (1989) Reversible axonal neuropathy from the treatment of AIDS and related disorders with 2′,3′-dideoxycytdine (ddC). *Muscle and Nerve* **12**: 856–860.

Eidelberg D, Sotrel A, Vogel H *et al.* (1986) Progressive polyradiculopathy in acquired immune deficiency syndrome. *Neurology* **36**: 912–916.

Evenhouse M, Haas E, Snell E *et al.* (1987) Hypotension in infection with the human immunodeficiency virus. *Annals of Internal Medicine* **107**: 598–599.

Follezou JY, Smadja D, Baulac M, Chauveine L and Laplane D (1987) Paralysie faciale isolée associée à l'infection HIV. *Presse Medicale* **16**: 357–358.

Freeman R, Roberts MS, Friedman LS and Broadbridge C (1990) Autonomic function and human immunodeficiency virus infection. *Neurology* **40**: 575–580.

Fuller GN, Jacobs JM and Guiloff RJ (1990) Axonal atrophy in painful peripheral neuropathy in AIDS. *Acta Neuropathologica* **81**: 198–203.

Fuller GN, Jacobs JM and Guiloff RJ (1993) Nature and incidence of peripheral nerve syndromes in HIV infection. *Journal of Neurology, Neurosurgery and Psychiatry* **56**: 372–381.

Gastaut JL, Gastaut JF, Pélissier JF *et al.* (1989) Neuropathies périphériques au cours de l'infection par le virus de l'immunodéficience humaine. *Revue Neurologique* **145**: 451–459.

Gherardi R. Labargy F, Mhiri C *et al.* (1989) Necrotizing vasculitis and HIV replication in peripheral nerves (letter). *New England Journal of Medicine* **321**: 685–686.

Giala M, Cone L, Cohen N *et al.* (1988) Responses of neurologic complications of AIDS to 3′-azido-3′-deoxythymidine and 9(1,3-dihydroxy-2-propoxymethyl)guanine. I. Clinical features. *Reviews of Infectious Diseases* **10**: 250–256.

Gibbels E and Diederich N (1988) Human immunodeficiency virus (HIV)-related chronic relapsing inflammatory demyelinating polyneuropathy with multifocal unusual onion bulbs in sural nerve biopsy. *Acta Neuropathologica* **75**: 529–534.

Glass JD and Erozan YS (1993) Rapid diagnosis of cytomegalovirus polyradiculitis in a patient with acquired immunodeficiency syndrome. *Annals of Neurology* **34**: 239.

Gold JE, Jimenez E and Zalusky R (1988) Human immunodeficiency virus related lymphoreticular malignancies and peripheral neurologic disease. *Cancer* **61**: 2318–2324.

Goldstein JM, Ausim Azizi S, Booss J and Volmer TL (1993) Human immunodeficiency virus associated motor axonal polyradiculopathy. *Archives of Neurology* **50**: 1316–1319.

Gozlan J, Salord JM, Roullet E *et al.* (1992). Rapid detection of cytomegalovirus DNA in cerebrospinal fluid of AIDS patients with neurological disorders. *Journal of Infectious Diseases* **166**: 1416–1421.

Grafe MR and Wiley CA (1989) Spinal cord and peripheral nerve pathology in AIDS: the role of human immunodeficiency virus. *Annals of Neurology* **25**: 561–566.

Grimaldi LM, Luzi L, Martino GV *et al.* (1993) Bilateral eighth cranial nerve neuropathy in human immunodeficiency virus infection. *Journal of Neurology* **240**: 363–366.

Gulevich SJ, Kalmijn JA, Thal LJ *et al.* (1992) Sensory testing in human immunodeficiency virus type 1-infected men. *Archives of Neurology* **49**: 1281–1284.

Hagberg L, Boeric M, Svennerholm L *et al.* (1986) Guillain–Barré syndrome as an early manifestation of HIV central nervous system infection. *Scandinavian Journal of Infectious Diseases* **18**: 591–592.

Hall CD, Snyder CR, Messenheimer JA *et al.* (1991) Peripheral neuropathy in a cohort of human immunodeficiency virus infected patients: incidence and relationship to other nervous system dysfunction. *Archives of Neurology* **48**: 1273–1274.

Harle JR, Disdier P, Chouc PY and Weiller PJ (1988) Hypotension orthostatique dysautonomique au cours d'une infection par le virus de l'immunodéficience humaine. *Presse Medicale* **17**: 917–918.

Ho DD, Rota TR, Schooley RT *et al.* (1985) Isolation of HTLV III from cerebrospinal fluid and neural tissues of patients with neurologic syndromes related to the acquired immunodeficiency syndrome. *New England Journal of Medicine* **313**: 1493–1497.

Janssen RS, Saykin AJ, Kaplan JE *et al.* (1988) Neurological complications of human immunodeficiency virus infection in patients with lymphadenopathy syndrome. *Annals of Neurology* **23**: 49–55.

Jeantils V, Lemaitre M-O, Robert J *et al.* (1986). Subacute polyneuropathy with encephalopathy in AIDS with human cytomegalovirus pathogenicity. *Lancet* **ii**: 1039.

Kalayjian RC, Cohen ML, Bonomo RA and Flanigan TP (1993) Cytomegalovirus ventriculoencephalitis in AIDS. A syndrome with distinct clinical and pathologic features. *Medicine* **72**: 67–77.

Kieburtz DK, Giang DW, Schiffer RB *et al.* (1991) Abnormal vitamin $B_{12}$ metabolism in human immunodeficiency virus infection: association with neurological dysfunction. *Archives of Neurology* **48**: 312–314.
Kieburtz KD, Seidlin M, Lambert JS *et al.* (1992) Extended follow-up of peripheral neuropathy in patients with AIDS and AIDS related complex treated with dideoxyinosine. *Journal of Acquired Immune Deficiency Syndromes* **5**: 60–64.
Kim YS and Hollander H (1993) Polyradiculopathy due to cytomegalovirus: report of two cases in which improvement occurred after prolonged therapy and review of the literature. *Clin Infect Dis* **17**: 32–37.
Krech U (1973) Complement fixing antibodies against cytomegalovirus antibodies in different parts of the world. *Bulletin of the World Health Organization* **49**: 605–610.
Lacroix C, Vazeux R, Brousse N *et al* (1993) A neuropathological study of 10 HIV-infected children. *Revue Neurologique* **149**: 37–45.
Lange DJ, Britton CB, Younger DS *et al.* (1988) The neuromuscular manifestations of human immunodeficiency virus infection. *Archives of Neurology* **45**: 1084–1088.
Léger JM, Bouche P, Bolgert F *et al.* (1989) The spectrum of polyneuropathies in patients infected with HIV. *Journal of Neurology, Neurosurgery and Psychiatry* **52**: 1369–1374.
Léger JM, Henin D, Belec L *et al.* (1992) Lymphoma-induced polyradiculopathy in AIDS: two cases. *Journal of Neurology* **239**: 132–134.
Leonard JC and Tobin JO (1971) A report from various centers of polyneuritis associated with cytomegalovirus infection. *Quarterly Journal of Medicine* **40**: 435–442.
Leport C, Chaunu MP, Sicre J *et al.* (1987) Neuropathie périphérique en relation avec l'infection par le rétrovirus LAV/HTLV-III. *Presse Medicale* **16**: 55–58.
Lin-Greenberger A and Taneja-Uppal N (1987) Dysautonomia and infection with the human immunodeficiency virus. *Annals of Internal Medicine* **106**: 167.
Lipkin WI, Parry G, Kiprov DD and Abrams D (1985) Inflammatory neuropathy in homosexual men with lymphadenopathy. *Neurology* **35**: 1479–1483.
Mah V, Vartavarian LM, Akers MA *et al.* (1988) Abnormalities of peripheral nerve in patients with human immunodeficiency virus infection. *Annals of Neurology* **24**: 713–717.
Mahé A, Bruet A, Chabin E and Fendler JP (1989) Acute rhabdomyolysis coincident with primary HIV-1 infection (letter). *Lancet* **ii**: 1454–1455.
Marshall DW, Brey RL, Cahill WT *et al.* (1988) Spectrum of cerebrospinal fluid findings in various stages of human immunodeficiency virus infection. *Archives of Neurology* **45**: 954–958.
Miller RF and Sample SJ (1987) Autonomic neuropathy in AIDS. *Lancet* **ii**: 343–344.
Miller RG, Parry GJ, Plaeffl W *et al.* (1988) The spectrum of peripheral neuropathy associated with ARC and AIDS. *Muscle and Nerve* **11**: 857–863.
Miller RG, Storey JR and Greco CM (1990) Ganciclovir in the treatment of progressive AIDS related polyradiculopathy. *Neurology* **40**: 569–574.
Mishra BB, Sommers W, Koski CL *et al.* (1985) Acute inflammatory demyelinating polyneuropathy in the acquired immune deficiency syndrome. *Annals of Neurology* **18**: 131–132.
Montaner JSG, Schechter MT, Rachlis A *et al.* (1995) Didanoside compared with continued zidovudine therapy for HIV-infected patients with 200 to 500 CD4 cells/$mm^3$. *Annals of Internal Medicine* **123**: 561–571.
Newman NJ and Lessell S (1992) Bilateral optic neuropathies with remission in two HIV-positive men. *Journal of Clinical Neuro-ophthalmology* **12**: 1–5.
Pantaleo G, Graziosi C and Fauci AS (1993) The immunopathogenesis of human immunodeficiency virus infection. *New England Journal of Medicine* **328**: 327–335.
Persuy PH, Arnott G, Fortier B *et al.* (1988) Syndrome de Guillain–Barré d'évolution favorable dans un cas d'infection récente par le virus de l'immunodéficience humaine. *Revue Neurologique* **144**: 32–35.
Petito CK, Navia BA, Cho ES *et al.* (1985) Vacuolar myelopathy pathologically resembling subacute combined degeneration in patients with the acquired immunodeficiency syndrome. *New England Journal of Medicine* **312**: 874–879.
Piette AM, Tusseau F and Chapman A (1987) Symptomatologie aiguë contemporaine de la primo-infection par le virus HIV. Deux observations. *Presse Medicale* **16**: 346–348.
Rance NE, McArthur JC, Cornblath DR *et al.* (1988) Gracile tract degeneration in patients with sensory neuropathy and AIDS. *Neurology* **38**: 265–271.
Raphaël SA, Price ML, Lischner HW *et al.* (1991) Inflammatory demyelinating polyneuropathy in a child with symptomatic human immunodeficiency virus infection. *Journal of Pediatrics* **118**: 242–245.

Roizman B and Batterson W (1985) Herpesviruses and their replication. In: *Herpes viruses and their replication* (eds BN Fields *et al.*) *Virology*, pp. 496–526. New York: Raven Press.

Ronchi O, Grippo A, Ghidini P *et al.* (1992) Electrophysiologic study of HIV-1+ patients without signs of peripheral neuropathy. *Journal of the Neurological Sciences* **113**: 209–213.

Roullet E, Assuerus, Gozlan J *et al.* (1994) Cytomegalovirus multifocal neuropathy in AIDS: analysis of 15 consecutive cases. *Neurology* **44**: 2174–2182.

Sadun AA, Pepose JS, Madigan M *et al.* (1995) AIDS-related optic neuropathy: a histological, virological and ultrastructural study. *Graefes Archive for Clinical and Experimental Ophthalmology* **233**: 387–398.

Said G, Lacroix C, Andrieu JN *et al.* (1987) Necrotizing arteritis in patients with inflammatory neuropathy and human immunodeficiency virus infection. *Neurology* **37** (Suppl. 1): 176.

Said G, Lacroix-Ciaudo C, Fujimura H, Blas C and Faux N (1988) The peripheral neuropathy of necrotizing arteritis: a clinicopathological study. *Annals of Neurology* **23**: 461–465.

Said G, Lacroix C, Chemouilli P *et al.* (1991) Cytomegalovirus neuropathy in acquired immunodeficiency syndrome: a clinical and pathological study. *Annals of Neurology* **29**: 139–146.

Selik RM, Starcher ET and Curran JW (1987) Opportunistic diseases reported in AIDS patients: frequencies, associations, trends. *AIDS* **1**: 175–182.

Sillevis Smith PAE and Portegies P (1990) Fisher's syndrome associated with human immunodeficiency virus infection. *Clinical Neurology and Neurosurgery* **92**: 353–355.

Simpson D and Morgello S (1992) Rapid detection of cytomegalovirus DNA in cerebrospinal fluid of AIDS patients with neurological disorders. *Journal of Infectious Diseases* **166**: 1416–1421.

Singh BM, Levine S, Yarrish RL *et al.* (1986) Spinal cord syndromes in the acquired immune deficiency syndrome. *Acta Neurologica Scandinavica* **73**: 590–598.

Small PM, McPhaul LW, Sooy CD *et al.* (1989) Cytomegalovirus infection of the laryngeal nerve presenting as hoarseness in patients with acquired immunodeficiency syndrome. *Journal of the American Medical Association* **86**: 108–110.

Snider WD, Simpson DM, Nielsen S *et al.* (1983) Neurological complications of human immunedeficiency syndrome. *Annals of Neurology* **14**: 403–418.

So YT and Olney RK (1994) Acute lumbosacral polyradiculopathy in acquired immunodeficiency syndrome: experience in 23 patients. *Annals of Neurology* **35**: 53–58.

Soubeyrand J, Niamkey E, Tea D *et al.* (1989) Liquide céphalo-rachidien et virus de l'immunodéficience humaine. *Semaine Hopiteaux Paris* **65**: 2781–2786.

Stricker RB, Sanders KA, Owen WF *et al.* (1992) Mononeuritis multiplex associated with cryoglobulinemia in HIV infection. *Neurology* **42**: 2103–2105.

Tyor WR, Glass JD, Griffen JW *et al.* (1992) Cytokine expression in the brain during the acquired immunodeficiency syndrome. *Annals of Neurology* **31**: 349–360.

Van-den-Berg LH, Sadiq SA, Lederman S and Latov N (1992) The gp120 glycoprotein of HIV-1 binds to sulfatide and to the myelin associated glycoprotein. *Journal of Neuroscience Research* **33**: 513–518.

Vendrell J, Heredia C, Pujol M *et al.* (1987) Guillain-Barré syndrome associated with seroconversion for anti-HTLV-III (abstract). *Neurology* **37**: 544.

Villa A, Foresti V and Confalonieri F (1987) Autonomic neuropathy and HIV infection. Lancet **i**: 915.

Vinters HV, Kwok MK, Ho HW *et al.* (1989) Cytomegalovirus in the nervous system of patients with the acquired immune deficiency syndrome. *Brain* **112**: 245–268.

Vishnubhakat SM and Beresford R (1988) Prevalence of peripheral neuropathy in HIV disease: prospective study of 40 patients. *Neurology* **38**: 350.

Wechsler AF and Ho DD (1989) Bilateral Bell's palsy at the time of HIV seroconversion. *Neurology* **39**: 747–748.

Wolf DG and Spector SA (1992) Diagnosis of human cytomegalovirus central nervous system disease in AIDS patients by DNA amplification from cerebrospinal fluid. *Journal of Infectious Diseases* **166**: 1412–1415.

Yarchoan R, Berg G, Prouwers P *et al.* (1987) Response of human immunodeficiency virus associated neurological disease to 3′-azido-3′-deoxythymidine. *Lancet* **i**: 132–134.

Yarrish RL (1987) Cytomegalovirus infection in AIDS. In: *AIDS and other manifestations of HIV infection* (eds GP Wormser, RE Stahl and EJ Bottone), pp. 478–517. Park Ridge, New Jersey: Noyes Publications.

# 8

# *Muscle Disease*

Different patterns of muscle disorders, including inflammatory and non-inflammatory myositis, pyomyositis and myopathy related to treatment with zidovudine occur in patients with HIV infection. Because of the large number of aetiologies of muscle disorders seen in this context, different paraclinical investigations of patients with weakness or muscle pain must be carried out to identify treatable causes of muscle involvement (Simpson and Wolfe, 1991).

## INFLAMMATORY MYOSITIS IN HIV-INFECTED PATIENTS

### Clinical data

Of a personal series of 275 HIV-infected patients investigated for weakness or neuropathy since 1983, inflammatory myositis was present in muscle biopsy specimens of 37 patients. Clinical manifestations of HIV-associated inflammatory myositis usually did not differ from those observed in patients with idiopathic polymyositis (Stern *et al.*, 1987; Lacroix *et al.*, 1991). Usually patients complain of myalgias and proximal weakness with difficulty in climbing stairs and muscle atrophy. At the beginning of the illness, myalgias occur after effort and eventually spontaneously. Myalgias are almost constant in HIV myositis (Dalakas *et al.*, 1986; Berman *et al.*, 1988; Simpson and Bender, 1988). In patients with HIV myositis, muscle tenderness is common upon palpation (Bailey *et al.*, 1987, Stern *et al.*, 1987; Nordstrom *et al.*, 1989). Atrophy, mostly of proximal muscles, was observed in one-third of our patients, whereas distal or generalized muscle atrophy was present in another one-third of patients (Dalakas *et al.*, 1986; Berman *et al.*, 1988; Gabbai *et al.*, 1990; Lacroix *et al.*, 1991). The other patients did not present with atrophy (Stern *et al.*, 1987). The HIV-related inflammatory myositis of one of our patients was revealed by a unilateral calf hypertrophy, which was followed several months later by atrophy of this group of muscles, while the opposite calf increased in volume and subsequently underwent muscle atrophy; 5 years later, he developed hypertrophy of the thigh and the muscle biopsy disclosed a subacute myositis. In a few patients distal weakness was associated with facial and axial impairments (Simpson and Bender, 1988). Of the patients in our series 10% had normal muscle strength. Dysphagia is uncommon. Occasional cases of dermatomyositis have been reported in HIV-infected patients (Stern *et al.*, 1987; Dalakas and Pezeshkpour, 1988). Inflammatory myositis was isolated in 13 of our patients; in addition four patients had granulomatous angiitis, four patients CMV polyradiculoneuropathy and 16 patients HIV polyneuropathy. The date of the onset of myositis during HIV infection is extremely variable. Myositis has been reported as the presenting symptom of HIV infection in three patients of our series (Dalakas and Pezeshkpour, 1988; Simpson and Bender, 1988). Inflammatory myopathy occurred later in the course of HIV infection in six other patients and in 27 of our patients with a $CD4^+$ T-cell count below 100 $mm^{+3}$, as well as in several cases previously reported (Bailey et al., 1987; Stern et al., 1987; Nordstrom *et al.*, 1989).

**Laboratory data**

Serum creatine kinase levels are increased in most patients and periodic evaluation is useful to monitor treatment (Dalakas *et al.*, 1986; Bailey *et al.*, 1987; Laraki *et al.*, 1990). In a series of nine patients with AIDS who complained of fatigue, Miller *et al.* (1991) did not find any difference in muscles compared with control patients using phosphorus magnetic resonance spectroscopy.

**Pathology**

Morphological abnormalities observed in this context are similar to those found in idiopathic polymyositis. Fibre necrosis was present in all our 37 patients as in many reported cases (Figure 8.1) (Dalakas *et al.*, 1986; Stern *et al.*, 1987; Simpson and Bender, 1988). Mononuclear cell infiltration of muscle fibres and interstitial infiltrates was usual (Figure 8.2). Inflammatory cells comprised lymphocytes, predominantly of the CD8 type, and macrophages. We did not find any MGCs in perimysial infiltrates in agreement with Bailey *et al.* (1987). Eight patients (21%) had associated vasculitis including four with granulomatous angiitis (Said *et al.*, 1988). Four patients had fibrosis (Figure 8.3) (Stern *et al.*, 1987). Sixteen AIDS patients (42%) had associated muscle siderosis (Gherardi *et al.*, 1991; Lacroix and Said, 1992). Immunocytochemistry disclosed HIV p24 and gp41 antigens in interstitial macrophages, in agreement with other studies (Chad *et al.*, 1990; Illa *et al.*, 1991). In patients with HIV myositis the predominant inflammatory cells were macrophages and $CD8^+$ T cells, suggesting that HIV myositis is a T-cell-mediated and MHC class I-restricted cytotoxic process (Illa *et al.*, 1991). We were unable to find HIV particles in muscle fibres by electron microscopy, in agreement with Simpson and Bender (1988) and Chad *et al.* (1990).

**Treatment**

Disabling forms of HIV inflammatory myopathy may require corticosteroids, especially when myositis develops in non-immunodepressed patients.

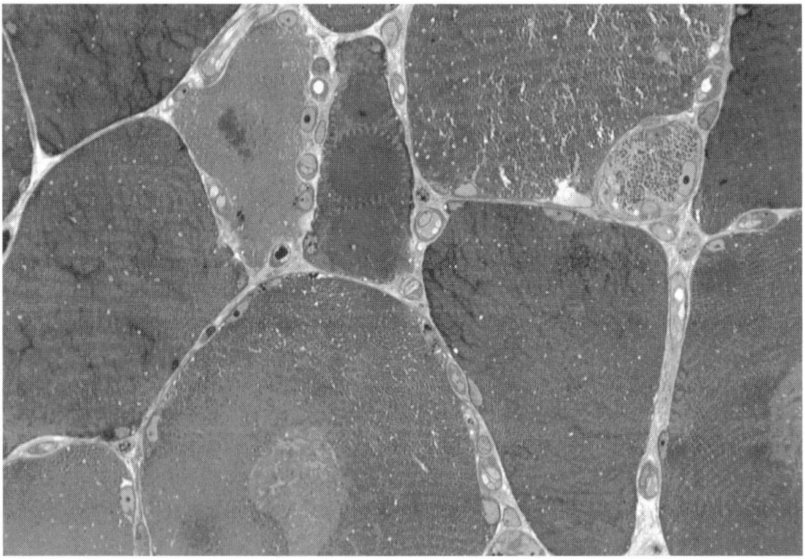

**Figure 8.1** HIV myositis in a patient who developed progressive proximal weakness. Note marked abnormalities of muscle fibres including small angulated fibres and central core abnormalities. (1-μm thick section of a plastic-embedded specimen; thionin blue; ×2600).

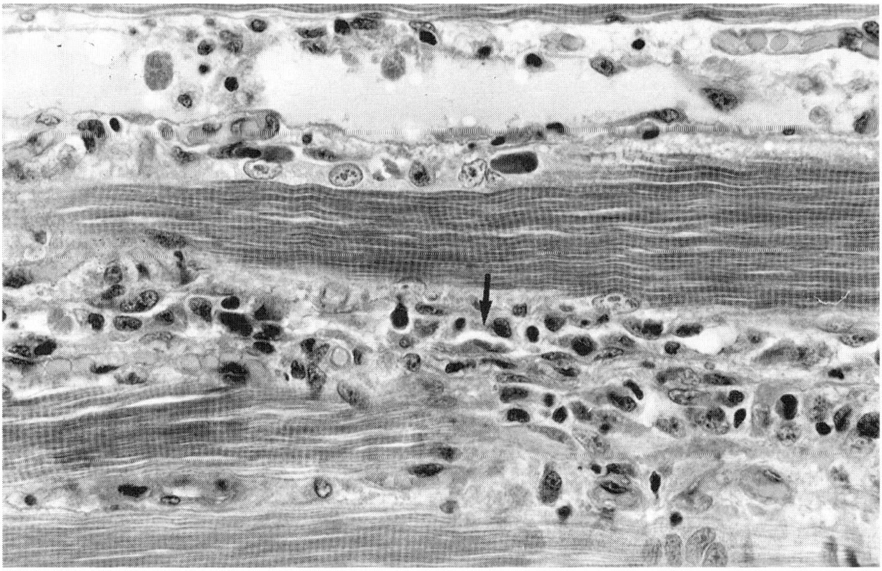

**Figure 8.2** Quadriceps muscle of a patient with hypertrophic HIV myositis. Many fibres are necrotic or infiltrated by mononuclear cells (arrow). (Paraffin section; H&E; ×1060).

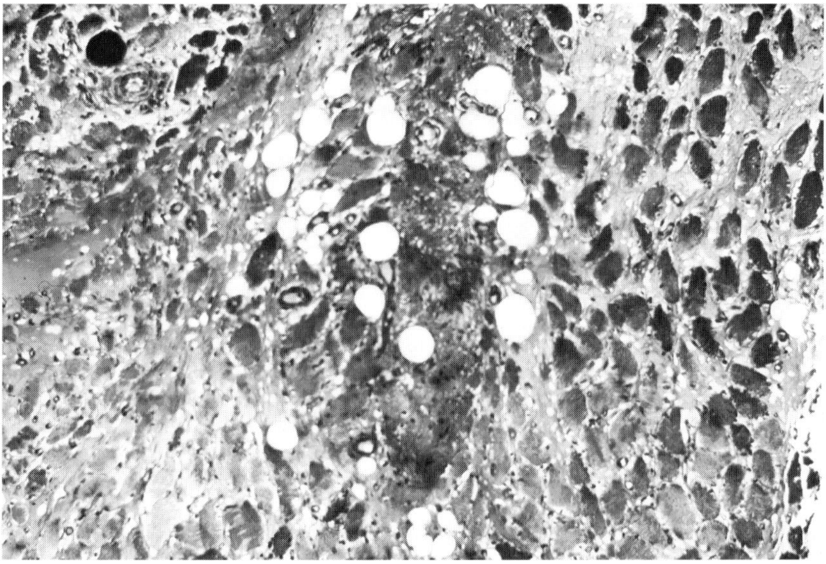

**Figure 8.3** Deltoid muscle of a patient with HIV myositis: note the intense fibrosis (stained in blue-green) between the muscle fibres. (Paraffin section; Masson's trichrome; ×690).

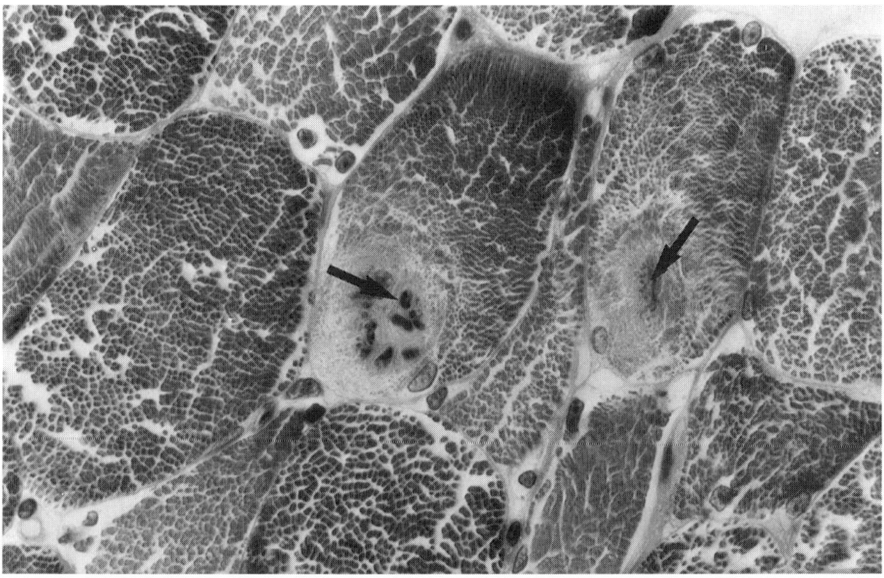

**Figure 8.4** Peroneus brevis muscle of a patient with an associated HIV neuropathy: rod bodies are present in some muscle fibres (arrows). (Paraffin section; H&E; ×1680).

Improvement of both clinical manifestations and creatine kinase (CK) levels are thus achieved in most cases (Dalakas and Pezeshkpour, 1988; Simpson, 1988; Lacroix *et al.*, 1991). However, some patients may have transient response to prednisone and rapidly develop ARC or AIDS (Dalakas and Pezeshkpour, 1988). There are also some anecdotal reports on the efficacy of plasma exchange, treatment with zidovudine (Simpson, 1988) or intravenous injection of immunoglobulins (Viard *et al.*, 1992).

## HIV-ASSOCIATED NON-INFLAMMATORY MYOPATHY

### Rod myopathy and loss of thick filaments

In some patients with HIV infection, slowly progressive proximal-muscle weakness and wasting occurred and muscle biopsy showed accumulation of rod bodies (nemaline), predominantly in type I muscle fibres (Dalakas *et al.*, 1987). In most cases patients with nemaline myopathy were HIV seropositive without profound immunosuppression (Dalakas *et al.*, 1987; Simpson and Bender, 1988). We observed rod bodies in 10 patients in association with HIV myositis or neuropathy. Rod bodies originate in Z-disc disruption when actin filaments are dissociated (Figure 8.4). These rare abnormalities in adults are not specific for HIV infection but suggest a possible role for HIV in lesions of myofilaments in the absence of inflammation. Similar myopathies with loss of thick filaments associated with rod bodies have been described in two HIV-seropositive patients (Gonzales *et al.*, 1988). In addition we observed cytoplasmic bodies in many muscle biopsies of patients with HIV neuropathy (Lacroix *et al.*, 1991).

### Muscle siderosis

In many patients with distal sensory neuropathy or CMV-related neuropathy who underwent nerve and muscle biopsy, we found iron deposits in many muscle specimens. All these patients were immunocompromised with a $CD4^+$ T-cell count under 100 $mm^{-3}$ (Lacroix and Said, 1992). Most patients who had abnormal iron deposits in muscle on histological examination complained of spontaneous muscle pains and weakness. Neurological examination showed normal or decreased muscle strength and often muscle tenderness, but it is impossible to know if iron deposits play any role in the occurrence of muscle pains. Iron deposits are located in the perimysium around blood vessels, mononuclear cells, endothelial cells and necrotic or apparently normal muscle fibres (Figure 8.5) (Lacroix and Said, 1992). We suggest that muscle siderosis is due to macrophage dysfunction in immunosuppressed patients, causing the accumulation of iron produced during the turnover of myoglobin from muscle fibres (Lacroix and Said, 1992). Other authors have suggested the possibility of erythrophagocytosis in the muscle (Gherardi *et al.*, 1991);

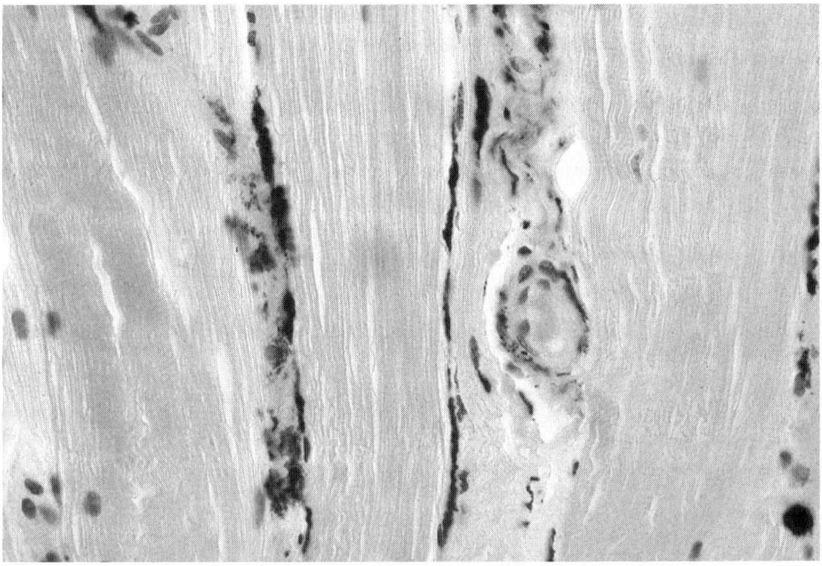

**Figure 8.5** Muscle siderosis in a patient with a CD4$^{+}$ T-cell count of 10/ml, who complained of myalgias; many iron deposits are stained in blue. (Paraffin section; Perls; ×2755).

however, this cannot account for the selective localization of iron deposits in muscle fibres.

**Other non-inflammatory muscular disorders**

Recurrent myoglobinuria has been reported in one HIV-seropositive patient (Lange *et al.*, 1988). We have observed an HIV-infected patient with mild immunosuppression who had a massive rhabdomyolysis associated with elevation of CK up to 200 000 UI/ml and renal insufficiency requiring haemodialysis. The muscle biopsy showed isolated necrotic fibres. In patients with AIDS and proximal wasting, selective atrophy of type II muscle fibres has also been reported (Dalakas *et al.*, 1989). Neurogenic muscular atrophy was present in most of the patients with HIV or CMV-related neuropathy. Two cases of myasthenia gravis syndrome associated with HIV infection have been described (Nath *et al.*, 1990; Martini *et al.*, 1991). Some authors have suggested that an HIV-related wasting syndrome, also called slim disease, is a myopathy when it occurs in the absence of diarrhoea or malabsorption, because all the patients showed mild abnormalities of muscle biopsies and some patients improved with prednisone (Simpson *et al.*, 1990). This syndrome looks rather heterogeneous, whereas muscle wasting and loss of weight are very common in the late stages of AIDS. The myocardium might be involved during HIV infection (Cohen *et al.*, 1986).

## ZIDOVUDINE MYOPATHY

Zidovudine, which is used in the treatment of HIV infection, inhibits reverse transcriptase and thus replication of the virus (Yarchoan *et al.*, 1989). Several months after the beginning of treatment of HIV-infected patients with zidovudine (AZT), many patients manifested proximal weakness and wasting associated with mild elevation of CK levels (Bessen *et al.*, 1988; Gorard *et al.*, 1988; Dalakas *et al.*, 1989). Clinical and biological presentations were similar to HIV myositis, except for CK levels which were, on average, lower than in patients with HIV myositis. All the patients who developed this myopathic syndrome were taking daily doses of AZT of 1 g or more for several months (Pinching *et al.*, 1990; Lacroix *et al.*, 1991). In a personal series of patients taking high doses of zidovudine, as many as 10% of them developed symptoms of myopathy within a few months (unpublished observations). In our experience

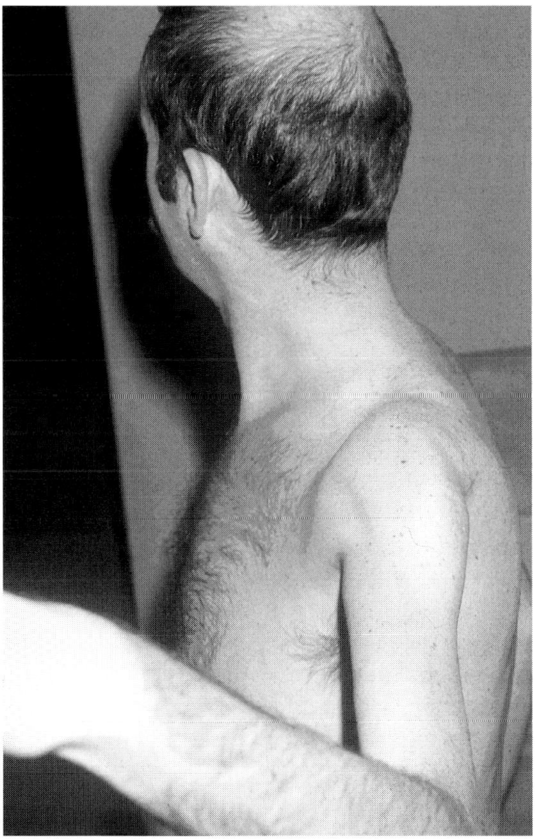

**Figure 8.6** A patient who developed a severe proximal myopathy while being treated with large doses of zidovudine and who improved after withdrawal of the drug. Note the marked amyotrophy of periscapular muscles.

AZT myopathy is often heralded by loss of weight, which is sometimes very rapid and spectacular (Figure 8.6). The myopathy develops between 6 and 24 months after the beginning of treatment with AZT, with an average of 10 months (Bessen *et al.*, 1989; Gertner *et al.*, 1989; Mhiri *et al.*, 1991). The myopathy occurred earlier in a few patients (Gertner *et al.*, 1989; Dalakas *et al.*, 1990) or occasionally later (Gorard *et al.*, 1988). The daily dose of zidovudine was around 1200 mg in most patients (Bessen *et al.*, 1988; Helbert *et al.*, 1988; Gertner *et al.*, 1989; Lacroix *et al.*, 1991), occasionally lower (Mhiri *et al.*, 1991; Lane *et al.*, 1993). The patients were at different stages of HIV infection and all were in good general condition when they started to lose weight and complain of muscular symptoms (Bessen *et al.*, 1988; Gorard *et al.*, 1988; Panegyres *et al.*, 1988). Muscle atrophy, which was present in 6/9 patients that we followed, was predominantly proximal in the upper limbs of two patients and lower limbs of two others; some patients had difficulty in standing from a sitting position or in walking (Gorard *et al.*, 1988). Three patients complained of myalgia and tenderness in proximal muscles (Mhiri *et al.*, 1991). In three patients the serum CK level was within normal limits but decreased after withdrawal of the drug (Panegyres *et al.*, 1988). This finding, and the wide range of normal values of CK levels, argues for the systematic assessment of serum CK activity: baseline levels should be determined before starting treatment with AZT, for comparison with later evaluations. After total withdrawal of zidovudine, all patients improved within 4 weeks, as in most reported cases (Said *et al.*, 1989; Chalmers *et al.*, 1991; Manji *et al.*, 1993). Reduction of the daily dose by half was not sufficient for symptomatic improvement in our experience. A washout period is necessary. In a few cases the patients received corticosteroid therapy (Bessen *et al.*, 1988; Pinching *et al.*, 1990). Zidovudine could be reintroduced 3 or 4 months later at lower doses. Only one patient relapsed 1 year after AZT was resumed.

Pathological findings were not specific. Muscle biopsy showed fibre necrosis, dissolution of myofibrils, vesiculations (Figure 8.7a) and glycogen accumulation. Inflammatory infiltrates were less important than in HIV myositis. In agreement with many authors, we found scattered ragged red fibres on Gomori's trichrome associated with dystrophic mitochondria, which sometimes contained paracrystalline inclusions on electron microscopy (Mhiri *et al.*, 1991; Pezeshkpour *et al.*, 1991). In our experience, typical ragged red fibres, of the type observed in mitochondrial myopathies, and mitochondrial paracrystalline inclusions on electron microscopic examination are rather scarce in the so-called AZT myopathy (Figure 8.7b). AZT myopathy may be difficult or impossible to differentiate from HIV myositis (Dalakas *et al.*, 1990). Some authors even think that AZT is not responsible for the myopathy (Simpson, 1988). The mitochondrial abnormalities in muscle specimens and the thymidine-like pharmacological side-effects of zidovudine (Yarchoan *et al.*, 1989) suggest inhibition of mitochondrial DNA polymerase by the drug (Arnaudo *et al.*, 1991; Mhiri *et al.*, 1991; Pezeshkpour *et al.*, 1991; Herzberg *et al.*, 1992). Some authors have found tubuloreticular inclusions in endothelial cells,

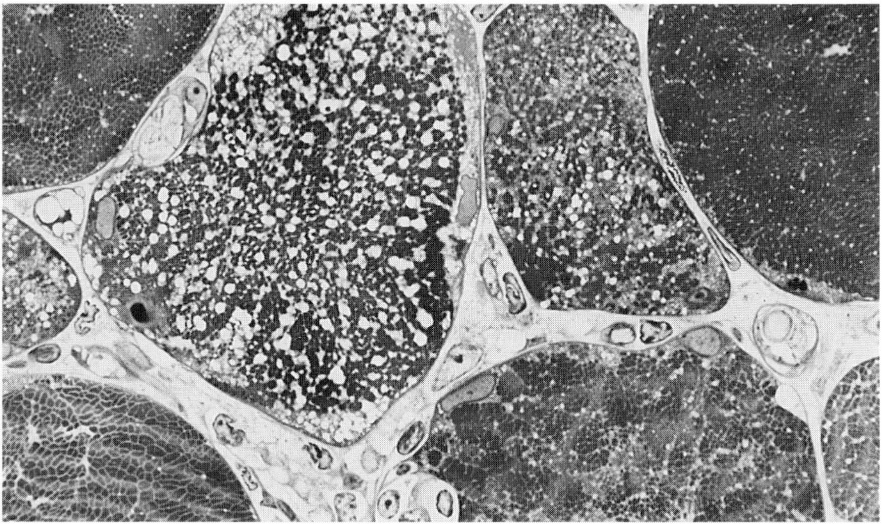

**(a)**

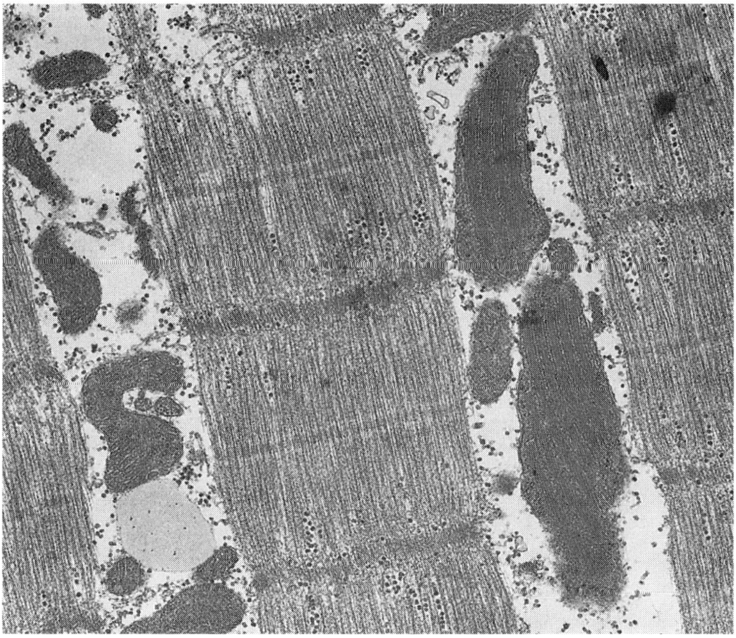

**(b)**

**Figure 8.7** Zidovudine myopathy. (a) Microvesiculations in most muscle fibres. (1-μm thick section; thionin blue; ×1700). (b) Electron micrograph of a muscle sample from the patient shown in Figure 8.6, showing numerous enlarged mitochondria with paracrystalline inclusions. (Uranyl acetate and lead citrate; ×18 000.)

vesicular changes, lipid storage or muscle carnitine deficiency in the muscle specimens of patients with zidovudine myopathy but not in those with HIV myositis (Panegyres *et al.*, 1990; Pezeshkpour *et al.*, 1991; Lane *et al.*, 1993; Dalakas *et al.*, 1994). The mechanism of AZT myopathy remains unclear. In two of our patients, who improved after withdrawal of the drug, HIV p24 antigen-positive mononuclear cells were found in muscle specimens by immunolabelling. An underlying HIV myositis may play a role in the development of AZT myopathy (Berger *et al.*, 1991; Lane *et al.*, 1993). Since the use of lower doses of zidovudine, AZT myopathy has become much less common (Till and MacDonell, 1990).

When zidovudine myopathy is suspected, the drug must be withdrawn for 1 month and clinical examination and CK assays performed again at the end of this period. Most patients with AZT myopathy improve within 1 month after withdrawal of AZT. If the patient does not improve the role of HIV myopathy is likely to be predominant (Said *et al.*, 1989; Chalmers *et al.*, 1991). Treatment with AZT can be started again at lower doses.

A single case of rhabdomyolysis attributed to 2′,3′-dideoxyinosine has been reported, probably secondary to dideoxyinosine-induced hypokalaemia concomitant with HIV myositis and dideoxyinosine-related toxic neuropathy (Doronzo *et al.*, 1993).

Massive rhabdomyolysis occurs in HIV patients. We have observed three patients with massive isolated rhabdomyolysis, which required haemodialysis in one (Figure 8.8).

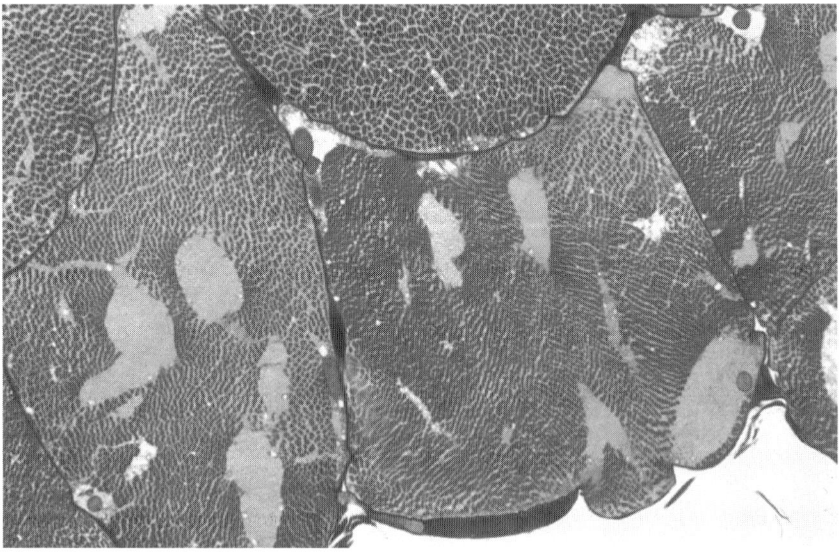

**Figure 8.8** Rhabdomyolysis showing many vacuoles secondary to destruction of myofibrils in an HIV-infected patient. (1-μm thick section; thionin blue; ×2700.)

## OPPORTUNISTIC INFECTION OF MUSCLES

### Pyomyositis

Pyomyositis is a common infection of muscles in non-immunocompromised patients in Africa. In industrialized countries, pyomyositis occurs virtually only in HIV-infected patients (Victor *et al.*, 1989). Clinically, pyomyositis is characterized by association of weakness, spontaneous muscle pains and often extreme tenderness of muscles upon palpation. Fever, shivering, excessive sweating and loss of weight are common. Subcutaneous and muscular nodules, which are extremely painful upon palpation, are suggestive of the diagnosis. Biopsy or needle aspiration of a nodule can be diagnostic. In one of the two patients with AIDS and pyomyositis we investigated, the diagnosis was made only by the demonstration of abscesses after biopsy of painful nodules. Microscopic examination showed massive interstitial infiltration with polymorphonuclear cells and relatively little destruction of muscle fibres. CT of the legs showed several muscle abscesses. The patient improved and muscle tenderness disappeared gradually under treatment with antibiotics. The nodules persisted for 4 weeks. CT performed 1 month later showed massive reduction of muscle abscesses. Pyomyositis usually occurs in patients during the late stages of HIV infection (Raphael *et al.*, 1989; Blumberg and Stephen, 1990; Christin and Sarosi, 1992).

### Toxoplasmosis

*Toxoplasma gondii* is the most frequent opportunistic infection of the CNS in patients with AIDS (Anders *et al.*, 1986). Cardiac toxoplasmosis seems to be common in patients with AIDS but only at a subclinical level (Hoffman *et al.*, 1990). Toxoplasmic cysts were present in the myocardium of only one of our 85 HIV-infected patients examined at autopsy (Lacroix *et al.*, 1991). However, toxoplasmosis of skeletal muscles is a rare finding in biopsy or autopsy specimens: no case was found in a series of 92 HIV-infected patients examined at autopsy (Wrzolek *et al.*, 1990). We have had the opportunity to see two patients with toxoplasmosis affecting skeletal muscles. One of them had symptoms of diffuse polymyositis, with fever and elevated CK levels. Muscle biopsy showed fibre necrosis associated with *T. gondii* cysts (Figure 8.9). Some cysts and free microorganisms were present in the muscle biopsy of another patient who had an HIV-related neuropathy. Skeletal muscle toxoplasmosis was observed in five patients in another series, three of whom were symptomatic (Gherardi *et al.*, 1992).

## VASCULITIS

Different patterns of vasculitis may be observed in HIV-infected patients and inflammatory lesions can also affect muscle blood vessels. Whereas vasculitic lesions of nerve blood vessels induce ischaemic damage to nerve fibres, lesions

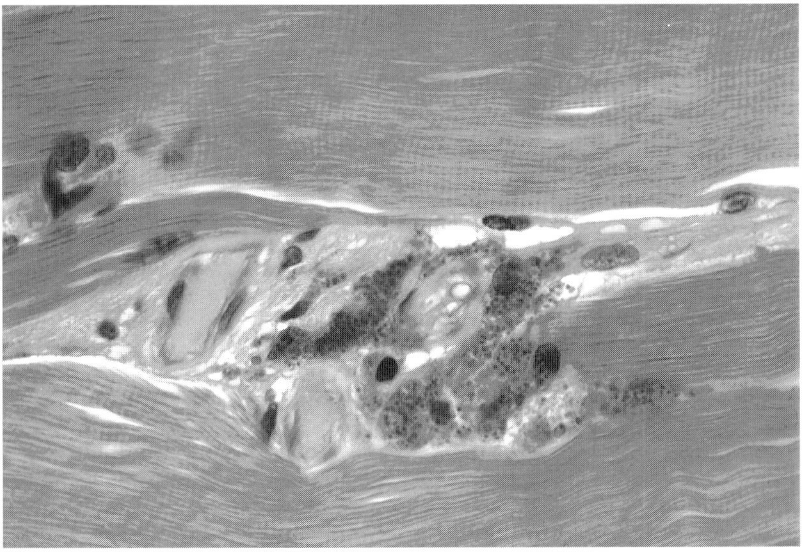

**Figure 8.9** Muscle toxoplasmosis in an AIDS patient showing cysts and free parasites associated with siderosis. (Paraffin section; H&E; ×685.)

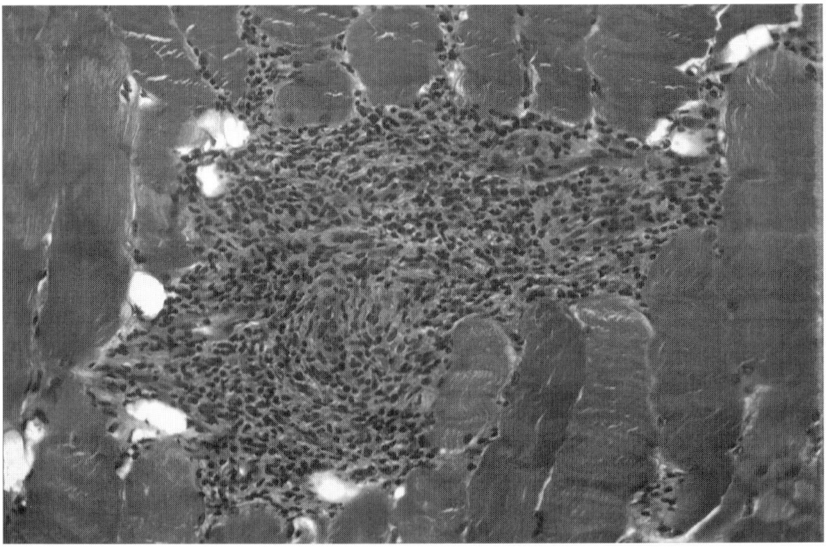

**Figure 8.10** Granulomatous angiitis in a muscle biopsy of a patient with HIV infection and a $CD4^{+}$ T-cell count of 350 $mm^{-3}$. (Paraffin section; H&E; ×1370.)

of muscle blood vessels are usually silent. Simultaneous sampling of muscle in the context of ischaemic–inflammatory neuropathy increases the yield of biopsy because of the demonstration of specific vasculitic lesions in muscle specimens (Said *et al.*, 1988). We and others have observed a wide range of abnormalities of blood vessels in muscle biopsy specimens (Kaye, 1989). Vasculitic lesions of muscle blood vessels include the following.

**Necrotizing arteritis** (see Chapter 7)

**Lymphomatoid granulomatosis**

Lymphomatoid granulomatosis, also called angiocentric lymphocytic process, has been observed in muscle (Calabrese *et al.*, 1989; Lacroix *et al.*, 1991), peripheral nerve (Lacroix *et al.*, 1991; Gherardi *et al.*, 1993) or the CNS (Kaye, 1989). Eight of our patients were found to have lymphomatoid granulomatosis in muscle specimens (Figure 8.10). The biopsy was performed for muscle pains in two patients, mononeuritis multiplex in two patients and distal sensory neuropathy in three patients; the last patient was a child with similar lesions in the CNS and PNS at autopsy. Some patients had associated HIV myositis. The $CD4^+$ T-cell count ranged from 16 to 1000 $mm^{-3}$. Inflammatory infiltrates were present around and in the walls of different vessels. Cells comprised lymphocytes, including a few $CD4^+$ and many $CD8^+$ T cells, some B cells and macrophages. In a patient who had massive polyclonal secretion of immunoglobulin, many plasma cells were present in the infiltrates. Three patients had the same lesions in epineurial vessels of the nerve biopsy specimen. We detected HIV gp41 antigen in a few macrophages in the muscle specimen of one patient. Some patients improved dramatically with steroids.

**Other types of vasculitis**

Non-specific microvasculitis is common in muscle specimens of patients with HIV myositis or neuropathy.

## REFERENCES


Anders K, Steinsapir KD, Iverson DJ *et al.* (1986) Neuropathologic findings in the acquired immunodeficiency syndrome (AIDS). *Clinical Neuropathology* **5**: 1–20.

Arnaudo E, Dalakas M, Shanske S *et al.* (1991) Depletion of muscle mitochondrial DNA in AIDS patients with zidovudine-induced myopathy. *Lancet* **337**: 508–510.

Bailey RO, Turok DI, Jaufmann BP and Singh JK (1987) Myositis and acquired immunodeficiency syndrome. *Human Pathology* **18**: 749–751.

Berger JR, Shelbert R, and Gregorius JB (1991) Exacerbation of HIV-associated myopathy by zidovudine. *AIDS* **4**: 229–230.

Berman A, Espinoza LR, Diaz JD *et al.* (1988) Rheumatic manifestations of human immunodeficiency virus infection. *American Journal of Medicine* **85**: 59–64.

Bessen LJ, Greene JB, Louie E, Seitzman P and Weinberg H (1988) Severe polymyositis-like syndrome associated with zidovudine therapy of AIDS and ARC. *New England Journal of Medicine* **318**: 708.

Blumberg H and Stephen D (1990) Pyomyositis and human immunodeficiency virus infection. *Southern Medical Journal* **83**: 1092–1095.

Calabrese LH, Estes M, Yen-Lieberman *et al.* (1989) Systemic vasculitis in association with human immunodeficiency virus infection. *Arthritis and Rheumatism* **32**: 569–576.
Chad DA, Smith TW, Blumenfield A *et al.* (1990) Human immunodeficiency virus (HIV)-associated myopathy: immunocytochemical identification of an HIV antigen (gp 41) in muscle macrophages. *Annals of Neurology* **28**: 579–582.
Chalmers AC, Greco CM and Miller RG (1991) Prognosis in AZT myopathy. *Neurology* **41**: 1181–1184.
Christin L and Sarosi G (1992) Pyomyositis in North America: case reports and review. *Clinical Infectious Diseases* **15**: 668–677.
Cohen IS, Anderson DW, Virmani R *et al.* (1986) Congestive cardiomyopathy in association with the acquired immunodeficiency syndrome. *New England Journal of Medicine* **15**: 628–629.
Dalakas MC and Pezeshkpour GH (1988) Neuromuscular diseases associated with human immunodeficiency virus infection. *Annals of Neurology* **23** (Suppl.): S38–S48.
Dalakas MC, Pezeshkpour GH, Gravell M and Sever JL (1986) Polymyositis associated with AIDS retrovirus. *Journal of the American Medical Association* **256**: 2381.
Dalakas MC, Pezeshkpour GH and Flaherty M (1987) Progressive nemaline (rod) myopathy associated with HIV infection. *New England Journal of Medicine* **317**: 1602–1603.
Dalakas MC, Wichman A and Sever J (1989) SIDA et système nerveux. *Journal of the American Medical Association* **14**: 791–796.
Dalakas MC, Illa I, Pezeshkpour GH *et al.* (1990) Mitochondrial myopathy caused by long term zidovudine therapy. *New England Journal of Medicine* **322**: 1098–1105.
Dalakas MC, Leon-Monzon ME, Bernardini I, Gahl WA and Jay CA (1994) Zidovudine-induced mitochondrial myopathy is associated with muscle carnitine deficiency and lipid storage. *Annals of Neurology* **35**: 482–487.
Doronzo R, Geremia L, Sacilotto G *et al.* (1993) 2′,3′-Dideoxyinosine-induced acute rhabdomyolisis. *Clinical Neuropathology* **12** (Suppl. 1): S45.
Gabbai AA, Schmidt B, Castelo A *et al.* (1990) Muscle biopsy in AIDS and ARC: analysis of 50 patients. *Muscle and Nerve* **13**: 541–544.
Gertner E, Thurn JR, Williams DN *et al.* (1989). Zidovudine associated myopathy. *American Journal of Medicine* **86**: 814–818.
Gherardi R, Mhiri C, Baudrimont M *et al.* (1991) Iron pigment deposits, small vessel vasculitis, and erythrophagocytosis in the muscle of human immunodeficiency virus-infected patients. *Human Pathology* **22**: 1187–1194.
Gherardi R, Baudrimont M, Lionnet F *et al.* (1992) Skeletal muscle toxoplasmosis in patients with acquired immunodeficiency syndrome: a clinical and pathological study. *Annals of Neurology* **32**: 535–542.
Gherardi R, Bélec L, Mhiri C *et al.* (1993) The spectrum of vasculitis in human immunodeficiency-virus infected patients. A clinicopathologic evaluation. *Arthritis and Rheumatism* **36**: 1164–1174.
Gonzales MF, Olney RK, So YT *et al.* (1988) Subacute structural myopathy associated with human immunodeficiency virus infection. *Archives of Neurology* **45**: 585–587.
Gorard DA, Henry K and Guiloff RJ (1988) Necrotizing myopathy and zidovudine. *Lancet* **i**: 1050.
Helbert M, Fletcher T, Peddle B *et al.* (1988) Necrotizing myopathy and zidovudine. *Lancet* **ii**: 689–690.
Herzberg NH, Zorn I, Zwart R *et al.* (1992) Major growth reduction and minor decrease in mitochondrial enzyme activity in cultured human muscle cells after exposure to zidovudine. *Muscle and Nerve* **15**: 706–710.
Hoffman P, Michiels JF, Saint-Paul MC *et al.* (1990) La localisation cardiaque de la toxoplasmose. *Semaine Hopiteaux Paris* **66**: 135–138.
Illa I, Nath A and Dalakas M (1991) Immunocytochemical and virological characteristics of HIV-associated inflammatory myopathies: similarities with seronegative polymyositis. *Annals of Neurology* **29**: 474–481.
Kaye BR (1989) Rheumatologic manifestations of infection with human immunodeficiency virus (HIV). *Annals of Internal Medicine* **111**: 158–167.
Lacroix C and Said G (1992) Muscle siderosis in AIDS: a marker for macrophage dysfunction? *Journal of Neurology* **239**: 46–48.
Lacroix C, Chemouilli P and Said G (1991) Manifestations musculaires au cours de l'infection HIV. In: *Manifestations Neurologiques et Infections Rétrovirales. SIDA et Autres Rétroviroses* (eds G. Said and AG Saimot), pp. 145–158. Paris: Pradel.
Lane RJ, McLeane KA, Moss J and Woodrow DF (1993) Myopathy in HIV infection: the role of

zidovudine and the significance of tubuloreticular inclusions. *Neuropathology and Applied Neurobiology* **19**: 406–413.

Lange DJ, Britton CB, Hays AP and Younger DS (1988) Human immunodeficiency virus infection and neuromuscular disease. In: *Peripheral Neuropathies 1988. What is Significantly New?* (eds JP Assal and C Lilger), pp. 465–492. Padova: Liviana Press.

Laraki R, Lebas J, Baudrimont M *et al.* (1990) L'atteinte musculaire au cours de l'infection par le virus de l'immunodéficience humaine. *Annales de Medicine Interne* **141**: 187–192.

Manji H, Harrison MJG, Round JM *et al.* (1993) Muscle disease, HIV and zidovudine: the spectrum of muscle disease in HIV-infected individuals treated with zidovudine. *Journal of Neurology* **240**: 479–488.

Martini L, Vion P, Le Gangneux E *et al.* (1991) Sida et myasthénie: une association exceptionnelle. *Revue Neurologique* **147**: 395–397.

Mhiri C, Baudrimont M, Bonne G *et al.* (1991) Zidovudine myopathy: a distinctive disorder associated with mitochondrial dysfunction. *Annals of Neurology* **29**: 606–614.

Miller RG, Carson BA, Moussari RS *et al.* (1991) Fatigue and myalgia in AIDS patients. *Neurology* **41**: 1603–1607.

Nath A, Kerman RH, Novak IS and Wolinsky JS (1990) Immune studies in human immunodeficiency virus infection with myasthenia gravis: a case report. *Neurology* **40**: 581–583.

Nordstrom DM, Petropolis AA, Giorno R *et al.* (1989) Inflammatory myopathy a~d acquirud immunodeficiency syndrome. *Arthritis and Rheumatism* **32**: 475–479.

Panegyres PK, Tan N, Kakulas BA, Armstrong JA and Hollingsworth P (1988) Necrotizing myopathy and zidovudine. *Lancet* **i**: 1050–1051.

Panegyres PK, Papadimitriou JM, Hollingsworth PN *et al.* (1990) Vesicular changes in the myopathies of AIDS. Ultrastructural observations and their relationship to zidovudine treatment. *Journal of Neurology, Neurosurgery and Psychiatry* **53**: 649–655.

Pezeshkpour G, Illa I and Dalakas M (1991) Ultrastructural characteristics and DNA immunocytochemistry in human immunodeficiency virus and zidovudine-associated myopathies. *Human Pathology* **22**: 1281–1288.

Pinching AJ, Helbert M and Peddle B (1990) Clinical experience with zidovudine in patients with acquired immune deficiency syndrome and immune deficiency-related complex. *Journal of Infection* **18** (Suppl.): 33–40.

Raphael S, Wolson BJ, Parker P *et al.* (1989) Pyomyositis in a child with acquired immunodeficiency syndrome. Patient report and brief review. *AJDC* **143**: 779–781.

Said G, Lacroix-Ciaudo C, Fujimura H, Blas C and Faux N (1988) The peripheral neuropathy of necrotizing arteritis: a clinico-pathologic study. *Annals of Neurology* **23**: 461–465.

Said G, Saimot AG, Matheron S, Chemouilli Ph and Kernbaum S (1989) Zidovudine myopathy: clinicopathologic aspects. Presented at a conference on Neurological and Neuropsychological complications of HIV infection, Québec, Abstract CM11.

Simpson DM (1988) Myopathy associated with human immunodeficiency virus (HIV) but not with zidovudine. *Annals of Internal Medicine* **88**: 842.

Simpson DM and Bender AN (1988) Human immunodeficiency virus-associated myopathy: analysis of 11 patients. *Annals of Neurology* **24**: 79–84.

Simpson DM and Wolfe DE (1991) Neuromuscular complications of HIV infection and its treatment. *AIDS* **5**: 917–926.

Simpson DM, Bender AN, Farraye J *et al.* (1990) Human immunodeficiency virus wasting syndrome may represent a treatable myopathy. *Neurology* **40**: 535–538.

Stern R, Gold J and Dicarlo EF (1987) Myopathy complicating the acquired immune deficiency syndrome. *Muscle and Nerve* **10**: 318–322.

Till M and MacDonell KB (1990) Myopathy with human immunodeficiency virus type-1 (HIV-1) infection: HIV-1 or zidovudine? *Annals of Internal Medicine* **113**: 492–494.

Viard JP, Vittecoq D, Lacroix C and Bach JF (1992) Response of HIV-1 associated polymyositis to intravenous immunoglobulin. *American Journal of Medicine* **92**: 580–581.

Victor G, Branley J, Opal SM and Mayer KH (1989) Pyomyositis in a patient with the acquired immunodeficiency syndrome (letter). *Archives of Internal Medicine* **149**: 705–709.

Wrzolek MA, Sher JH, Kozlowski PB and Rao C (1990) Skeletal muscle in AIDS: an autopsy study. *Muscle and Nerve* **13**: 508–515.

Yarchoan R, Mitsuya H, Myers CE and Broder S (1989) Clinical pharmacology of 3′-azido-2′,3′-dideoxythymidine (zidovudine) and related dideoxynucleosides. *New England Journal of Medicine* **321**: 726–738.

# Index